Recent Advances in Imaging with PET, CT, and MR Techniques

Editors

HABIB ZAIDI
ABASS ALAVI
DREW A. TORIGIAN

PET CLINICS

www.pet.theclinics.com

Consulting Editor
ABASS ALAVI

October 2020 • Volume 15 • Number 4

ELSEVIER

1600 John F. Kennedy Boulevard • Suite 1800 • Philadelphia, Pennsylvania, 19103-2899

http://www.pet.theclinics.com

PET CLINICS Volume 15, Number 4
October 2020 ISSN 1556-8598, ISBN-13: 978-0-323-75787-4

Editor: John Vassallo (j.vassallo@elsevier.com)
Developmental Editor: Casey Potter

PET Clinics (ISSN 1556-8598) is published quarterly by Elsevier Inc., 360 Park Avenue South, New York, NY 10010-1710. Months of issue are January, April, July, and October. Periodicals postage paid at New York, NY, and additional mailing offices. Subscription prices per year are $247.00 (US individuals), $422.00 (US institutions), $100.00 (US students), $279.00 (Canadian individuals), $475.00 (Canadian institutions), $100.00 (Canadian students), $275.00 (foreign individuals), $475.00 (foreign institutions), and $140.00 (foreign students). To receive student and resident rate, orders must be accompanied by name of affiliated institution, date of term, and the signature of program/residency coordinator on institution letterhead. Orders will be billed at individual rate until proof of status is received. Foreign air speed delivery is included in all Clinics subscription prices. All prices are subject to change without notice. POSTMASTER: Send address changes to PET Clinics, Elsevier Health Sciences Division, Subscription Customer Service, 3251 Riverport Lane, Maryland Heights, MO 63043. **Customer Service: 1-800-654-2452 (U.S. and Canada); 314-447-8871 (outside U.S. and Canada). Fax: 314-447-8029. E-mail: journalscustomerservice-usa@elsevier.com (for print support); journalsonlinesupport-usa@elsevier.com (for online support).**

Reprints. For copies of 100 or more of articles in this publication, please contact the Commercial Reprints Department, Elsevier Inc., 360 Park Avenue South, New York, NY 10010-1710. Tel.: 212-633-3874; Fax: 212-633-3820; E-mail: reprints@elsevier.com.

PET Clinics is covered in MEDLINE/PubMed (Index Medicus).

Contributors

CONSULTING EDITOR

ABASS ALAVI, MD, MD (Hon), PhD (Hon), DSc (Hon)
Professor of Radiology, Division of Nuclear Medicine, Department of Radiology, Hospital of the University of Pennsylvania, Perelman School of Medicine, University of Pennsylvania, Philadelphia, Pennsylvania, USA; Department of Pediatric Hematology-Oncology, University of California, Davis, Sacramento, California, USA

EDITORS

HABIB ZAIDI, PhD
Division of Nuclear Medicine and Molecular Imaging, Geneva University Hospital, Geneva University Neurocenter, Geneva University, Geneva, Switzerland; Department of Nuclear Medicine and Molecular Imaging, University of Groningen, University Medical Center Groningen, Groningen, the Netherlands; Department of Nuclear Medicine, University of Southern Denmark, Odense, Denmark

ABASS ALAVI, MD, MD (Hon), PhD (Hon), DSc (Hon)
Professor of Radiology, Division of Nuclear Medicine, Department of Radiology, Hospital of the University of Pennsylvania, Perelman School of Medicine, University of Pennsylvania, Philadelphia, Pennsylvania, USA; Department of Pediatric Hematology-Oncology, University of California, Davis, Sacramento, California, USA

DREW A. TORIGIAN, MD
Department of Radiology, University of Pennsylvania, Philadelphia, Pennsylvania, USA

AUTHORS

HOJJAT AHMADZADEHFAR, MD, MSc
Department of Nuclear Medicine, Klinikum Westfalen, Dortmund, Germany

ABASS ALAVI, MD, MD (Hon), PhD (Hon), DSc (Hon)
Professor of Radiology, Division of Nuclear Medicine, Department of Radiology, Hospital of the University of Pennsylvania, Perelman School of Medicine, University of Pennsylvania, Philadelphia, Pennsylvania, USA; Department of Pediatric Hematology-Oncology, University of California, Davis, Sacramento, California, USA

MAHSA AMIRRASHEDI, PhD (Candidate)
Department of Medical Physics and Biomedical Engineering, Tehran University of Medical Sciences, Research Center for Molecular and Cellular Imaging, Tehran University of Medical Sciences, Tehran, Iran

MOHAMMAD REZA AY, PhD
Department of Medical Physics and Biomedical Engineering, Tehran University of Medical Sciences, Research Center for Molecular and Cellular Imaging, Tehran University of Medical Sciences, Tehran, Iran

ABHIJIT BHATTARU, UGS
Department of Radiology, Hospital of the
University of Pennsylvania, Philadelphia,
Pennsylvania, USA

AUSTIN J. BORJA, BA
Department of Radiology, Hospital of the
University of Pennsylvania, Perelman School of
Medicine at the University of Pennsylvania,
Philadelphia, Pennsylvania, USA

DONALD WESLEY CAIN, MD
Diagnostic Neuroradiology Fellow, Department
of Radiology, University of Colorado Anschutz
Medical Center, Aurora, Colorado, USA

RHANDERSON CARDOSO, MD
Cardiovascular Fellow, Division of Cardiology,
Johns Hopkins Hospital, Baltimore, Maryland,
USA

THOMAS Q. CHRISTENSEN, MS
Department of Clinical Engineering, Region of
Southern Denmark, Esbjerg, Denmark

NIKOS EFTHIMIOU, PhD
PET Research Centre, Faculty of Health
Sciences, University of Hull, Hull, United
Kingdom; Department of Radiology, Perelman
School of Medicine, University of
Pennsylvania, Philadelphia, Pennsylvania, USA

FARAZ FARHADI, BS
Department of Radiology and Imaging
Sciences, National Institutes of Health, Clinical
Center, Bethesda, Maryland, USA

**ALI GHOLAMREZANEZHAD, MD, FEBNM,
DABR**
Department of Radiology, Keck School of
Medicine of USC, University of Southern
California, Los Angeles, California, USA

RINA GHORPADE, MD
Department of Radiology, Hospital of the
University of Pennsylvania, Philadelphia,
Pennsylvania, USA

ALI GUERMAZI, MD, PhD
Department of Radiology, Boston University
School of Medicine, Boston, Massachusetts,
USA

**POUL FLEMMING HØILUND-CARLSEN,
MD, DMSc, Prof (Hon)**
Department of Nuclear Medicine, Odense
University Hospital, Department of Clinical
Research, University of Southern Denmark,
Odense, Denmark

DEBANJAN HALDAR, BS
Department of Radiology, Hospital of the
University of Pennsylvania, Philadelphia,
Pennsylvania, USA

EMILY C. HANCIN, MS, BA
Department of Radiology, Hospital of the
University of Pennsylvania, Lewis Katz School
of Medicine at Temple University, Philadelphia,
Pennsylvania, USA

SØREN HESS, MD
Department of Radiology and Nuclear
Medicine, Hospital Southwest Jutland,
University Hospital of Southern Denmark,
Esbjerg, Denmark; Department of Regional
Health Research, Faculty of Health Sciences,
University of Southern Denmark, Odense,
Denmark

ELIZABETH C. JONES, MD, MPH, MBA
Department of Radiology and Imaging
Sciences, National Institutes of Health, Clinical
Center, Bethesda, Maryland, USA

PETER JOYCE, MD
Department of Radiology, Keck School of
Medicine of USC, University of Southern
California, Los Angeles, California, USA

SANAZ KATAL MD
Department of Nuclear Medicine/PET-CT,
Kowsar Hospital, Shiraz, Iran

MOHSEN KHOSRAVI, MD
Department of Radiology, Thomas Jefferson
University, Philadelphia, Pennsylvania, USA

BENJAMIN KOA, BS
Department of Radiology, Hospital of the
University of Pennsylvania, Drexel University
College of Medicine, Philadelphia,
Pennsylvania, USA

AJAY KOHLI, MD
Department of Radiology, University of
Pennsylvania, Hospital of the University of
Pennsylvania, Philadelphia, Pennsylvania, USA

THORSTEN M. LEUCKER, MD, PhD
Assistant Professor of Medicine, Division of
Cardiology, Johns Hopkins Hospital,
Baltimore, Maryland, USA

ASHKAN A. MALAYERI, MD
Department of Radiology and Imaging
Sciences, Clinical Center, National Institutes of
Health, Bethesda, Maryland, USA

NAVDEEP SINGH MANHAS, BS
California University of Science and Medicine,
California, USA

XUAN MIAO, BA
Department of Radiology, Hospital of the
University of Pennsylvania, Philadelphia,
Pennsylvania, USA

NANCY MOHSEN, MD
Associate Professor, Department of Radiology,
University of Pennsylvania, Hospital of the
University of Pennsylvania, Philadelphia,
Pennsylvania, USA

MICHAEL A. MORRIS, MD, MS
Department of Radiology and Imaging
Sciences, National Institutes of Health, Clinical
Center, Bethesda, Maryland, USA; Department
of Computer Science and Electrical
Engineering, University of Maryland, Baltimore
County, Baltimore, Maryland, USA

PAWEŁ MOSKAL, PhD
Marian Smoluchowski Institute of Physics,
Jagiellonian University, Kraków, Poland

ANDREW B. NEWBERG, MD
Departments of Radiology, and Integrative
Medicine and Nutritional Sciences, Thomas
Jefferson University, Philadelphia,
Pennsylvania, USA

MOOZHAN NIKPANAH, MD
Department of Radiology and Imaging
Sciences, Clinical Center, National Institutes of
Health, Bethesda, Maryland, USA

SAYURI PADMANHABHAN, UGS
Department of Radiology, Hospital of the
University of Pennsylvania, Philadelphia,
Pennsylvania, USA

NEENA PASSI, MD
Cardiology Fellow, University of Pennsylvania,
Hospital of the University of Pennsylvania,
Philadelphia, Pennsylvania, USA

VALERIA POTIGAILO, MD
Visiting Associate Professor, Department of
Radiology, University of Colorado Anschutz
Medical Center, Aurora, Colorado, USA

JINA PRAKPOOR, MD
Department of Radiology, University of
Pennsylvania, Hospital of the University of
Pennsylvania, Philadelphia, Pennsylvania, USA

CHAMITH RAJAPAKSE, PhD
Department of Radiology, Hospital of the
University of Pennsylvania, Philadelphia,
Pennsylvania, USA

WILLIAM Y. RAYNOR, BS
Department of Radiology, Hospital of the
University of Pennsylvania, Drexel University
College of Medicine, Philadelphia,
Pennsylvania, USA

**MONA-ELISABETH REVHEIM, MD, PhD,
MHA**
Department of Radiology, Hospital of the
University of Pennsylvania, Philadelphia,
Pennsylvania, USA; Division of Radiology and
Nuclear Medicine, Oslo University Hospital,
Institute of Clinical Medicine, Faculty of
Medicine, University of Oslo, Oslo, Norway

CHAITANYA ROJULPOTE, MD
Department of Radiology, Hospital of the
University of Pennsylvania, Philadelphia,
Pennsylvania, USA; Department of Internal
Medicine, The Wright Center for Graduate
Medical Education, Scranton, Pennsylvania,
USA

BABAK SABOURY, MD, MPH
Department of Radiology and Imaging
Sciences, National Institutes of Health, Clinical
Center, Bethesda, Maryland, USA; Department
of Computer Science and Electrical
Engineering, University of Maryland, Baltimore
County, Baltimore, Maryland, USA;
Department of Radiology, Hospital of the
University of Pennsylvania, Philadelphia,
Pennsylvania, USA

SANA SALEHI, MD
Department of Radiology, Keck School of
Medicine of USC, University of Southern
California, Los Angeles, California, USA

SIAVASH MEHDIZADEH SERAJ, MD
Department of Radiology, Hospital of the
University of Pennsylvania, Philadelphia,
Pennsylvania, USA

EWA Ł. STĘPIEŃ, PhD
Marian Smoluchowski Institute of Physics,
Jagiellonian University, Kraków, Poland

THOMAS J. WERNER, MS
Department of Radiology, Hospital of the
University of Pennsylvania, Philadelphia,
Pennsylvania, USA

HABIB ZAIDI, PhD
Division of Nuclear Medicine and Molecular
Imaging, Geneva University Hospital, Geneva
University Neurocenter, Geneva University,
Geneva, Switzerland; Department of Nuclear
Medicine and Molecular Imaging, University of
Groningen, University Medical Center
Groningen, Groningen, the Netherlands;
Department of Nuclear Medicine, University of
Southern Denmark, Odense, Denmark

VINCENT ZHANG, BA
Department of Radiology, Hospital of the
University of Pennsylvania, Philadelphia,
Pennsylvania, USA

Contents

limits dissemination of total-body PET in hospitals and even in research clinics. The J-PET tomography system is based on axially arranged low-cost plastic scintillator strips. It constitutes a realistic cost-effective solution of a total-body PET for broad clinical applications. High sensitivity of total-body J-PET and triggerless data acquisition enable multiphoton imaging, opening possibilities for multitracer and positronium imaging, thus promising quantitative enhancement of specificity in cancer and inflammatory disease assessment.

Presented and discussed are challenges that had to be addressed for generation of the first long axial field-of-view (LAFOV) PET static and dynamic images. A brief comparison between the two main "schools of thought" behind the development of the only two implemented scanners at the time of writing is given. Although both aim to achieve the best possible quantitative static PET images and high-quality dynamic time-activity curves, their methods are different and reflect their history and future. As the benefits of the LAFOV are appealing to many, some popular strategies for cost management are briefly presented.

Total-body PET scans will initiate a new era for the PET clinic. The benefits of 40-fold effective sensitivity improvement provide new capabilities to image with lower radiation dose, perform delayed imaging, and achieve improved temporal resolution. These technical features are detailed in the first of this 2-part series. In this part, the clinical impacts of the novel features of total-body PET scans are further explored. Applications of total-body PET scans focus on the real-time interrogation of systemic disease manifestations in a variety of practical clinical contexts. Total-body PET scans make clinical systems biology imaging a reality.

Fused PET/computed tomography has demonstrated success in the detection and quantification of atherosclerotic plaques. Recently, total-body PET imaging has demonstrated increased sensitivity and specificity in atherosclerosis. This article reviews the literature regarding this novel imaging technique. Moreover, evidence that has pointed toward 18F-sodium fluoride as the radiotracer of choice over 18F-fluorodeoxyglucose for evaluation of plaque burden is discussed. Finally, a global disease assessment is introduced as an adjunct tool for vascular PET imaging.

In recent years, ^{18}F-Sodium Fluoride (NaF)-PET/CT has seen its role in the detection and management of osteoporosis increase. This article reviews the extent of this application in the literature, its efficacy compared with other comparable imaging tools, and how total-body PET/CT combined with global disease assessment can revolutionize measurement of total osteoporotic disease activity. NaF-PET/CT eventually can be the modality of choice for metabolic bone disorders, especially with these advances in technology and computation.

PET with 18F-fluorodeoxyglucose (FDG) is used to assess a wide array of inflammatory and neoplastic disorders. FDG-PET has shown particular utility in the evaluation of disorders of the central nervous system (CNS). Although fused PET/computed tomography (CT) is frequently used across the globe for these diseases, recent evidence has pointed to PET/magnetic resonance (MR) imaging as a more sensitive and specific molecular imaging modality. This article reviews the literature regarding the advantages of PET/MR imaging compared with PET/CT imaging, especially in CNS disease. It also introduces a new concept for PET-based evaluation of patients with neurodegenerative disorders: global disease assessment.

Cardiac PET/MR imaging is an integrated imaging approach that requires less radiation than PET/computed tomography and combines the high spatial resolution and morphologic data from MR imaging with the physiologic information from PET. This hybrid approach has the potential to improve the diagnostic and prognostic evaluation of several cardiovascular conditions, such as ischemic heart disease, infiltrative diseases such as sarcoidosis, acute and chronic myocarditis, and cardiac masses. Herein, the authors discuss the strengths of PET and MR imaging in several cardiovascular conditions; the challenges and potential; and the current data on the application of this powerful hybrid imaging modality.

18F-Fluorodeoxyglucose PET has been used to evaluate a wide array of inflammatory and neoplastic pathologies. MR imaging has great soft tissue resolution and high accuracy for detection of edema. Combining PET with MR imaging offers substantial advantages in musculoskeletal imaging. Specifically, evidence demonstrates the potential of imaging of bone marrow, soft tissue, and synovia by PET/MR imaging. Because of inherent limitations of ^{1}H-MR to image cortical bone, there are some challenges; however, the use of 18F-sodium fluoride for PET/MR imaging could change the landscape. This article reviews the literature regarding PET/MR imaging in identification and management of many musculoskeletal diseases.

PET/computed tomography scans and PET/MR imaging have been applied in imaging tumors of the musculoskeletal system for their ability to provide information about metabolic activity. However, applications of these imaging modalities are now being extended to nononcologic musculoskeletal pathologies, such as osteoarthritis, rheumatoid arthritis, and osteoporosis. This article aims to explore the alternative uses of these imaging modalities in oncologic and nononcologic musculoskeletal pathologies. It also discusses the various strengths and some weaknesses that are seen in particular situations.

During the past decades, the role of fludeoxyglucose (FDG)-PET and hybrid PET/computed tomography (CT) has been established clinically in the diagnostic workup of a multitude of infectious and inflammatory disorders. In recent years, the fusion of MR imaging to PET has also been increasingly explored, and this may be especially useful in musculoskeletal and gastrointestinal inflammatory diseases due to exceptional soft tissue contrast and reduced radiation dose. This article outlines the current potential for hybrid molecular imaging in the musculoskeletal system and the gastrointestinal tract with special focus on the potential for fused PET/CT/MR imaging.

Detecting inflammation is among the most important aims of medical imaging. Inflammatory process involves immune system activity and local tissue response. The role of PET with fludeoxyglucose F 18 has been expanded. Systemic vasculitides and cardiopulmonary inflammatory disorders constitute a wide range of diseases with multisystemic manifestations. PET with fludeoxyglucose F 18 is useful in their diagnosis, assessment, and follow-up. This article provides an overview of the current status and potentials of hybrid molecular imaging in evaluating cardiopulmonary and vascular inflammatory diseases focusing on the potential for PET with fludeoxyglucose F 18/MR imaging and PET/CT scans.

PET CLINICS

PROGRAM OBJECTIVE

The goal of the *PET Clinics* is to keep practicing radiologists and radiology residents up to date with current clinical practice in positron emission tomography by providing timely articles reviewing the state of the art in patient care.

TARGET AUDIENCE

Practicing radiologists, radiology residents, and other health care professionals who provide patient care utilizing radiologic findings.

LEARNING OBJECTIVES

Upon completion of this activity, participants will be able to:

1. Review the role and clinical relevance of medical imaging techniques, instrumentation, and application in clinical and research settings.
2. Discuss recent development and advancement in multimodality medical imaging instrumentation, image reconstruction, and analysis techniques.
3. Recognize the challenges and opportunities for multimodality medical imaging instrumentation and innovative clinical applications.

ACCREDITATION

The Elsevier Office of Continuing Medical Education (EOCME) is accredited by the Accreditation Council for Continuing Medical Education (ACCME) to provide continuing medical education for physicians.

The EOCME designates this journal-based CME activity for a maximum of 14 *AMA PRA Category 1 Credit*(s)™. Physicians should claim only the credit commensurate with the extent of their participation in the activity.

All other health care professionals requesting continuing education credit for this enduring material will be issued a certificate of participation.

DISCLOSURE OF CONFLICTS OF INTEREST

The EOCME assesses conflict of interest with its instructors, faculty, planners, and other individuals who are in a position to control the content of CME activities. All relevant conflicts of interest that are identified are thoroughly vetted by EOCME for fair balance, scientific objectivity, and patient care recommendations. EOCME is committed to providing its learners with CME activities that promote improvements or quality in healthcare and not a specific proprietary business or a commercial interest.

The planning committee, staff, authors and editors listed below have identified no financial relationships or relationships to products or devices they or their spouse/life partner have with commercial interest related to the content of this CME activity:

Hojjat Ahmadzadehfar, MD, MSc; Abass Alavi, MD, MD (Hon), PhD (Hon), DSc (Hon); Mahsa Amirrashedi, PhD (Candidate); Mohammad Reza Ay, PhD; Abhijit Bhattaru, UGS; Austin J. Borja, BA; Donald Wesley Cain, MD; Rhanderson Cardoso, MD; Regina Chavous-Gibson MSN, RN; Thomas Q. Christensen, MS; Nikos Efthimiou, PhD; Faraz Farhadi, BS; Ali Gholamrezanezhad, MD, FEBNM, DABR; Rina Ghorpade, MD; Ali Guermazi, MD, PhD; Poul Flemming Høilund-Carlsen, MD, DMSc, Prof (Hon); Debanjan Haldar, BS; Emily C. Hancin, MS, BA; Søren Hess, MD; Elizabeth C. Jones MD, MPH, MBA; Peter Joyce, MD; Sanaz Katal, MD; Mohsen Khosravi, MD; Benjamin Koa, BS; Ajay Kohli, MD; Thorsten M. Leucker, MD, PhD; Ashkan A. Malayeri, MD; Navdeep Singh Manhas, BS; Xuan Miao, BA; Nancy Mohsen, MD; Michael A. Morris, MD, MS; Paweł Moskal, PhD; Andrew B. Newberg, MD; Moozhan Nikpanah, MD; Sayuri Padmanhabhan, UGS; Neena Passi, MD; Valeria Potigailo, MD; Jina Prakpoor, MD; Chamith Rajapakse, PhD; William Y. Raynor, BS; Mona-Elisabeth Revheim, MD, PhD, MHA; Chaitanya Rojulpote, MD; Babak Saboury, MD, MPH; Sana Salehi, MD; Siavash Mehdizadeh Seraj, MD; Ewa Ł. Stępień, PhD; John Vassallo; Vignesh Viswanathan; Thomas J. Werner, MS; Habib Zaidi, PhD; Vincent Zhang, BA.

The planning committee, staff, authors and editors listed below have identified financial relationships or relationships to products or devices they or their spouse/life partner have with commercial interest related to the content of this CME activity:

Drew A. Torigian, MD: consultant/advisor for and owns stock in Quantitative Radiology Solutions LLC.

UNAPPROVED/OFF-LABEL USE DISCLOSURE

The EOCME requires CME faculty to disclose to the participants:

1. When products or procedures being discussed are off-label, unlabelled, experimental, and/or investigational (not US Food and Drug Administration [FDA] approved); and
2. Any limitations on the information presented, such as data that are preliminary or that represent ongoing research, interim analyses, and/or unsupported opinions. Faculty may discuss information about pharmaceutical agents that is outside of FDA-approved labelling. This information is intended solely for CME and is not intended to promote off-label use of these medications. If you have any questions, contact the medical affairs department of the manufacturer for the most recent prescribing information.

TO ENROLL

To enroll in the *PET Clinics* Continuing Medical Education program, call customer service at 1-800-654-2452 or sign up online at http://www.theclinics.com/home/cme. The CME program is available to subscribers for an additional annual fee of USD 235.00

METHOD OF PARTICIPATION

In order to claim credit, participants must complete the following:

1. Complete enrolment as indicated above.
2. Read the activity.
3. Complete the CME Test and Evaluation. Participants must achieve a score of 70% on the test. All CME Tests and Evaluations must be completed online.

CME INQUIRIES/SPECIAL NEEDS

For all CME inquiries or special needs, please contact elsevierCME@elsevier.com.

Preface

Recent Advances in Imaging with PET, Computed Tomography, and MR Techniques

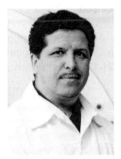

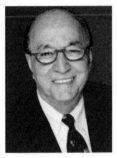

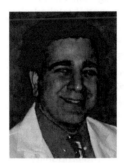

Habib Zaidi, PhD   Abass Alavi, MD   Drew A. Torigian, MD

Editors

This is an exciting time for multimodality medical imaging in the era of precision medicine. The history of medical imaging is very rich with boundless sensational developments performed by pioneers in the field. These developments cover all imaging techniques and modalities, including x-ray computed tomography (CT), MR imaging, and PET, and their combination on advanced hybrid imaging devices, such as PET/CT and PET/MR imaging.

Recent developments in medical imaging techniques, instrumentation, and clinical applications have created a need for a review of their role and clinical relevance in clinical and research settings. Likewise, the number of papers related to these subjects published in peer-reviewed journals and presented at various conferences and symposia has been increasing steadily, which motivated the compilation of the enclosed reviews as a snapshot of the dynamically changing field of multimodality medical imaging. This issue presents recent advances in CT, MR imaging, and PET imaging techniques, particularly total-body PET imaging instrumentation and reconstruction strategies, and summarizes state-of-the-art clinical applications of novel imaging technologies. This special issue is thus distinct from previous ones in the sense that it focuses particularly on total-body PET imaging and PET/MR imaging. Future prospects and suggestions for further research are also discussed.

The first contribution by Drs Potigailo, Kohli, Prakpoor and colleagues focuses on reviewing recent advances in anatomical CT and MR imaging modalities, including modern emerging functional (perfusion and vascular) imaging techniques. The following article by Drs Amirrashedi, Zaidi, and Ay provides a comprehensive review of preclinical PET scanners developed in academic and corporate settings with a particular emphasis on innovations in instrumentation and conceptual designs. The concept of newly introduced total-body PET imaging achieved by extending the axial field-of-view up to 2 m, which improves substantially the sensitivity, thus allowing dose reduction, faster imaging, improved temporal resolution, and dynamic imaging, is discussed by Drs Saboury, Morris, Farhadi and colleagues. The cost of this system is the major drawback for wider clinical adoption of this technology. In this regard, the following contribution by Drs Moskal and Stępień describes J-PET, a cost-effective solution for total-body PET through the use of axially arranged low-cost plastic scintillator strips. Addressing the challenges of image reconstruction for long axial field-of-view PET scanners and dynamic imaging is systematically tackled in the contribution by Efthimiou. The clinical applications of total-body PET imaging in various fields and particularly in atherosclerosis and osteoporosis are covered in 3 comprehensive

https://doi.org/10.1016/j.cpet.2020.08.002
1556-8598/20/© 2020 Published by Elsevier Inc.

pet.theclinics.com

articles (Drs Saboury, Morris, Nikpanah and colleagues; Drs Borja, Rojulpote, Hancin and colleagues; and Drs Zhang, Koa, Borja and colleagues). The emergence of PET/MR imaging-triggered much worthwhile methodological research. This in turn spurred the exploration of the clinical potential of this novel imaging modality. As such, the clinical applications of PET/MR imagingin exploring the central nervous system (Drs Borja, Hancin, Khosravi and colleagues), cardiovascular diseases (Drs Cardoso and Leucker), and musculoskeletal diseases (Drs Hancin, Borja, Nikpanah and colleagues) are elegantly reviewed. Last, but not least, 3 articles (Drs Manhas, Salehi, Joyce and colleagues; Drs Katal, Gholamrezanezhad, Nikpanah and colleagues; Drs Nikpanah, Katal, Christensen, and colleagues) provide in-depth appraisal of the role of multimodality imaging (PET/CT/MR imaging) in musculoskeletal and inflammatory diseases.

The development of advanced multimodality medical imaging instrumentation and related image reconstruction and analysis techniques as well as associated clinical applications have been very rapid and exciting, and there is every reason to believe the field will move forward more swiftly in the near future with the advent of novel crystals and photodetector technologies and the unlimited imagination of active scientists. There is no shortage of challenges and opportunities for multimodality medical imaging instrumentation and innovative clinical applications nowadays. We hope that, in this limited space, we were able to provide a flavor of recent advances in instrumentation and potential applications in clinical and research settings. We would like to thank all the authors who contributed these articles and hope that these contributions will be beneficial to readers.

Habib Zaidi, PhD
Division of Nuclear Medicine and
Molecular Imaging
Geneva University Hospital
Geneva CH-1211, Switzerland

Abass Alavi, MD
Department of Radiology
Hospital of the University
of Pennsylvania
Philadelphia, PA 19104, USA

Drew A. Torigian, MD
Department of Radiology
University of Pennsylvania
Philadelphia, PA 19104, USA

E-mail addresses:
Habib.Zaidi@hcuge.ch (H. Zaidi)
Abass.Alavi@pennmedicine.upenn.edu (A. Alavi)
Drew.Torigian@pennmedicine.upenn.edu
(D.A. Torigian)

Recent Advances in Computed Tomography and MR Imaging

Valeria Potigailo, MD[a], Ajay Kohli, MD[b], Jina Prakpoor, MD[b], Donald Wesley Cain, MD[a], Neena Passi, MD[c], Nancy Mohsen, MD[b],*

KEYWORDS

- Functional MRI • Neurovascular imaging • MR enterography • MR elastography
- Artificial intelligence

KEY POINTS

- Neuroradiology is at the forefront of functional and structural imaging with an increasing number of noninvasive methods that study brain activation, and enable detailed characterization of brain architecture and vessel wall pathology.
- Implementation of noninvasive vascular and cerebral perfusion imaging techniques has reshaped clinical paradigms in diagnosis and treatment of stroke and cerebrovascular disease.
- Recent advances in abdominal imaging include development of standardized guidelines for interpretation of MR enterography in Crohn disease, and performance and interpretation of MR defecography.
- Magnetic resonance elastography has become a useful adjunct in the evaluation of hepatic fibrosis.
- Application of artificial intelligence methodology is proving advantageous in disease classification, image interpretation, and workflow optimization.

BODY IMAGING

Many of the most recent advances in computed tomography (CT) and MR imaging applications in abdominopelvic imaging have come in the form of the development and acceptance of standardized multidisciplinary guidelines for the performance, interpretation, and reporting of findings in a way that focuses on clinically relevant questions that can be widely applied across imaging institutions. They have also leveraged technological advances in high-resolution fast imaging techniques with MR imaging.

Magnetic Resonance Elastography

Conditions that result in the development of hepatic fibrosis have been increasing in prevalence. These conditions include obesity, hepatitis B, hepatitis C, and alcoholism. Hepatic fibrosis, resulting in impaired hepatocyte function and exchange between hepatocytes and portal blood, contributes both to the development of irreversible portal hypertension and to the microenvironmental changes that favor the occurrence of hepatocellular carcinoma.[1] The degree of hepatic fibrosis is an important factor in determining prognosis, clinical progression or regression, treatment options, and treatment response, in patients with chronic

a Department of Radiology, University of Colorado Anschutz Medical Center, 12401 East 17th Avenue, Leprino, Mail Stop L954, Aurora, CO 80045, USA; b Department of Radiology, University of Pennsylvania, Hospital of the University of Pennsylvania, 1 Silverstein Suite 130, 3400 Spruce Street, Philadelphia, PA 19104, USA; c University of Pennsylvania, Hospital of the University of Pennsylvania, 3400 Spruce Street, Philadelphia, PA 19104, USA
* Corresponding author.
E-mail address: nancy.mohsen@pennmedicine.upenn.edu

PET Clin 15 (2020) 381–402
https://doi.org/10.1016/j.cpet.2020.07.001

liver disease.[1-3] For example, patients with F3 fibrosis have a markedly increased risk of developing hepatocellular carcinoma. Although liver biopsy is widely considered to be the gold standard in assessing liver fibrosis, it is limited by small sample size and sampling error, owing to the inherent geographic heterogeneity of liver involvement.[3,4] Although the complication risk is small, with reported complications estimated at 3% with a mortality of 0.03%, clinicians are reluctant to take on this risk in asymptomatic patients.[4,5] Therefore, a fast, accurate, noninvasive, cost-effective, and reproducible technique is needed in assessing the extent of hepatic fibrosis. Magnetic Resonance Elastography (MRE) of the liver is now available with multiple MR manufacturers and has evolved as a noninvasive imaging technique that meets all of these criteria.[3]

Application of any liver elastography technique arises from the understanding that the severity of hepatic fibrosis correlates to the degree of liver stiffness. Therefore, in the appropriate patient setting, quantitating liver stiffness correlates to the degree of fibrosis.[3,6,7] Fibrosis however is not the only cause of increased liver stiffness. Biliary obstruction, acute inflammation, and venous congestion from right heart dysfunction are all causes of increased liver stiffness emphasizing the importance of appropriate patient selection.[3,6] Certain limitations and pitfalls do exist (**Box 1**).

Technique

Mechanical waves are generated in the liver by a passive acoustic driver placed on the patient's abdomen, which transmits a vibration (usually at 60 Hz) generated by an active driver located outside the room and connected by tubing.[3,6] The liver is imaged in 2 to 4 consecutive 14-second breath-holds, phase contrast sequences (usually modified gradient echo sequences with a cyclic motion encoding gradient [MEG] applied across the z-axis). The entire examination takes 1 minute or less. A wave map of the liver is generated (which can be presented in gray scale or color rendering). The faster these waves propagate through the tissue, the longer the wavelength and the stiffer the tissue. From the wave map, an inversion algorithm is used to calculate a stiffness map called an elastogram.

Image interpretation

First evaluation of the source image is needed to determine that there is adequate signal to obtain a reliable elastogram. Wave maps should be reviewed to determine that a reliable consistent wave pattern is visible propagating through the liver and is not excessively motion degraded. Liver stiffness is measured in kilopascals, drawing regions of interest (ROI) in the elastograms. ROI should only be measured where there is adequate wave amplitude and should not be closer than one-half wavelength to the liver margin to avoid edge effects (**Fig. 1**). Large vessels, gallbladder fossa, and regions of artifact should also be avoided. ROI measurement of less than 2.5 kPa is normal, and greater than 5 kPa correlates to F4 fibrosis or cirrhosis (**Table 1**).

Advantages

MRE samples large regions of the liver, which is advantageous in a geographically inhomogeneous process, such as hepatic fibrosis. Transient elastography and shear wave elastography both perform with ultrasound sample points within the liver, whereas MR provides the largest surface area sampling of the liver compared with any other technique. MRE is not affected by obesity in contrast to shear wave elastography. Perihepatic ascites and bowel interposition between the liver and abdominal wall also do not affect MRE.

Limitations/pitfalls

Major limitations to this technique include patient inability to breath-hold greater than 14 seconds, resulting in unreliable motion degraded images, and iron overload, which creates significant artifact and signal loss because of susceptibility invalidating findings.[8] Limitations of all hepatic elastography techniques include patient-related factors that may result in increased liver stiffness in the absence of fibrosis. These factors include acute exacerbations of hepatitis with acute liver function test elevation, congestive heart failure, recent feeding (because of transient increased

---

Box 1
Magnetic resonance elastography technical limitations/pitfalls

MR elastography will not be reliably performed with Gradient recalled echo sequences in patients with hepatic iron deposition

Patient inability to breath-hold will result in excess image noise and nondiagnostic images

ROI measurements near the liver edge may have spurious results. Measurements on the elastogram should be made greater than one-half wavelength from liver margin to avoid spurious results from edge effects

Avoid ROI measurement in gallbladder fossa, or large vessels

Liver stiffness maybe increased in the setting of acute inflammation, extrahepatic cholestasis, congestive heart failure

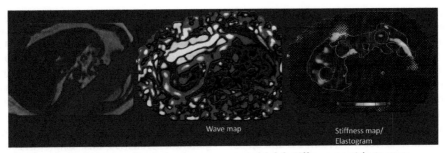

Fig. 1. MRE (*left*) magnitude image, (*center*) color wave map, (*right*) stiffness map/elastogram.

portal blood flow), extrahepatic cholestasis, and deep inspiration because of increased intraabdominal pressure, which may result in elevated liver stiffness that is not secondary to fibrosis.[6,8,9]

Alternatives

Shear wave elastography and fibroscan are ultrasound-based techniques that only provide limited spot measurements at limited depth in the liver. These ultrasound elastography techniques are suboptimal in the setting of obese patients, bowel interposition, and perihepatic ascites because of increased distance of liver from the transducer, obscuration by bowel gas, and much smaller sample size. These techniques however are superior in the setting of iron overload because they are not affected by signal loss and susceptibility artifact seen with MR imaging.

Magnetic Resonance Enterography in the Monitoring of Small Bowel Crohn Disease

Bowel imaging has greatly benefited from the development of fast imaging techniques. When used in conjunction with ileocolonoscopy, CT and MR enterography can identify proximal small bowel inflammation, including areas of purely intramural inflammation, not accessible to the endoscopist. Although imaging with both CT and MR enterography is an important adjunct in the evaluation of patients with Crohn disease, MR is gaining wider application, because of several inherent advantages. Given that Crohn disease patients are often young and require repeated imaging over the course of a lifetime, the lack of ionizing radiation with MR imaging is a notable benefit. Moreover, advances in fast imaging techniques, including steady state free precession (SSFP), reduce limitations in interpretation caused by bowel motion. We now are able to image through the same bowel segments multiple times throughout the course of an examination, limiting the mischaracterization of peristalsis as luminal narrowing. Finally, the widespread use of diffusion-weighted imaging improves confidence in identifying diseased bowel segments.

Until recently, the imaging protocols and interpretation of these studies have been quite variable between readers and institutions.[10] Recent advances in the standardization of language and consensus recommendations were developed by representatives of the Society of Abdominal Radiology in conjunction with Society of Pediatric Radiology, and the American Gastroenterological Association.[10] These recommendations, published in March 2018, focus on the systematic evaluation and reporting of CT and MR enterography in the setting of Crohn disease. The guidelines emphasize assessment for 4 major categories of complication on each examination. Namely, active inflammation as evidenced by asymmetric wall thickening, mural edema/increased T2 signal, and hyperenhancement, with or without narrowing. Stricture is specifically defined as luminal narrowing with unequivocal proximal bowel dilation greater than 3 cm, with or without active inflammation.[10] Penetrating disease includes sinus tracts, fistula, abscess, and free perforation, excluding perianal disease, which should be discussed separately. Last, the radiologist must note the presence or absence of perianal fistula, as well as mesenteric venous thrombus, avascular necrosis, primary sclerosing cholangitis, pancreatitis, cholelithiasis, and nephrolithiasis that are

Table 1 Kilopascal values for magnetic resonance elastography interpretation at 60 Hz	
Elastogram ROI Measurement in Kilopascals	**Degree of Fibrosis**
<2.5	None
2.5–2.9	Normal or inflammation
2.9–3.5	F1-F2 (stage 1–2 fibrosis)
3.5–4	F2-F3 (stage 2–3 fibrosis)
4–5	F3-F4 (stage 3–4 fibrosis)
>5	F4 (stage 4 fibrosis or cirrhosis)

commonly associated with Crohn disease. Image interpretation relies on characterization of major features, including wall thickness, mural enhancement, mural edema, and diffusion restriction. Although it was previously thought that patients with Crohn either had active inflammatory, stricturing, or penetrating fistulizing disease, it is now understood that there is a spectrum with patients manifesting features of one or all of these over the course of their illness[10,11] (**Tables 2** and **3**).

Before imaging, the patient ingests 1.5 L of oral Breeza or Volumen over a span of 45 minutes, divided into 0.5 L every 15 minutes, to achieve optimal bowel distention.[12] The patient is placed prone on the MR imaging table if they can tolerate this positioning; otherwise, they can be imaged supine.[13,14] Stepwise cinematic SSFP thick slice imaging through the small bowel can be performed to obtain additional information regarding bowel motion because inflamed/diseased segments will show decreased peristalsis. After cinematic imaging, imaging of the abdomen and pelvis is performed utilizing large field-of-view coronal T2-weighted imaging of the abdomen and pelvis, axial T2-weighted imaging, fat-saturated T2-weighted sequence in at least one plane, and diffusion-weighted imaging. Finally, 3D dynamic contrast-enhanced imaging performed in the coronal plane is obtained[13,14] (**Figs. 2** and **3**).

Pitfalls

It is important for the radiologist to be aware that normal jejunum will show increased nonfocal restricted diffusion relative to normal ileum, and similarly, nondistended bowel may appear to have restricted diffusion.[10] Achieving adequate bowel distension is essential, and the radiologist's awareness of this pitfall is paramount to avoiding it. Diffusion alone should not be used to determine active inflammation, but in the setting of enhancement and increased t2 signal, correlates to severe inflammation at endoscopy.

Limitations

Patients unable to tolerate or complete the oral contrast preparation to achieve adequate small bowel distention may have limited results with this technique. Also, patients who are unable to breath-hold, are unable to follow instructions, or are claustrophobic may be better candidates for CT enterography.

Dynamic Imaging of the Pelvic Floor/Magnetic Resonance Defecography

Pelvic floor failure is an often overlooked problem that currently affects 23% of women in the United States.[15] The pathophysiology is incompletely understood, but appears to be multifactorial, including a combination of chronically increased pelvic pressure, anatomic damage from prior surgeries or vaginal deliveries, chronic constipation and straining, and hormonal factors related to menopause, resulting in varying degrees of muscle laxity and ligamentous failure at the pelvic floor.[15,16] Prevalence increases with age, with numbers expected to peak as the Baby Boomer generation reaches their sixth decade. Patients will commonly present with symptoms of increased pelvic pressure, chronic constipation, a sensation of obstructed defecation, and/or incontinence (fecal or urinary).[17,18]

MR defecography has emerged as a tool in the assessment of pelvic floor dysfunction in patients with symptoms of pelvic organ prolapse or obstructed defecation. Aided by the recent adoption of standard guidelines for the performance and interpretation of these studies by the European Society of Genitourinary Radiology, this technique is emerging as a fast, comfortable, comprehensive examination, which does not require the special equipment or ionizing radiation needed for standard fluoroscopic imaging. The examination is performed privately in the MR imaging scanner, as opposed to the fluoroscopy suite, eliminating the psychological barrier of having to defecate in front of staff. In contrast to fluoroscopic defecography, MR defecography is capable of assessing the anatomy and function of the pelvic floor musculature and organs, including all 3 compartments of the pelvic floor, both at rest and under physiologic stress. Traditionally, many clinicians have relied on physical examination to determine need for surgery, sometimes only focusing on the symptomatic compartment, resulting in overly targeted interventions, which do not take into account the full extent of the patient's disease. MR imaging defecography often identifies unsuspected multicompartmental involvement and correctly characterizes enteroceles, which are often mischaracterized as rectoceles on physical examination, significantly altering the planned surgical intervention and facilitating a more comprehensive surgical approach.

Technique

- Rectal injection of 180 to 250 mL ultrasound gel
- Supine 3-plane static fast spin echo/turbo spin echo T2-weighted imaging of the pelvis is performed to provide anatomic evaluation of the floor
- Midline multislice sagittal steady-state or balanced state free precession performed

Table 2
Active inflammation (known Crohn)

Severity	Luminal Narrowing	T2 Signal	Ulcers	Wall Thickness	Diffusion	Enhancement
				Note*** Only measure loops distended with enteric contrast. Measuring thickest portion of most inflamed loop		Note*** Increased signal/attenuation relative to normal small bowel segments • Segmental mural hyperenhancement in the absence of wall thickening is nonspecific
Mild	None	No to minimal increase	None	3-5 mm		Mild hyperenhancement
Severe	Yes	Increased intramural T2 signal (T2 FS)	Present	>10 mm	High signal on high B-value diffusion	Marked mural hyperenhancement

With permission: adapted from: "Consensus Recommendations for Evaluation, Interpretation, and Utilization of Computed Tomography and Magnetic Resonance Enterography in Patients With Small Bowel Crohn's Disease" Bruining et al., Radiology Vol. 286, No. 3: 776-799; Copyright RSNA, 2018.

Table 3
Crohn inflammation magnetic resonance/computed tomographic enterography findings

Finding	Criteria
Segmental mural hyperenhancement	Asymmetric-mesenteric border more involved Stratified-hyperenhancement of inner wall Homogeneous-transmural hyperenhancement
Wall thickening	Mild: 3-5 mm Moderate: 5-9 mm Severe: ≥10 mm
Intramural edema	Hyperintense signal on T2-weighted MR imaging cannot comment on CT
Stricture	Reserve term for luminal narrowing *with unequivocal upstream dilation >3 cm* (describe length and location for potential subsequent intervention)
Ulceration	Small focal breaks in the luminal bowel surface with focal extension of air or contrast into the inflamed bowel wall (do not extend beyond bowel wall)

With permission: adapted from: "Consensus Recommendations for Evaluation, Interpretation, and Utilization of Computed Tomography and Magnetic Resonance Enterography in Patients With Small Bowel Crohn's Disease" Bruining et al. Radiology Vol. 286, No. 3: 776-799 Copyright RSNA, 2018.

during Kegel, strain, and defecation (see **Box 2**)

Advance coaching of the patient on the 3 maneuvers required is critical to obtaining a diagnostic study. Supine static T2 FSE imaging of the pelvis is performed to provide anatomic evaluation of the floor. Subsequent midline multislice sagittal steady-state or balanced state free precession performed during Kegel, strain, and defecation assesses function. The study is only considered diagnostic if movement of the pelvic floor and abdominal wall is seen during Kegel and strain.[15] Schawkat and colleagues[16] in 2018 reported that left lateral decubitus positioning may be helpful in patients unable to defecate supine. Some controversy in the literature remains on whether supine positioning may underestimate prolapse compared with the sitting position, which Khatri and colleagues[19] discuss eloquently, raising the need for a well-designed comparison study.

Anatomic landmarks, including the pubococcygeal line (PCL), H (hiatus), and M line (pelvic floor descent), are evaluated at rest and during defecation to assess pelvic floor muscular function for laxity or dyssynergy.[15,17–20] Hiatal enlargement indicates pelvic floor laxity, and added M line enlargement beyond 2 cm with defecation indicates descending perineum.[15,19,20] Decreased hiatus with decreased anorectal angle during defecation indicates pelvic floor dyssynergy.

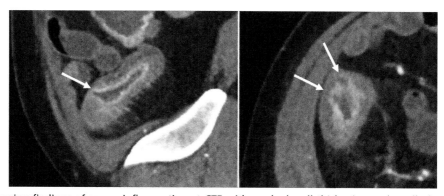

Fig. 2. Imaging findings of severe inflammation at CTE with marked wall thickening and small ulcerations on sagittal (*left, arrow*) and axial images (*right, arrows*). (With permission: Published in: "Consensus Recommendations for Evaluation, Interpretation, and Utilization of Computed Tomography and Magnetic Resonance Enterography in Patients With Small Bowel Crohn's Disease" Bruining et al. Radiology Vol. 286, No. 3: 776-799 Copyright RSNA, 2018.)

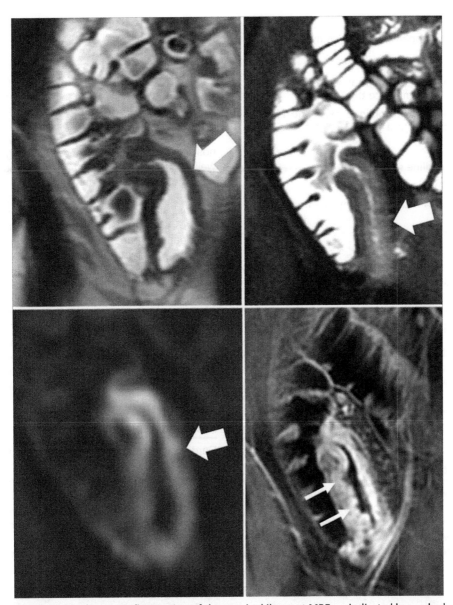

Fig. 3. Imaging findings of severe inflammation of the terminal ileum at MRE, as indicated by marked wall thickening (*top left, arrow*), intramural edema or hyperintensity on a T2-weighted image with fat saturation (*top right, arrow*), increased intramural signal on high b-value diffusion-weighted images (*bottom left, arrow*), and small ulcerations on gadolinium-enhanced images (*bottom right, small white arrows*). (With permission; Published in: "Consensus Recommendations for Evaluation, Interpretation, and Utilization of Computed Tomography and Magnetic Resonance Enterography in Patients With Small Bowel Crohn's Disease" Bruining et al. Radiology Vol. 286, No. 3: 776-799 Copyright RSNA, 2018.)

Static imaging further evaluates the pelvic floor for anatomic defects, such as muscular asymmetry or levator muscle hernias, as well as nonmuscular pathologic condition, such as endometriosis[20] (**Figs. 4–6**).

Pelvic organ prolapse is graded as mild, moderate, or severe in each of the 3 pelvic compartments. Grading is based on measuring the lowest point of the pelvic organ (that is, bladder, vaginal apex, anorectal junction) below the PCL in increments of 3 cm starting 1 cm below the PCL[15] (**Figs. 7–9**).

Rectoceles are defined as anterior focal outpouchings of the rectal wall and are graded based on measurement in the anteroposterior dimension from the anterior margin of the rectal wall to a line extended superiorly from the anterior wall of the anal canal (**Fig. 10**).

INNOVATIONS IN CARDIOTHORACIC IMAGING

Cardiac disease remains the leading cause of morbidity and mortality worldwide and is prevalent across nearly all income groups.[21] Recent advances in CT and MR imaging have helped diagnose and prognosticate various cardiac diseases, allowing for earlier intervention and prevention of adverse outcomes.

Risk Stratification of Cardiovascular Disease

There have been numerous technical developments in CT technology, including increasing coverage with wider detectors, retrospective and prospective electrocardiogram-triggering, current modulation, high- and low-voltage scanning, reconstruction techniques, including iterative reconstruction as well as increased temporal and spatial resolution that have decreased radiation, and many more. Because of these advancements, cardiac CT has emerged as a highly effective and very safe modality to assess cardiac anatomy and pathology. In fact, SCOT HEART, a multicenter study, showed that the addition of CT coronary angiography was able to not only clarify the diagnosis but also change planned investigations as well as treatments, potentially reducing the risk of future myocardial infarction.[22]

For patients with high risk of coronary disease, CT analysis allows for determination of high-risk features of plaque (such as low attenuation, spotty calcifications, napkin ring sign). Furthermore, for patients with symptomatic intermediate disease, fractional flow reserve (FFR), which allows for the determination of flow-specific analysis within the coronary arteries, has been shown to have good correlation with invasive FFR and increases the overall specificity of ischemia-causing lesions.[23] In addition, for asymptomatic intermediate-risk patients, a noninvasive calcium score CT scan helps recategorize patients as either high or low risk for CAD, thus improving personalized treatment.

Structural Heart

Cardiac CT has also become a critical tool in the evaluation of patients with structural abnormalities of the heart. It is particularly helpful in planning minimally invasive techniques for valvular diseases, such as transcatheter aortic valve replacement (TAVR), as well as transcatheter mitral valve replacement, which are becoming standard of care over more invasive surgical techniques.[24]

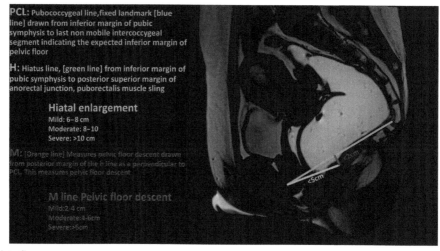

Fig. 4. Pelvic floor.

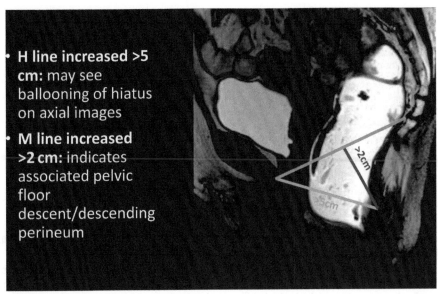

Fig. 5. Pelvic floor laxity.

Recent guidelines have extended approval for TAVR in patients with lower surgical risk, shifting the paradigm in management strategy. With more patients becoming eligible for TAVR, focus has now shifted to optimizing patient selection to improve survival and quality-of-life outcomes. Cardiac CT has thus become an indispensable tool, because anatomic analysis is now at the forefront of patient selection and procedural planning.

Advancements in cardiac CT have allowed for improved visualization of key anatomic structures impacted by TAVR, including the coronary ostia, the aortic root, left ventricular outflow tract, and anterior mitral leaflet. With improved visualization, more detailed measurements are enabled allowing

for more accurate valve sizing and better execution of valve deployment. Determination of the origin of coronary heights in relation to valvular prosthesis is an important factor in determining a patient's candidacy for TAVR, and this can be easily assessed by CT. Tube modulation is an important technique in tailoring spatial resolution to visualize important preprocedural details, such as annular sizing and risk stratification, to assess for left ventricular outflow obstruction. In addition to cardiac measurements, advanced CT imaging of chest, abdomen, and pelvis allows for tailoring of access point as well as fluoroscopic angle measurement. The utility of advanced CT does not end at the placement of a valve prosthesis. Imaging of

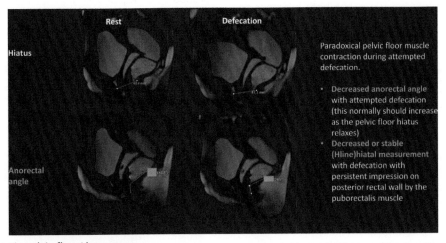

Fig. 6. Spastic pelvic floor/dyssynergy.

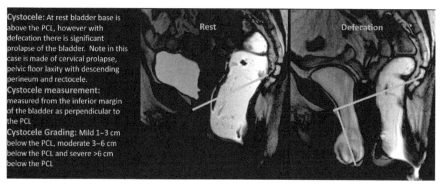

Cystocele: At rest bladder base is above the PCL, however with defecation there is significant prolapse of the bladder. Note in this case is made of cervical prolapse, pelvic floor laxity with descending perineum and rectocele.
Cystocele measurement: measured from the inferior margin of the bladder as perpendicular to the PCL
Cystocele Grading: Mild 1–3 cm below the PCL, moderate 3–6 cm below the PCL and severe >6 cm below the PCL

Rest

Defecation

Fig. 7. Anterior compartment.

prosthetic valve dysfunction using CT is becoming an important supplement to echocardiograms, especially for the evaluation of acute complications (such as valvular abscess) or subacute to chronic complications (such as valvular leaks).[25]

Tissue Characteristics

Until recently, the workhorse for cardiac MR imaging was the evaluation of late gadolinium enhancement (LGE), which only allows for the evaluation of localized areas of tissue damage. Unfortunately, this is most helpful when there is irreversible replacement fibrosis. A major MR breakthrough is the ability to also assess tissues that demonstrate earlier fibrosis.

This is where the utility of T1 mapping shows most promise. The intrinsic T1 time of a tissue acts as a marker for the presence and extent of myocardial disease. Furthermore, comparing T1 pretimes and posttimes allows for the calculation of extracellular cellular volume (ECV), which is a determinant of myocardial fibrosis in reference to left ventricular volume. There is a significant correlation between biopsy-proven collagen volume fraction to T1 and ECV values.[26]

Similarly, T2 mapping allows for the assessment of inflammation within the myocardium. Studies have shown that T2 mapping is the only useful CMR parameter for the assessment of biopsy-proven myocarditis for patients with symptoms longer than 10 to 14 days.[27] There are no vendor-specific reference values for T1 and T2 values currently, limiting the standardization and implementation of these modalities across institutions (**Figs. 11** and **12**).

Dual-Energy Computed Tomography

Acute pulmonary embolism (PE) is a common complication of venous thromboembolism and represents the third-leading cause of cardiovascular-related death in the United States.[28] These emboli commonly originate in the veins of the lower extremities, although they may also originate elsewhere, and travel hematogenously to obstruct the pulmonary arterial

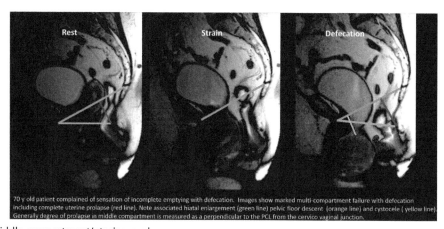

Rest   Strain   Defecation

70 y old patient complained of sensation of incomplete emptying with defecation. Images show marked multi-compartment failure with defecation including complete uterine prolapse (red line). Note associated hiatal enlargement (green line) pelvic floor descent (orange line) and cystocele (yellow line). Generally degree of prolapse in middle compartment is measured as a perpendicular to the PCL from the cervico vaginal junction.

Fig. 8. Middle compartment/uterine prolapse.

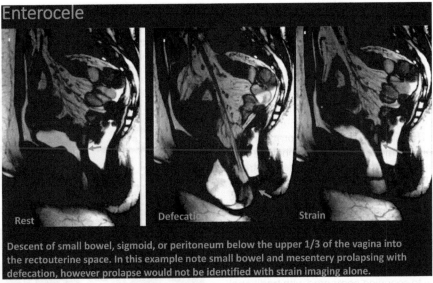

Fig. 9. A 60 year old patient with prior hysterectomy and incomplete evacuation with small bowel mesentery and small bowel loops herniating below the PCL with defecation. Also note large associated cystocele.

vasculature to varying degrees. Accurate and timely diagnosis is key to successful treatment.

In the past decade, pulmonary multidetector computed tomography (MDCT) angiography has been widely regarded as the gold standard in the diagnosis of PE, with risk stratification algorithms and D-dimer as adjuncts for stratifying its use. Traditional MDCT angiography has been limited in only being able to provide morphologic information without additional functional information on pulmonary perfusion.[29–31] To meet this need, there has been implementation of dual-energy

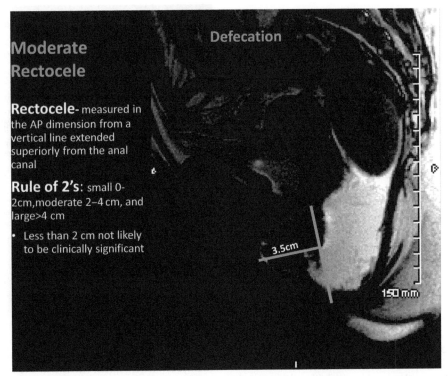

Fig. 10. A 60 year old female with sensation of incomplete evacuation and pelvic pressure. Note anterior protrusion of the rectal wall displacing the vagina anteriorly.

computed tomographic (DE-CT) angiography, which, via perfusion mapping, is able to increase sensitivity for the detection of PE compared with MDCT angiography alone and adds particular value for the identification of small peripheral PEs[31,32] (**Figs. 13–15**).

Technique

The aim of DE-CT protocols is to inform assessment of both pulmonary artery morphology and parenchyma perfusion from a single contrast-enhanced CT. DE-CT is based on concurrent acquisition at low and high radiographic energies, or voltages, which enables evaluation of absorption differences of the contrast medium, usually iodine, between the 2 voltages.[33] DE-CT angiography generally uses a high-concentration iodine injection that is injected rapidly, followed by a longer delay to scanning compared with traditional computed tomography angiography (CTA), in order to enable the iodine to disperse through the parenchyma.[31,34] Commercially available software is then used for postprocessing to reconstruct an iodine map overlay on traditional MDCT images. The iodine enhancement has been demonstrated to correspond to lung blood volume, and as such, these maps visualize perfusion deficits of pulmonary parenchyma[35] (see **Figs. 13–15**).

Advantages

Compared with traditional CTA, there is no significant increase in radiation exposure.[36] The degree of perfused blood volume can be quantified and used for objective risks stratification of the PE via objective measures of thrombus burden and right heart strain through the right-to-left ventricular ratio. In addition to functional information, DE-CT provides high-resolution anatomic and perfusion detail of the pulmonary parenchyma that is also useful in the evaluation of emphysema, pulmonary nodule, and ground-glass opacities.[31] Furthermore, identification of pulmonary perfusion deficits has been shown to be predictive of all-cause mortality irrespective of whether a clot is seen on CT, making these findings useful beyond the realm of PE diagnosis.[37]

Limitations

Artifacts from motion or the high concentration of iodine may result in false negative or false positive findings, and DE-CT is subject to artifact in patients of large body habitus. Postprocessing of DE-CT images also requires additional time and reader experience for interpretation.

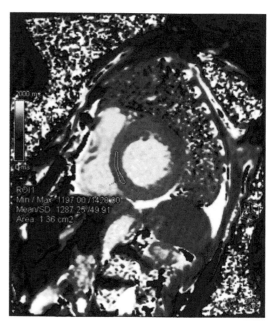

Fig. 11. A T1 map with an ROI analysis. There was clinical concern for amyloid, and the native T1 value was diffusely elevated and measured 1270 ms at the septum (normal values, 950–1050 milliseconds), which helped arrive at the diagnosis of chronic myocarditis, changing patient's therapeutic management.

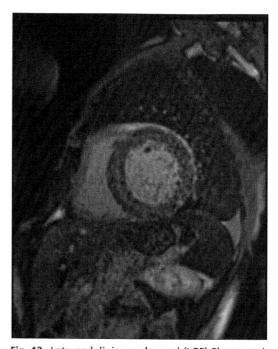

Fig. 12. Late gadolinium enhanced (LGE) Phase sensitive inversion recovery (PSIR) image demonstrated midmyocardial enhancement within the septum and lateral to inferolateral walls, which represented areas of fibrosis.

NEURORADIOLOGY
Functional MR Imaging and Magnetoencephalography

Functional MR imaging (fMR imaging) is a noninvasive method for evaluation of brain activity and localization of brain functions. In clinical practice, it is most widely used for preoperative planning with language, motor, and visual cortex localization, epilepsy workup, and evaluation of neurocognitive, psychiatric, and posttraumatic disorders (**Fig. 16**).[38] Not infrequently, fMR imaging can replace intraoperative cortical stimulation mapping[39] and/or Wada testing.[40] This approach can not only save time and resources but also limit potential procedural complications.

The fundamental principle of fMR imaging is based on the presence of neurovascular coupling, which is a relationship between localized neuronal activity and a hemodynamic response within that specific brain region. Neuronal activation induces a transient spike in blood flow, delivery of oxygenated blood, and, eventually, a drop in the deoxyhemoglobin concentration. This, subsequently, causes a small spike of T2* signal, which can be imaged giving rise to blood oxygen level dependent (BOLD) contrast technique[41] used in fMR imaging.

There are 2 types of fMR imaging: task-based (fMR imaging) and resting state (rs-fMR imaging). The task-based approach takes advantage of the BOLD contrast difference between the task/paradigm administration and rest period, whereas the rs-fMR imaging relies on spontaneous or "resting state" brain activity. Although task-based fMR imaging is more commonly used in clinical practice, rs-fMR imaging is gaining more acceptance as we develop more precise analysis methods and improve our understanding of the resting state brain networks, also known as connectomes. The potential benefits of rs-fMR imaging include decreased scan times, ability to analyze multiple connectomes and brain activation regions in a retrospective manner, and relative independence from the patient's functional status.[42]

Magnetoencephalography (MEG) is another noninvasive technique that interrogates human brain activity and function. This method may be used as a complementary or at times alternative method to fMR imaging. MEG is designed to receive and process infinitesimal amounts of induced magnetic fields created by an inherent intracellular movement of charged ions/electric currents. The most important benefit of MEG is its superior temporal and spatial resolution compared with fMR imaging. MEG also provides direct evaluation of brain activity, whereas fMR

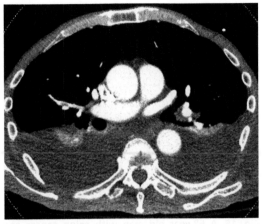

Fig. 13. A 68-year old man with colon cancer and known deep venous thrombosis. Axial sections demonstrate subtle subsegmental filling defects in the right mid lung.

imaging indirectly estimates brain activity from oxygen consumption and CO_2 production. Furthermore, MEG is not limited by motion artifacts and can be used safely and effectively in children.[43]

Diffusion Tensor/Kurtosis/Spectrum Imaging and Fiber Tractography

Diffusion tensor imaging (DTI) is used for localization and evaluation of the white matter tracts in the brain, spinal cord and, occasionally, cranial nerves. DTI is commonly obtained in concert with fMR imaging to assist with preoperative planning and epilepsy surgery (**Fig. 17**). DTI is a diffusion-weighted imaging technique based on the

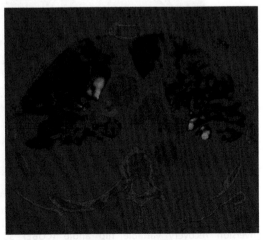

Fig. 14. A 68-year old man with colon cancer and known deep venous thrombosis. Axial perfusion map shows a corresponding wedge-shaped perfusion deficit increasing confidence for PE.

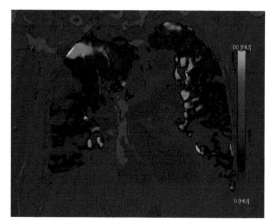

Fig. 15. A 68-year old man with colon cancer and known deep venous thrombosis. Coronal perfusion map shows same wedge-shaped perfusion defect in right mid lung. Coronal section of a perfusion image of DE-CT demonstrates wedge-shaped perfusion deficits within the right upper and middle lobes.

mathematical tensor model used to characterize the anisotropy, magnitude, and orientation of the moving water protons. This technique quantifies the direction and magnitude of water diffusivity and estimates the location and orientation of the white matter tracts. The data are commonly represented in the form of functional anisotropy (FA) and mean diffusivity maps and may be further processed into 3-dimensional (3D) fiber tractography.[44,45]

Several additional emerging diffusion MR techniques, such as diffusion kurtosis and diffusion spectrum imaging, have the benefit of improved fiber tract resolution and visualization of the intravoxel crossing fibers.[46,47]

Arterial Spin Labeling

Arterial spin labeling (ASL) is a perfusion MR imaging technique that eliminates the need for exogenous contrast tracer, which is otherwise required in the conventional dynamic susceptibility contrast, or dynamic contrast-enhanced MR perfusion techniques. ASL allows for quantitative analysis of cerebral blood flow (CBF) and is commonly used for evaluation of tumor perfusion, cerebrovascular diseases, dementia/cognitive disorders, epilepsy, and infection[48,49] (**Fig. 18**). It is also gaining acceptance as a tool for measurement of functional brain activation.[50] Typically, an echo planar imaging sequence or 3D gradient and spin echo is used with an off-resonance RF pulse that magnetizes or "labels" the arterial blood proximal to the ROI.[51] Tissue perfusion/CBF is then estimated by subtracting the static images from the magnetized images.

Cerebral Vessel Wall Imaging

Vessel wall (VW)-MR imaging is an elegant noninvasive angiographic MR imaging technique that provides detailed visualization of the vascular wall and is used as an adjunct to conventional MR

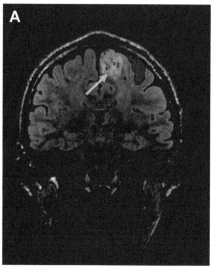
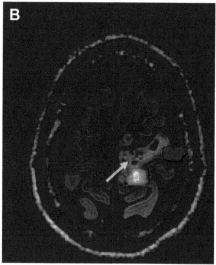

Fig. 16. fMR imaging. Right hand finger tapping motor task fMR imaging in a patient with left superior frontal dysembryoplastic neuroepithelial tumor (DNET). BOLD fMR imaging overlaid on structural fluid attenuated inversion recovery variable flip angle (CUBE) 3D sequence coronal (*A*) and axial (*B*) reconstructions demonstrating left cerebral hand motor cortex activations (*pink*) slightly overlapping the superolateral aspect of the lesion (*white arrow*). Left foot motor cortex activation (*green*) is also seen to slightly overlap the posterior aspect of the lesion (*white arrow*) (*B*). The patient declined resection in part because of proximity to eloquent motor cortex.

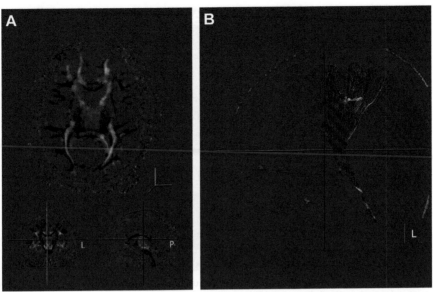

Fig. 17. DTI and tractography. (*A*) Combined FA and directional map of DTI demonstrating cerebral white matter tracts in the same patient with left frontal DNET. Color hue indicates direction: red, right to left; green, antero-posterior; blue, superior to inferior. (*B*) 3D fiber tractography of the corticospinal tract derived from the source DTI data demonstrates slightly reduced tract representations in the area of the left frontal DNET. The patient had no sensory or motor deficit. L, left; P, posterior.

angiography, CTA, or digital subtraction angiography, which assesses the vascular lumen. VW-MR imaging may be indicated in cases of challenging or inconspicuous intracranial atherosclerotic plaques, vasculitis, reversible cerebral vasoconstriction syndrome, or arterial dissection.[52] This technique requires high spatial and contrast resolution, which can be achieved by using higher magnetic fields (3 T vs 1.5 T), black blood, or other blood/brain/cerebrospinal fluid suppression techniques and a combination of 2-dimensional and 3D techniques (**Fig. 19**).

Magnetic Resonance Black Blood Thrombus Imaging

MR black blood thrombus imaging (MRBTI) is a noninvasive black blood imaging technique initially developed for segmentation of myocardium and blood pool in cardiovascular imaging. It was recently adopted by the Neuroradiology community to improve visualization and early detection of cerebral venous thrombosis, which often presents a diagnostic challenge when using conventional MR venography. MRBTI typically uses a double inversion recovery T1 measurement turbo spin-echo/fast-spin echo and double-inversion recovery short tau inversion recovery sequence to suppress the signal from moving blood. This technique allows for direct thrombus visualization in

contradistinction to conventional MR venography that evaluates vascular lumen.[53]

Susceptibility Weighted Imaging and Quantitative Susceptibility Mapping

Susceptibility weighted imaging (SWI) is an MR imaging technique that exploits intrinsic differences in magnetic susceptibility of tissues and compounds. For example, calcium hydroxyapatite demonstrates diamagnetic properties and will have an opposite signal on filtered phase images compared with the paramagnetic iron/hemosiderin deposition (**Figs. 20** and **21**). SWI also shows great sensitivity for detecting small volumes of blood products and has an ability to differentiate between arterial and venous vessels.[54]

Although conventional SWI is a qualitative technique, quantitative susceptibility mapping (QSM) is a postprocessing tool that computes a map of tissue magnetic susceptibility values. Clinically, a combination of SWI and QSM is increasingly used for evaluation of vascular malformations, traumatic brain injury, multiple sclerosis, and stroke.[55]

Artificial Intelligence

In health care, 2 major categories of Artificial Intelligence (AI) are being implemented: machine learning (ML) and natural language processing (NLP).

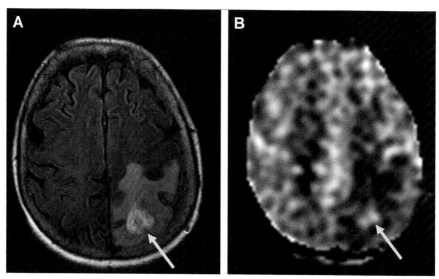

Fig. 18. ASL in a patient with left parietal glioblastoma multiforme. FLAIR image (*A*) demonstrating centrally hyperintense mass (*arrow*) in the left parietal lobe with surrounding vasogenic edema. ASL image (*B*) demonstrating hyperintense hyperperfusion correlating with tumor (*arrow*).

ML makes predictions and/or decisions from structured data, for example, imaging studies, by using mathematical models built from several types of datasets. In order to understand unstructured data, NLP analyzes inputs such as clinical notes and converts them to a form that can then be further analyzed using ML.[56] AI methodology has been applied to enhance image interpretation, workflow dynamics, disease classification, prediction of pathologic condition, and response to treatment. More recently, AI research has been focusing on the clinical decision support chain, protocol selection, and image acquisition/improvement[57] (**Fig. 22**).

Perfusion Computed Tomography

Perfusion computed tomography (CTP) is a contrast-enhanced CT technique that provides a noninvasive, qualitative, and quantitative assessment of cerebrovascular perfusion. After the scan is acquired, a time-attenuation curve is generated and multiple perfusion parameters, such as cerebral blood volume (CBV), cerebral blood flow (CBF), mean transit time (MTT), and time to peak (TTP), are calculated and displayed as color maps. These calculations are based on the central volume theory: CBF = CBV/MTT (**Fig. 23**).

One of the main goals of CTP is to differentiate a potentially salvageable brain tissue (penumbra) from an irreversibly damaged brain tissue (core infarct), which can help triage stroke patients into thrombectomy/thrombolysis versus conservative treatment. Other common indications for the use of CTP include evaluation of cerebrovascular reserve, vasospasm, and tumor angiogenesis.[58]

Dual-Energy Computed Tomography

Spectral or dual-energy CT is a CT technique that uses 2 distinct photon energy spectra for evaluation

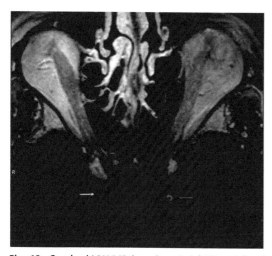

Fig. 19. Cerebral VW-MR imaging: Axial T1-weighted volume isotropic turbo spin echo acquisition (VISTA) VW image demonstrating severe stenosis and smooth circumferential enhancement of the left cavernous internal carotid artery in a patient with acute vasculitis (*red arrow*). There is also mild smooth circumferential VW enhancement without stenosis of the visualized right cavernous ICA (*white arrow*).

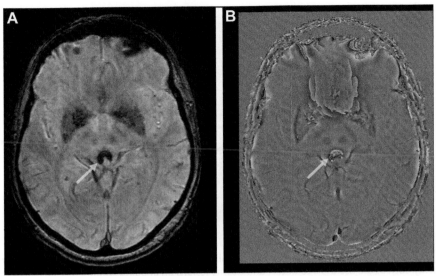

Fig. 20. SWI calcium. Axial susceptibility-weighted angiography (SWAN) image demonstrating hypointense susceptibility signal in the pineal gland (*A*) with hyperintensity on the associated filtered phase image (*B*), denoting diamagnetic calcium in this patient with physiologic pineal calcifications (*arrow*).

of materials with different photoelectric energies/K-edges and, therefore, different radiographic attenuation profiles. The 2 most commonly used tube voltages are 80 kVp and 140 kVp.[59] The closer the K-edge of the studied material to the tube voltage used, the greater the contrast. For example, the K-edge of iodine is 33.2 keV, and its attenuation will be greater at 80 kVp than at 140 kVp, allowing for the clinically important material decomposition imaging that can differentiate intracranial hematoma from contrast staining, mineral deposition, or metal fragments.

Additional clinical applications of DE-CT include virtual monoenergetic and weighted average images, which simulate conventional nonenhanced CT and obviate additional scan time and radiation.

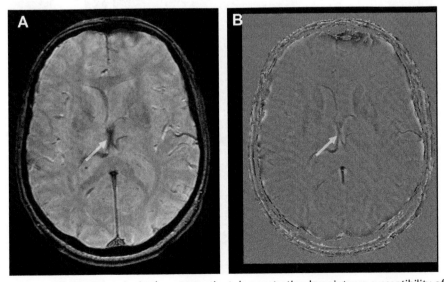

Fig. 21. SWI vein. Axial SWAN images in the same patient demonstrating hypointense susceptibility of the internal cerebral veins (*A*) with hypointensity on the associated filtered phase image (*B*), denoting paramagnetic blood products within the vessels (*arrow*). Note: Appearance or "color" of blood and calcium is magnet specific but can be correlated with intensity of cortical veins.

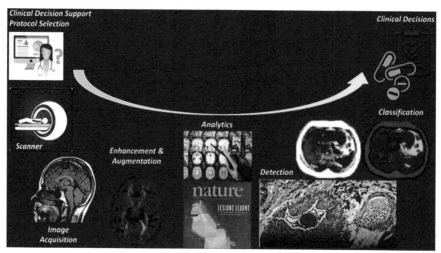

Fig. 22. AI. Imaging value chain. Although most AI applications have focused on the downstream (or right) side of this pathway, such as the use of AI to detect and classify lesions on imaging studies, it is likely that there will be earlier adoption for the tasks on the upstream (or left) side, where most of the costs of imaging are concentrated. (*From* "Applications of Deep Learning to Neuro-Imaging Technique. Guangming Zhu, Bin Jiang, Liz Tong, Yuan Xie, Greg Zaharchuk, and Max Wintermark* Front Neurol. 2019; 10: 869"; Figure 2; with permission.)

Furthermore, metal artifact reduction, subtraction of mural calcifications, or embolization coil material can be achieved with DE-CT providing superior visualization of the vessel and adjacent anatomy[60] (**Fig. 24**).

Micro-Computed Tomography

Microfocus, or microscopic CT, is a noninvasive CT technique that achieves histologic levels of spatial resolution measuring in microns compared with millimeters for the standard CT scanner. Greater

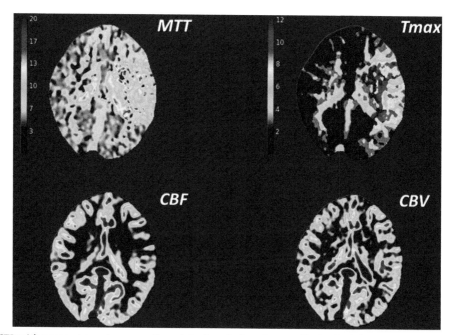

Fig. 23. CTP with parametric color maps. Unmatched perfusion abnormality in the left MCA territory with a large area of increased MTT and Tmax (penumbra) and a smaller area of decreased CBF and CBV (core infarct) in the peripheral cortical and subcortical left frontal and parietal lobes. These findings suggest a potential benefit of reperfusion therapy.

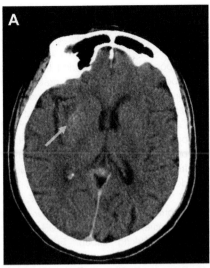 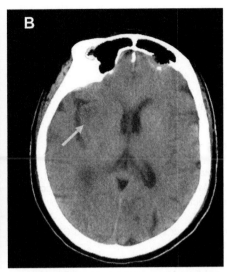

Fig. 24. DE-CT. Patient with right MCA infarct status post thrombectomy. (*A*) Single-energy CT scan demonstrates nonspecific hyperdensity in the right basal ganglia in the region of the infarct (*white arrow*), suggestive of contrast staining versus hemorrhage. (*B*) DE-CT acquired at 140 kV and 80 kV with 70 keV shows resolution of hyperdensity confirming contrast staining (*white arrow*). (Images courtesy of Carina W. Yang, MD and Saad A. Ali, MD; University of Chicago Medicine.)

resolution is accomplished by using a fixed radiographic source and an adjustable detector height, resulting in decreased source to image distance. Limitations of this technique are long acquisition times (minutes to hours), high sensitivity to motion, and increased radiation dose.[61] For these reasons, most current clinical applications include ex vivo sample imaging (breast tissue, endarterectomy specimen)[62] and virtual fetal autopsies.[63]

SUMMARY

A wide range of technological advances have been made in Neuroradiology over the past several years. The use of functional imaging, including fMR imaging, MEG, and functional arterial spin labeling, has become commonplace in clinical practice, enhancing the ability to localize eloquent brain and prevent potentially devastating surgical complications in patients undergoing tumor or epilepsy surgery. Several new elegant noninvasive angiographic methods, such as MRBTI and VWMRI, have improved diagnostic accuracy when facing challenging intracranial vascular diseases. Perfusion CT has reshaped the approach to diagnosis and treatment of stroke patients, whereas micro-CT has increased CT resolution to histologic levels. These imaging methods, combined with the power of AI, will continue to advance the knowledge of human anatomy and physiology and enhance the value of Neuroimaging in patient care.

In addition, in abdomino-pelvic imaging, standardization of imaging protocols and interpretation is now promoting the dissemination of clinically relevant and reproducible imaging data to the practicing specialist. The application of functional imaging has become more widespread, particularly in the evaluation of pelvic floor dysfunction, and inflammatory bowel disease.

One of the most promising areas of innovation within cardiovascular CT imaging is the application of ML to further automate diagnoses. For supervised ML, where data sets have been labeled with outcomes or classes, the qualification of coronary artery calcium, epicardial and thoracic fat pad analysis, and its determinant to coronary artery calcium disease as well as derivation of coronary CTA FFR, have a significant potential to be automated and aid the clinician in diagnosis.[64]

Furthermore, deep learning has great potential in the assessment of cardiac anatomy within cardiac MR imaging. Using neural networks, it is now possible to automatically segment right and left ventricular endocardium and epicardium to allow for the fully automated assessment of cardiac mass and function, including ejection fraction (for which MR remains the gold standard).[65]

Although the potential for AI applications in health care holds a great deal of promise, there are many challenges, particularly finding large data sets, data heterogeneity, as well as establishing ground truth within medical images, which is often one of the most significant challenges. However, once these challenges are addressed, AI may herald a new era of innovation within all of radiology subspecialties, not just within cardio-vascular imaging.

DISCLOSURE

The authors have nothing to disclose.

REFERENCES

1. Stasi C, Milani S. Non-invasive assessment of liver fibrosis: between prediction/prevention of outcomes and cost-effectiveness. World J Gastroenterol 2016; 22(4):1711–20.
2. Bataller R, Brenner DA. Liver fibrosis. J Clin Invest 2005;115:209–18.
3. Venkatesh S, Ehman R. Magnetic resonance elastography of liver. Magn Reson Imaging Clin N Am 2014;22:433–46.
4. Regev A, Berho M, Jeffers LJ, et al. Sampling error and intraobserver variation in liver biopsy in patients with chronic HCV infection. Am J Gastroenterol 2002;97:2614–8.
5. Piccinino F, Sagnelli E, Pasquale G, et al. Complications following percutaneous liver biopsy. A multi-centre retrospective study on 68,276 biopsies. J Hepatol 1986;2:165–73.
6. Friedrich-Rust M, Poynard T, Castera L. Critical comparison of elastography methods to assess chronic liver disease. Nat Rev Gastroenterol Hepatol 2016; 13:402–11.
7. Su LN, Guo SL, Li BX, et al. Diagnostic value of magnetic resonance elastography for detecting and staging of hepatic fibrosis: a meta-analysis. Clin Radiol 2014;69:e545–52.
8. Sirli R, Sporea I, Bota S, et al. A comparative study of non-invasive methods for fibrosis assessment in chronic HCV infection. Hepat Mon 2010; 10:88–94.
9. Stasi C, Piluso A, Arena U, et al. Evaluation of the prognostic value of liver stiffness in patients with hepatitis C virus treated with triple or dual antiviral therapy: a prospective pilot study. World J Gastroenterol 2015;21:3013–9.
10. Bruining DH, Zimmerman EM, Loftus EV Jr, et al. Consensus recommendations for evaluation, interpretation, and utilization of computed tomography and magnetic resonance enterography in patients with small bowel Crohn's disease. Radiology 2018; 286:776–96.
11. Kaushal P, Somwaru AS, Charabaty A, et al. MR enterography of inflammatory bowel disease with endoscopic correlation. Radiographics 2017;37:1, 116-131.
12. Bekendam MIJ, Puylaert CAJ, Phoa SKSS, et al. Shortened oral contrast preparation for improved small bowel distension at MR enterography. Abdom Radiol (N Y) 2017;42:2225–32.
13. Martin D, Kalb B, Miller F, et al, Committee on Body Imaging (Abdominal) (ACR Committee responsible for sponsoring the draft through the process). ACR–SAR–SPR practice parameter for the performance of magnetic resonance (MR) enterography. 2015.
14. Grand DJ, Guglielmo FF, Al-Hawary MM. MR enterography in Crohn's disease: current consensus on optimal imaging technique and future advances from the SAR Crohn's disease-focused panel. Abdom Imaging 2015;40(5):953–64.
15. El Sayed RF, Alt CD, Maccioni F, et al. Magnetic resonance imaging of pelvic floor dysfunction - joint recommendations of the ESUR and ESGAR Pelvic Floor Working Group. Eur Radiol 2017;27(5): 2067–85.
16. Schawkat K, Pfister B, Parker H, et al. Dynamic MRI of the pelvic floor: comparison of performance in supine vs left lateral body position. Br J Radiol 2018; 91(1092):20180393.
17. García del Salto L, de Miguel Criado J, Aguilera del Hoyo LF, et al. MR imaging–based assessment of the female pelvic floor. Radiographics 2014;34(5): 1417–39.
18. Gupta AP, Pandya PR, Nguyen M, et al. Use of dynamic MRI of the pelvic floor in the assessment of anterior compartment disorders. Curr Urol Rep 2018;19:112.
19. Khatri G, de Leon AD, Lockhart ME. MR imaging of the pelvic floor. Magn Reson Imaging Clin N Am 2017;25(3):457–80.
20. Bitti GT, Argiolas GM, Ballicu N, et al. Pelvic floor failure: MR imaging evaluation of anatomic and functional abnormalities. Radiographics 2014;34:2, 429-448.
21. Gandhi MM, Lampe FC, Wood DA. Incidence, clinical characteristics, and short-term prognosis of angina pectoris. Br Heart J 1995;73:193–8.
22. The SCOT-HEART investigators. CT coronary angiography in patients with suspected angina due to coronary heart disease (SCOT-HEART): an open-label, parallel-group, multicentre trial. Lancet 2015; 385(9985):2383–91.
23. Renker M, Schoepf UJ, Becher T, et al. Computed tomography in patients with stable angina pectoris : measurement of fractional flow reserve. Herz 2017;42:51–7.
24. Commissioner, Office of the. FDA expands indication for several transcatheter heart valves to patients at low risk for death or major complications associated with open-heart surgery. U.S. Food and Drug Administration, FDA. Available at: www.fda.gov/news-events/press-announcements/fda-expands-indication-several-transcatheter-heart-valves-patients-low-risk-death-or-major.

25. Faure ME, Swart LE, Dijkshoorn ML, et al. Advanced CT acquisition protocol with a third generation dual-source CT scanner and iterative reconstruction technique for comprehensive prosthetic heart valve assessment. Eur Radiol 2018;28:2159–68.

26. Nakamori S, Dohi K, Ishida M, et al. Native T1 mapping and extracellular volume mapping for the assessment of diffuse myocardial fibrosis in dilated cardiomyopathy. JACC Cardiovasc Imaging 2018; 11(1):48–59.

27. Lurz P, Luecke C, Eitel I, et al. Comprehensive cardiac magnetic resonance imaging in patients with suspected myocarditis: the MyoRacer-Trial. J Am Coll Cardiol 2016;67(15):1800–11.

28. Pipavath SN, Godwin JD. Acute pulmonary thromboembolism: a historical perspective. AJR Am J Roentgenol 2008;191(3):639–41.

29. Toplis E, Mortimore G. The diagnosis and management of pulmonary embolism. Br J Nurs 2020; 29(1):22–6.

30. Remy-Jardin M, Pistolesi M, Goodman LR, et al. Management of suspected acute pulmonary embolism in the era of CT angiography: a statement from the Fleischner Society. Radiology 2007;245(2): 315–29.

31. Lu GM, Zhao Y, Zhang LJ, et al. Dual-energy CT of the lung. AJR Am J Roentgenol 2012;199(5 Suppl): S40–53.

32. Lu GM, Wu SY, Yeh BM, et al. Dual-energy computed tomography in pulmonary embolism. Br J Radiol 2010;83(992):707–18.

33. Ohana M, Jeung MY, Labani A, et al. Thoracic dual energy CT: acquisition protocols, current applications and future developments. Diagn Interv Imaging 2014;95(11):1017–26.

34. Nance JW Jr, Henzler T, Meyer M, et al. Optimization of contrast material delivery for dual-energy computed tomography pulmonary angiography in patients with suspected pulmonary embolism. Invest Radiol 2012;47(1):78–84.

35. Thieme SF, Graute V, Nikolaou K, et al. Dual energy CT lung perfusion imaging–correlation with SPECT/CT. Eur J Radiol 2012;81(2):360–5.

36. Henzler T, Fink C, Schoenberg SO, et al. Dual-energy CT: radiation dose aspects. AJR Am J Roentgenol 2012;199(5 Suppl):S16–25.

37. Takx RAP, Henzler T, Schoepf UJ, et al. Predictive value of perfusion defects on dual energy CTA in the absence of thromboembolic clots. J Cardiovasc Comput Tomogr 2017;11(3):183–7.

38. Orringer D, Vago D, Golby A. Clinical applications and future directions of functional MRI. Semin Neurol 2013;32(04):466–75.

39. Bizzi A, Blasi V, Falini A, et al. Presurgical functional MR imaging of language and motor functions: validation with intraoperative electrocortical mapping. Radiology 2008;248(2):579–89.

40. Binder JR. Functional MRI is a valid noninvasive alternative to Wada testing. Epilepsy Behav 2011; 20(2):214–22.

41. Logothetis NK. The underpinnings of the BOLD functional magnetic resonance imaging signal. J Neurosci 2003;23(10):3963–71.

42. Lv H, Wang Z, Tong E, et al. Resting-state functional MRI: everything that nonexperts have always wanted to know. Am J Neuroradiol 2018;39(8): 1390–9.

43. Hall EL, Robson SE, Morris PG, et al. The relationship between MEG and fMRI. Neuroimage 2014; 102:80–91.

44. Hijaz TA, Mccomb EN, Badhe S, et al. Tractography tutorial and introduction to major white matter. Neurographics 2019;9(1):62–74.

45. Jellison BJ, Field AS, Medow J, et al. Diffusion tensor imaging of cerebral white matter: a pictorial review of physics, fiber tract anatomy, and tumor imaging patterns. Am J Neuroradiol 2004;25(3):356–69.

46. Steven AJ, Zhuo J, Melhem ER. Diffusion kurtosis imaging: an emerging technique for evaluating the microstructural environment of the brain. Am J Roentgenol 2014;202(1):26–33.

47. Wedeen VJ, Wang RP, Schmahmann JD, et al. Diffusion spectrum magnetic resonance imaging (DSI) tractography of crossing fibers. Neuroimage 2008; 41(4):1267–77.

48. Petcharunpaisan S, Ramalho J, Castillo M. Arterial spin labeling in neuroimaging. World J Radiol 2010;2(10):384–98.

49. Haller S, Zaharchuk G, Thomas DL, et al. Arterial spin labeling perfusion of the brain: emerging clinical applications. Radiology 2016;281(2):337–56.

50. Steketee RME, Mutsaerts HJMM, Bron EE, et al. Quantitative functional arterial spin labeling (fASL) MRI - sensitivity and reproducibility of regional CBF changes using pseudo-continuous ASL product sequences. PLoS One 2015;10(7). https://doi.org/10.1371/journal.pone.0132929.

51. Grade M, Hernandez Tamames JA, Pizzini FB, et al. A neuroradiologist's guide to arterial spin labeling MRI in clinical practice. Neuroradiology 2015; 57(12):1181–202.

52. Mandell DM, Mossa-Basha M, Qiao Y, et al. Intracranial vessel wall MRI: principles and expert consensus recommendations of the American Society of Neuroradiology. Am J Neuroradiol 2017;38(2): 218–29.

53. Yang Q, Duan J, Fan Z, et al. Early detection and quantification of cerebral venous thrombosis by magnetic resonance black-blood thrombus imaging. Stroke 2016;47(2):404–9.

54. Ciraci S, Gumus K, Doganay S, et al. Diagnosis of intracranial calcification and hemorrhage in pediatric patients: comparison of quantitative susceptibility mapping and phase images of susceptibility-

weighted imaging. Diagn Interv Imaging 2017; 98(10):707–14.

55. Liu C, Li W, Tong KA, et al. Susceptibility-weighted imaging and quantitative susceptibility mapping in the brain. J Magn Reson Imaging 2015;42(1):23–41.

56. Jiang F, Jiang Y, Zhi H, et al. Artificial intelligence in healthcare: past, present and future. Stroke Vasc Neurol 2017;2(4):230–43.

57. Zhu G, Jiang B, Tong L, et al. Applications of deep learning to neuro-imaging techniques. Front Neurol 2019;10:1–13.

58. Wintermark M, Sincic R, Sridhar D, et al. Cerebral perfusion CT: technique and clinical applications. J Neuroradiol 2008;35(5):253–60.

59. Johnson TRC. Dual-energy CT: general principles. AJR Am J Roentgenol 2012;199(5 Suppl).

60. Machida H, Tanaka I, Fukui R, et al. Dual-energy spectral CT: various clinical vascular applications. Radiographics 2016;36(4):1215–32.

61. Hutchinson JC, Shelmerdine SC, Simcock IC, et al. Early clinical applications for imaging at microscopic detail: microfocus computed tomography (micro-CT). Br J Radiol 2017;90(1075):1–10.

62. Wintermark M, Jawadi SS, Rapp JH, et al. High-resolution CT imaging of carotid artery atherosclerotic plaques. Am J Neuroradiol 2008;29(5):875–82.

63. Lombardi S, Scola E, Ippolito D, et al. Micro-computed tomography: a new diagnostic tool in postmortem assessment of brain anatomy in small fetuses. Neuroradiology 2019;61(7):737–46.

64. Singh G, Al'aref SJ, Van Assen M, et al. Machine learning in cardiac CT: basic concepts and contemporary data. J Cardiovasc Comput Tomogr 2018;12: 192–201.

65. Winther HB, Hundt C, Schmidt B, et al. ν-Net: deep learning for generalized biventricular mass and function parameters using multicenter cardiac MRI data. JACC Cardiovasc Imaging 2018;11(7): 1036–8.

Advances in Preclinical PET Instrumentation

Mahsa Amirrashedi[a,b], Habib Zaidi[c,d,e,f], Mohammad Reza Ay, PhD[a,b],*

KEYWORDS

• Small-animal PET imaging • Preclinical PET scanner • Instrumentation • Design • Performance

KEY POINTS

- High-resolution PET scanners dedicated to preclinical studies facilitate the characterization of small details within the animal's body.
- Understanding the new trends in preclinical imaging will be helpful to further establish the crucial role of small-animal PET scanners in a wide spectrum of biomedical research activities.
- Detector material and design considerations are the most determinant factors affecting the PET scanner's overall performance.

INTRODUCTION

Because of anatophysiological similarities between human and animal species, the use of animal models, particularly vertebrate mammals, has dramatically revolutionized many fields of modern research in basic biology, translational medicine, pharmaceutical industry, and several other areas.[1–3] Among numerous imaging modalities devoted to murine model investigations, PET rekindled a considerable interest due to gleaning a wealth of quantitative information about biological processes at the molecular and cellular levels.[4] Salient progress and considerable advances in small-animal PET imaging has had and will continue to have a far more profound effect on drug development and biomedical research. Ideally, a PET scanner dedicated to small laboratory animals would have to promise high-enough resolving power coupled to optimum detection efficiency to ensure visualization of a small amount of radiotracer uptake within microstructures of the animal body. In the light of ever-increasing demands for devices with better resolvability, a higher level of sensitivity, and wide accessibility for noninvasive screening of small structures and physiologic processes in laboratory rodents, the number of dedicated preclinical PET scanners is increasing rapidly. Preclinical PET scanners are gaining in importance, whereas concerns are surfacing over the design aspects as well as costs associated with software products and hardware developments. To conquer these limitations and challenges, a variety of dedicated small-animal PET prototypes, as well as commercial scanners with different configurations, architectural designs, and diversified types of software were characterized and evaluated during recent years. Although extensive research has been carried out on individual scanners, a comprehensive comparative assessment of the performance of different preclinical PET scanners is missing. This article aims to review advances in preclinical PET with particular emphasis on instrumentation until early 2020.

a Department of Medical Physics and Biomedical Engineering, Tehran University of Medical Sciences, Tehran, Iran; b Research Center for Molecular and Cellular Imaging, Tehran University of Medical Sciences, Tehran, Iran; c Division of Nuclear Medicine and Molecular Imaging, Geneva University Hospital, Geneva CH-1211, Switzerland; d Geneva University Neurocenter, Geneva University, Geneva CH-1205, Switzerland; e Department of Nuclear Medicine and Molecular Imaging, University of Groningen, University Medical Center Groningen, Groningen 9700 RB, Netherlands; f Department of Nuclear Medicine, University of Southern Denmark, Odense 500, Denmark
* Corresponding author, Department of Medical Physics & Biomedical Engineering, Tehran University of Medical Sciences, School of Medicine, Poursina Street, Tehran, Islamic Republic of Iran.
E-mail address: mohammadreza_ay@sina.tums.ac.ir

PET Clin 15 (2020) 403–426
https://doi.org/10.1016/j.cpet.2020.06.003

BRIEF HISTORY OF PRECLINICAL PET SCANNERS

The early development of preclinical PET scanners dates back to mid-1990s when the first dedicated systems were developed following the same design principles used in human scanners. A more detailed history and characterization of the first animal scanners have been well-reviewed by Chatziioannou,[5] Goertzen and colleagues,[6] Levin and Zaidi,[7] and Tai.[8] However, to project the current trends and essential challenges in this era, a brief snapshot of the early designs adopted for animal studies is valuable. The first generation of specialized PET systems used large gantry apertures to accommodate medium-sized species, such as rhesus and squirrel monkeys as well as small rodents. The SHR-2000 scanner is one of the earliest designs explored by Hamamatsu (Hamamatsu, Japan)[9,10], which comprises Bismuth-Germinate (BGO) detectors arranged in four rings with 384 mm diameter and spatial resolution of 3 mm and 4.8 mm in the transaxial and axial directions, respectively. The viability of in vivo measurements in rat brain using a dual BGO block detector was initially reported by Rajeswaran and colleagues.[11] This was followed by the development of the first PET device dedicated to conscious brain imaging in rats.[12] This small tomograph, so-called RATPET, was based on 16 BGO detector blocks coupled to photomultiplier tubes (PMTs) arranged in a ringlike geometry with 115 mm diameter and 50 mm axial field-of-view (AFOV), which ultimately resulted in a transaxial resolution of 2.2 mm at the center of the field of view (CFOV).[12] The first Avalanche-photodiode (APD)-based scanner (Sherbrooke APD PET) consisted of 512 BGO crystals arranged in 2 rings such that the face-to-face distance between opposite detectors of the ring was 135 mm and the axial length was 10.5 mm. The scanner features a wobbling scheme and one-to-one coupling to improve the spatial resolution up to 2.1 mm at the CFOV. The first commercial platform adapted successfully for imaging small laboratory species are the microPET series developed by Concorde Microsystems Inc. (Knoxville, TN).[13] The first-generation microPET systems offered dedicated 4-ring versions for primates (P4) and rodents (R4) imaging with ring diameters of 261 and 148 mm, respectively.[14,15] Both configurations were composed of lutetium-oxyorthosilicate (LSO) scintillators forming a 78 mm axial length. The next-generation microPET series, including Focus-120, Focus-220, and the Inveon-DPET have also been marketed.[16–18] All microPET families developed by Siemens were based on

LSO/PSPMT detectors with further refinements in detector geometries, crystal dimensions, and electronics. The Inveon, the last design of the microPET series, is a trimodality platform offering the largest axial extension (127 mm), up to three-fold higher sensitivity (6.27%) in comparison to its predecessors.

The yttrium-aluminum-perovskite (YAP)-(S)PET scanner developed at the Universities of Ferrara and Pisa was a commercial model using four rotating heads with a 150 mm distance between opposite panels.[19] As its name implies, the scanner was based on YAP crystals. For simultaneous PET/SPECT imaging, one pair of the opposed detectors was set in coincidence mode to enable PET acquisition, whereas the second was operated as SPECT detectors equipped with low-energy high-resolution collimators. The use of PET or SPECT mode was also feasible. The reconstructed volumetric resolution in PET mode at the CFOV was 8.5 mm^3, with maximum absolute sensitivity of 1.87% for an energy window of 50 to 850 keV.

The only preclinical product marketed by Philips is the Mosaic-HP composed of pixelated lutetium-yttrium-orthosilicate (LYSO) crystals encoded by PMT-based readouts.[20] The transaxial FOV (TFOV) and axial FOV (AFOV) of the scanner were suitable for one-bed whole-body rodent imaging. The transaxial spatial resolution was 2.34 mm for a central point source with a 2.83% peak absolute photon sensitivity (385–665 keV).

Another fully engineered preclinical device (ClearPET) with adjustable rotating heads was manufactured by Raytest Isotopenmessgeraete GmbH (Mannheim, Germany). The scanner is made up of 20 rotating dual-layered LYSO/lutetium-YAP (LuYAP) detectors. The adjustable heads allowed forming TFOVs with 94 and 144 mm diameters and axial extension of 110 mm. The reconstructed spatial resolution and absolute photon sensitivity following NEMA-NU4 standards are 1.9 to 2 mm full-width at half maximum (FWHM) at 5 cm radial offset and 4.7% (100–750 keV), respectively.[21,22]

The FLEX Triumph is the first trimodality PET/SPECT/computed tomographic (CT) system introduced into the market by Gamma Medica-Ideas (Northridge, CA). The platform includes a 4-head SPECT subunit based on cadmium zinc telluride (CZT) detectors coplanar with the XO-CT scanner, integrated with the X-PET or LabPET8 subsystems. X-PET, the commercial version of Rodent Research PET (RRPET), is based on 16 BGO/PMT detector blocks, arranged in a pentagon shape to form a FOV with 200 mm width and 116 mm length. The large AFOV together with BGO-based crystals result in good sensitivity of

5.9% at CFOV when using 250 to 750 keV energy window.[23]

Another well-known family in the preclinical PET market is LabPET series commercialized by Gamma Medica/GE Healthcare.[24,25] LabPET family features phoswich detectors individually coupled to APD photodetectors. Three versions of the scanner, called LabPET4, LabPET8, and LabPET12, with an equivalent ring diameter of 162 mm and axial extensions of 37.5, 75, and 115 mm were released by the company.[24,26] The LabPET scanners comprise dual-layered tapered LYSO/ lutetium-gadolinium oxyorthosilicate (LGSO) phoswich detectors with side-by-side readout electronics to cope with the parallax-error associated with small ring diameters.

SEDECAL (Madrid, Spain) has also offered different commercial designs with finer crystal elements in comparison to the abovementioned systems. One of them incorporated LYSO/GSO crystals backed by PSPMTs known as Argus (eXplore Vista), whereas the second one (VrPET/ CT) is a coplanar PET/CT scanner based on V-shaped LYSO detector blocks arranged in a partial ring geometry with a rotating gantry.[27,28] The other coplanar design manufactured by the same company is the rPET-1 composed of 2 rotating planar heads with 45 mm AFOV and TFOV. In comparison to other versions of the rPET scanners with two double-block heads, the rPET-1 suffers from 2-fold lower sensitivity. The small crystal pitches used on the rPET-1 resulted in 1.4-mm spatial resolution at the CFOV following NEMA-NU4 protocols.[21] For the widest energy window available on the scanner (100–700 keV), the highest achievable sensitivity was 1%.

STATE-OF-THE-ART PRECLINICAL PET SCANNERS

The remarkable improvements in system designs and overall performance introduced by the different vendors resulted in the current generation preclinical PET scanners surpassing the previous generations in many aspects (**Fig. 1**, **Table 1**). Because of space constraints, the general features of each model (evaluated after 2012) is briefly discussed in this section. Detailed information about various designs along with system performance tests following NEMA NU 4-2008 procedure[22] are also summarized in **Tables 2** and **3**.

Recently, Mediso Medical Imaging Systems (Budapest, Hungary) came up with a wide range of multimodality in vivo solutions, including Nano-PET/CT, nanoScan PET/MR imaging, and Nano-PET/SPECT/CT platforms as well as other bimodal techniques, such as SPECT/CT and SPECT/MR imaging. Except for the magnet shielding in PET/MR imaging combination, the PET component in NanoScan family is identical, which consists of fine LYSO pixels arranged around a 180-mm ring enabling sequential PET and CT acquisitions via NanoPET/CT or in-line PET and MR imaging (1T) via nanoScan PET/MR imaging.[29,30] The AFOV and TFOV of the units are sufficiently large (95 and 123 mm, respectively) to encompass the entire body of rodents. Another specific and highly versatile design released by Mediso is the MultiScan LFER 150 PET/CT, which is particularly adapted for dynamic brain imaging in awake nonhuman primates (NHPs) in recumbent and sitting positions.[30,31]

The IRIS PET from Inviscan (Strasbourg, France) represents the latest generation of commercial small-animal scanners operating either in rotating or stationary modes.[32] In bimodal PET/CT mode, the PET module is placed at the back of the CT unit and could rotate around the scanned objects to acquire high-quality images in step and shoot modes with 95 mm coverage in the axial direction.[32]

The Albira triple-modality system is an integrated SPECT/PET/CT platform manufactured by Bruker Oncovision (Valencia, Spain) in the form of a single-, dual-, and triple-ring models.[33–35] All versions feature the same TFOV (80 mm) but different axial extensions (~46, 94.5, and 148 mm). The system is integrated with a high-resolution CT and SPECT subsystems sharing a common gantry. The SPECT detectors are based on (CsI(Na)) with adjustable FOVs and mounted in a coplanar configuration with the CT unit. Albira is the first revolutionary design commercially available based on monolithic LYSO detectors instead of pixelated crystals to circumvent parallax issue and achieve a highly uniform spatial resolution across the scanner FOV. The first generation of Albira was based on PSPMT readout, whereas the next-generation detectors were made up of LYSO crystals readout by high-density silicon photomultipliers (SiPMs) arrays (Si detectors), which in turn facilitates integration as a PET insert for simultaneous PET/MR imaging.[36,37] PET/CT Si78 is a new high-performance bimodal technology introduced by Bruker.[37] Si78-PET subsystem is identical to the Albira Si with an extended AFOV (up to 149–200 mm) and a seamless integration with a low-dose high-resolution CT subsystem. With 10-layered depth of interaction (DOI) encoding capability coupled to SiPM technology, Si detectors deliver supreme spatial resolution along the scanner's FOV for accurate quantification.

Unlike conventional PET scanners, MILabs VECTor (Utrecht, Netherlands) exploits a

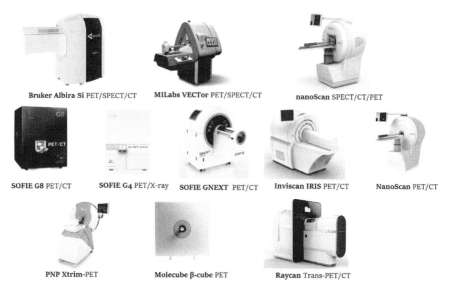

Fig. 1. Range of state-of-the-art PET scanners dedicated to preclinical imaging. *Courtesy of* the owner companies.

completely different concept for detecting annihilation photons. The scanner is equipped with 192 clustered pinholes collimator attached to 3 NaI(Tl)-based stationary heads generating a triangular shape to surround the object. Each pinhole has a diameter of 0.7 mm with 16° to 18° opening angle, making the detection of annihilation photons in single mode feasible.[38,39] Its specific design enables imaging of co-injected radiotracers to perform concurrent PET/SPECT acquisition with submillimeter spatial resolution.[40]

PETbox is a benchtop prototype built specifically for imaging laboratory mice with dual head detectors on a static gantry.[41] PETbox 4 is the upgraded version, made up of 4 stationary heads with a dimension of 5 × 10 cm² forming a TFOV of 44 mm and AFOV of 98 mm.[42] This compact low-cost design is well-suited for whole-body mouse imaging. Another central feature of the scanner is the use of BGO scintillators, which improves the scanner's detection capability for low-dose studies up to 18.1% with a default window of 150 to 650 keV.

BGO crystals have also been implemented on G-series (G4, G8, and GNEXT) commercialized by Sofie Biosciences (CA, USA).[43–45] As the name suggests, G4 is composed of 4 detector modules in a boxlike geometry, whereas the number of transaxial modules is increased up to 8 in its upgraded G8 version to effectively cover the gap areas. In addition, there are several hardware refinements that improve G8 performance in comparison to G4, including scintillator dimensions, light guide designs, and acquisition electronics.[43] Another key difference is the integration mode. G8 is a sequential integrated PET/CT, whereas G4 version is supplied with x-ray projection and optical photographic images to gather complementary anatomic templates for PET images. With submillimeter spatial resolution and peak absolute sensitivity of 9% at the CFOV, G8 is among the latest generation high-performance preclinical PET scanners. At the time of writing this review, Sofie unveiled the latest member of G-series family, GNEXT PET/CT, with DOI measurement capability by using LYSO/BGO phoswich detectors. By incorporating this unique feature, GNEXT achieves 12% sensitivity and less than 1 mm spatial resolution at the CFOV with 120 mm TFOV and axial length of 105 mm.[45]

Inliview-3000 is a trimodal SPECT/PET/CT imaging scanner developed at the Tsinghua University (China).[46] All subunits are mounted on the same gantry and sharing a common animal chamber. The scanner features the same LSO/PMT ring for either PET or SPECT imaging modes integrated with a cone-beam CT module. The PET unit has 50 and 100 mm TFOV and AFOV, respectively. Switching to SPECT acquisition is applicable by an add-on collimator with 50 elliptical pinholes. The average spatial resolution of the scanner operating in PET mode is 2.12 mm FWHM at the CFOV with 3.2% peak sensitivity for a 250 to 750 keV energy window.

β-cube from MOLECUBES (Gent, Belgium) is one of the most intuitive and unique bench-tops exploiting monolithic LYSO crystals coupled to SiPMs.[47,48] The system has a TFOV of 72 mm

Table 1
Design characteristics of PET scanners dedicated for preclinical studies

Scanner	Manufacturer	Scintillator	Crystal Dimensions (mm³)	Electronic	Crystal Pitch (mm)	Gantry Aperture (mm)	TFOV (mm)	AFOV (mm)	DOI Capability
microPET P4[6,14]	Siemens	LSO (8 × 8)	2.2 × 2.2 × 10	PSPMT	2.45	220	190	78	NO
microPET R4[6,15]	Siemens	LSO (8 × 8)	2.1 × 2.1 × 10	PSPMT	2.45	120	100	78	NO
microPET Focus-120[6,17]	Siemens	LSO (12 × 12)	1.51 × 1.51 × 10	PSPMT	1.59	120	100	76	NO
microPET Focus-220[6,16]	Siemens	LSO (12 × 12)	1.51 × 1.51 × 10	PSPMT	1.59	220	190	76	NO
Inveon-DPET[6,18,100]	Siemens	LSO (20 × 20)	1.51 × 1.51 × 10	PSPMT	1.59	120	100	127	NO
Mosaic-HP[6,20]	Philips	GSO	2 × 2 × 10	PMT	2.3	197[a]	128	119	NO
Argus(eXplore Vista)[6,27]	Sedecal	LYSO/GSO (13 × 13)/(20 × 20)	1.45 × 1.45 × 7/8	PSPMT	1.55	80	67	48	YES
ClearPET[6,21]	Raytest GmbH	LYSO/LuYAP (8 × 8)/(8 × 8)	2 × 2 × 10/10	PSPMT	2.3	135/220[a]	94/144	110	YES
rPET-1[21]	Sedecal	MLS	1.4 × 1.4 × 12	PSPMT	1.5	140[a]	45.6	45.6	NO
VrPET[28]	Sedecal	LYSO (30 × 30)	1.4 × 1.4 × 12	PSPMT	1.5	140[a]	86.6	45.6	NO
LabPET4[25]	Gamma Medica	LYSO/LGSO	2 × 2 × 11.9/13.3	APD	NA	162[a]	100	37	YES
LabPET8[6,24]	Gamma Medica	LYSO/LGSO	2 × 2 × 11.9/13.3	APD	NA	162[a]	100	75	YES
LabPET12[6,26]	Gamma Medica	LYSO/LGSO	2 × 2 × 11.9/13.3	APD	NA	162[a]	100	112.5	YES
X-PET[23]	Gamma Medica	BGO (8 × 8)	2.32 × 2.32 × 9.4	PMT	NA	165[a]	100	116	NO
NanoPET/CT[30,111]	Mediso	LYSO (39 × 81)	1.12 × 1.12 × 13	PSPMT	1.17	160	123	94.8	NO
NanoScan PET/MRI[29,111]	Mediso	LYSO (39 × 81)	1.12 × 1.12 × 13	PSPMT	1.17	160	120	94	NO
nanoScan (PET82S)[111]	Mediso	LYSO (29 × 29)	1.51 × 1.51 × 10	NA	NA	110	80	98.6	NO
LFER 150[59]	Mediso	LYSO (29 × 29)	1.51 × 1.51 × 10	NA	NA	260	200	150	NO
Albira[35]	Bruker	LYSO[b]	50 × 50 × 10	MAPMT	Monolithic	111	80	46	YES
Albira[33]	Bruker	LYSO[b]	50 × 50 × 10	MAPMT	Monolithic	111	80	94.5	YES
Albira[90]	Bruker	LYSO[b]	50 × 50 × 10	MAPMT	Monolithic	111	80	148	YES
Albira Si[36]	Bruker	LYSO[b]	50 × 50 × 10	SiPMs	Monolithic	NA	80	148	YES
PETbox[41]	UCLA	BGO (20 × 44)	2 × 2 × 5	PSPMT	2.2	50	44	96.8	NO
PETbox4[42]	UCLA	BGO (24 × 50)	1.82 × 1.82 × 7	PSPMT	1.9	50	45	95	NO

(continued on next page)

Table 1
(continued)

Scanner	Manufacturer	Scintillator	Crystal Dimensions (mm³)	Electronic	Crystal Pitch (mm)	Gantry Aperture (mm)	TFOV (mm)	AFOV (mm)	DOI Capability
G4[44]	Sofie Biosciences	BGO (24 × 50)	1.8 × 1.8 × 7	MAPMT	1.83	50	45	94	NO
G8[43]	Sofie Biosciences	BGO (26 × 26)	1.75 × 1.75 × 7.2	MAPMT	1.83	50	47.44	94.95	NO
GNEXT[45]	Sofie Biosciences	LYSO/BGO (8 × 8)/(8 × 8)	1.01 × 1.01 × 6.1 / 1.55 × 1.55 × 8.9	NA	NA	139	120	104	YES
ClairvivoPET[53]	Shimadzu	LYSO/LYSO (32 × 53)/ (32 × 54)	1.28 × 2.68 × 7	PMT	1.4 × 2.8	182	102	151	YES
TransPET-LH[50]	Raycan	LYSO	1.89 × 1.89 × 13	PSPMT	2.03	192[a]	130	53	NO
Trans-PET/CT X5[51]	Raycan	LYSO (13 × 13)	1.9 × 1.9 × 13	NA	NA	160	130	50	NO
Xtrim-PET[55]	Parto Negar Persia	LYSO (24 × 24)	2.1 × 2.1 × 10	SiPMs	2.1	166	100	50.3	NO
IRIS[32]	Inviscan SAS	LYSO (27 × 26)	1.6 × 1.6 × 12	MAPMT	1.69	100	80	95	NO
β-cubes[47]	Molecubes	LYSO[b]	25 × 25 × 8	MPPC	Monolithic	76[a]	72	130	YES
VECTor[39]	MILabs	NaI(Tl)[b]	NA	NA	Monolithic	NA	48	36	YES
MuPET[56]	University of Texas M.D. Anderson Cancer Center	LYSO (30 × 30)	1.24 × 1.4 × 9.5	PMT	NA	166	100	116	NO
Eplus-260[59]	Chinese Academy of Sciences	LYSO (16 × 16)	1.9 × 1.9 × 10	PSPMT	2	263[a]	190	64	NO
MiniEXPLORER[60]	EXPLORER Consortium and Siemens Medical solutions	LYSO (13 × 13)	4 × 4 × 20	PMT	NA	435[a]	320	457	NO
MiniEXPLORER II[61]	EXPLORER Consortium and Siemens Medical solutions	LYSO (6 × 7)	2.76 × 2.76 × 18.1	SiPMs	2.85	520[a]	NA	483	NO

Abbreviations: MLS, mixed lutetium silicate; NA, not available.
[a] Ring diameter.
[b] Monolithic crystal.

Table 2
Spatial resolution of preclinical PET scanners

Scanner	Radial FWHM (mm)	Volumetric Resolution (mm³)	Reconstruction Method
microPET P4[6]	2.29 at 5 mm	10.9 at 5 mm	FORE + FBP
microPET R4[6]	1.65 at center 2.13 at 5 mm	12.8 at 5 mm	FORE + FBP
microPET Focus-120[6]	1.18 at center 1.92 at 5 mm	6 at 5 mm	FORE + FBP
microPET Focus-220[6]	1.75 at 5 mm	5.35 at 5 mm	FORE + FBP
Inveon-DPET[6]	1.63 at 5 mm	6.33 at 5 mm	FORE + FBP
Mosaic-HP[6]	2.7 at center 2.32 at 5 mm	14.2 at 5 mm	3DRP
Argus(eXplore Vista)[6]	1.63 at 5 cm	NA	2DFBP
ClearPET[6,21]	1.94 at 5 mm 1.9 at 5 mm	12.16 at 5 mm	3DFBP
rPET-1[6]	1.4 at 5 mm	4 at 5 mm	SSRB + FBP
VrPET[6,21]	1.48 at center 1.52 at 5 cm	6.54 at 5 mm	SSRB + FBP
LabPET4[25]	1.42 at center	NA	MLEM + SRM
LabPET8[6]	1.7 at center 1.65 at 5 mm	7.5 at center	SSRB + FBP
LabPET12[26]	1.65 at 5 mm	NA	SSRB + FBP
X-PET[23]	2 at center	12 at center	FORE + FBP
NanoPET/CT[30]	1.03 at center	1.19 at center	SSRB + FBP
NanoScan PET/MRI[29]	1.28 at center 1.5 at 5 mm	1.8 at 5 mm	SSRB + FBP
LFER 150[31]	1.81at 5 cm	5.06 at 5 mm	FORE + FBP
Albira 1 ring	1.55 at center 1.65 at 5 mm	4.45 at center 5.52 at center	SSRB + FBP
Albira 2 ring[33]	1.78 at center 1.92 at 5 mm	7.5 at center 6.46 at 5 mm	SSRB + FBP
Albira 3 ring	1.55 at center	4.45 at center	SSRB + FBP
Albira Si[36]	0.89 at center	~ 1 within whole FOV	MLEM + DOI
PETbox[41]	1.61 at central coronal plane x 1.54 at central coronal plane y 2.61 anterior-posterior	6.63 at center	MLEM
PETbox4[42]	1.32 at center	3.4 at center	3D MLEM
G4[44]	~1.35 at center	NA	MLEM
G8[43]	<1 at center <1 at 5 mm	<1 at center <1 at 5 mm	MLEM
ClairvivoPET[53]	2.16 at 5 cm	13 at 5 mm	FORE + FBP
TransPET-LH[50]	0.95 at center	1 at center	3D OSEM
Trans-PET/CT X5[51]	2.11 at center	5.72 at center	SSRB + FBP
Xtrim-PET[55]	2.01 at 5 mm	6.81 at center	SSRB + FBP
IRIS[32]	1.05 at 5 mm	1.38 at 5 mm	3DMLEM
β-cubes[47]	1.06 at center	~1	3DFBP
VECTor[39]	NA	NA	NA

(*continued on next page*)

Table 2
(continued)

Scanner	Radial FWHM (mm)	Volumetric Resolution (mm³)	Reconstruction Method
MuPET[56]	1.25 at center 1.48 at 5 mm	1.34 at center 1.96 at 5 mm	SSRB + FBP
Eplus-260[59]	1.68 mm at 5 mm	3.71 at 5 mm	SSRB + OSEM + PSF
MiniEXPLORER[60]	3 at center	~ 27 at center	3D list mode OSEM + TOF
MiniEXPLORER II[61]	2.6 within 10 mm from center[a]	NA	FORE + FBP

Abbreviations: FBP, filtered back projection; FORE, fourier rebinning; MLEM, maximum-likelihood expectation maximization; NA, not available; OSEM, ordered subset expectation maximization; PSF, point spread function; SRM, system response matrix; SSRB, single-slice rebinning.
[a] Average spatial resolution within 10 mm CFOV based on NEMA NU 2-2012 standard.

and AFOV of 130 mm to easily accommodate small laboratory rodents in a compact and lightweight design. Regarding performance evaluation of the scanner, 1-mm³ volumetric resolution has been achieved due to 5-layered DOI capability of the monolithic detectors. The sensitivity for (435-588) and (255-765) keV energy windows are 5.7% and 12.4%, respectively.

The Trans-PET BioCaliburn is a highly modular and flexible preclinical PET series introduced by Raycan Technology (Suzhou, China) and available as LH, SH, and SH2 models with different AFOV and TFOV adapted to the user's requirements.[49,50] SH and SH2 modes have smaller TFOV (65 mm) in comparison to LH model (130 mm). The main difference between SH and SH2 models is the axial span of the detectors, which is twice for SH2 (106 mm). All models are constructed using LYSO arrays with 1.89 × 1.89 × 13 mm³ crystal size with ~1 mm spatial resolution at the CFOV. A newer bimodal imager manufactured by Raycan, referred to as Trans-PET/CT X5 system with optimization in the firmware, was recently installed and evaluated.[51,52] The system has 130 mm TFOV, similar to the LH model, with a shorter AFOV (50 mm) and full digital electronics.

Among all commercial systems, the largest AFOV (151 mm) belongs to ClairvivoPET manufacturer by Shimadzu (Kyoto, Japan).[53,54] The system is based on a dual-layered LYSO detection scheme arranged to form a TFOV with 102 mm diameter and equipped with ^{137}Cs transmission source for attenuation correction. Because of the large AFOV, the system outperforms most of the commercial series with an absolute sensitivity of 8.72% using a 250 to 750 keV energy window.[53]

Xtrim-PET is a cost-effective and high-modular porotype design based on SiPM technology from Parto Negar Persia (Tehran, Iran). The single-ring version of the scanner consists of 10 LYSO block detectors with 100 mm TFOV and 50.4 mm AFOV. The effective AFOV can be extended up to 195 mm for whole-body rodent imaging and multibed reconstruction. This compact and portable design offers ~2 mm spatial resolution and 2.99% peak detection efficiency at the CFOV for a 250 to 650 keV energy window.[55]

MuPET/CT developed at the University of Texas M.D. Anderson Cancer Center is a low-cost high-performance prototype based on PMT.[56] Of note in this design is the block-detector production methodology called slab-sandwich-slice. Each sandwich is made up of 13 attached LYSO slabs. After cutting sandwiches into slices, 13 slices were stacked together to make a block. In order to form a gap-free detection ring, the end crystals of each block are tapered with 6° to achieve 95% packing fraction. The system offers a 6.38% sensitivity for a 350 to 650 keV energy window.

SuperArgus PET/CT family, the latest version from SEDECAL, is the first real-time PET imager enabling on-line position adjustment using a time stamp technique. SuperArgus systems use state-of-the-art phoswich technology with expandable TFOV and AFOV to enable scanning objects with different size, ranging from mice to primates.[57]

Recently, four different configurations of preclinical PET models were designed by MR Solutions (UK) allowing standalone, simultaneous, and sequential PET/CT or PET/MR imaging. All the available models (MRS*PET/CT benchtop, MRS*PET/CT80, MRS*PET/CT120, MRS*PET/CT220) feature the same detector assemblies of multilayered (LSO/PMT) detectors with parallax-correcting capability and submillimeter (<0.8 mm) spatial resolution.[58]

Table 3
Results of NEMA-NU4 2008 performance evaluation along with energy and temporal resolutions for preclinical PET scanners

Scanner	TW (ns)	ER (%)	TR (ns)	Peak Absolute Sensitivity (%)[a]	NECR-Mice (kcps)	NECR-Rat (kcps)	SF-Mice (%)	SF-Rat (%)
microPET P4[6,14]	6	26	3.2	1.19 (350–650)	601[9]	173	5.2	16.7
microPET R4[6,15]	6	23	NA	2.06 (350–650)	618	164	9.3	22.2
microPET Focus-120[6,17]	6	18.3	NA	3.42 (350–650)	897	267	5.6	20.3
microPET Focus-220[6,16]	6	18.5	NA	2.28 (350–650)	763[9] (250–700)	359	7.2	19.3
Inveon-DPET[6,18,100]	3.4	14.6	1.22	6.72 (350–625)	1670	592	7.8	17.2
Mosaic-HP[6,20,69]	7	17	NA	2.83 (385–665)	555	244	5.4	12.7
Argus (eXplore Vista)[6,27]	7	26/33 (LYSO/GSO)	~1.3	4.32 (250–700)	117	40	21	34.4
ClearPET[6,21]	12	25/28 (LuYAP/LYSO)	2	4.7 (100–750) 3.03 (250–650)	73.4 (250–750) 73 (250–650)	NP	31 (250–650)	NP
rPET-1[21]	3.8	NA	NA	1 (100–700)	29.2 (250–650)	NP	24.2	NP
VrPET[6,28]	3.8	16.5	NA	1.56 (250–650) 0.94 (400–700) 2.22 (100–700)	74 (100–700)	31	11.5	23.3
LabPET4[25]	20	24/25	6.6 (LYSO/LYSO) 8.9 (LGSO/LYSO) 10.7 (LGSO/LGSO)	1.1 (250–650)	129	72	17	29
LabPET8[6,24,25]	20 22 10/15/20[b]	24/25	6.6 (LYSO/LYSO) 8.9 (LGSO/LYSO) 10.7 (LGSO/LGSO)	2.36 (250–650) 1.33 (250–650) 2.1 (250–650)	279 183 (250–650)	94 67	15.6 19	29.5 31
LabPET12[6,26]	20	19/20	7.1 (LYSO/LYSO) 8.3 (LGSO/LYSO) 9.2 (LGSO/LGSO)	5.4 (250–650)	362	156	16	29.3
X-PET[23]	12	NA	NA	5.9 (250–750) 9.3 (350–650)	106 (250–750)	49	7.9	21
NanoPET/CT[30]	5	19	1.5–3.2	7.7 (250–750)	430	130	15	30
	5	19	1.5–3.2	8.4 (250–750)	406	119	17.30	34

(continued on next page)

Table 3
(continued)

NanoScan PET/MRI[29]

Scanner	TW (ns)	ER (%)	TR (ns)	Peak Absolute Sensitivity (%)[a]	NECR-Mice (kcps)	NECR-Rat (kcps)	SF-Mice (%)	SF-Rat (%)
LFER 150[31]	5	3.3–5.4	NA	3.3 (400–600) 5.4 (250–750)	NP	398 (400–600)	NP	14
Albira 1ring	5	18	NA	2 (358–664) 2.5 (255–767)	16.9 (358–664)	12.8	7.5	13
Albira 2 ring[33]	5	18	NA	4.18 (358–664) 5.3 (255–767)	72 (255–767)	42	9.8	21.8
Albira 3 ring	5	18	NA	6.3 (358–664)	NA	NA	NA	NA
Albira Si[36]	NA	15	NA	9 (256–767)	576 (256–767)	330	NA	NA
PETbox[41]	20	20.1	4.1	3.99 (150–650)	20 (150–650) 18.2 (250–650)	NP	21.3 (150–650) 14.3 (250–650)	NP
PETbox4[42]	20	18	4.1	18.1 (150–650)	35	NP	28	NP
G4[44]	20	18	NA	14 (150–650)	NP	NP	NP	NP
G8[51]	20	19.3	NA	9 (350–650) 17.8 (150–650)	44 (350–650)	NP	11	NP
ClairvivoPET[53,54]	10	NA	NA	8.7 (250–750)	415 (250–750)	NP	17.7	NA
TransPET-LH[50]	5	13	1.5	2.4 (250–750) 2.04 (350–650)	110 (250–750) 62 (350–650)	40 25	11 8.4	19.3 17.7
Trans-PET/CT X5[51]	5	15	NA	1.7 (350–650)	126 (350–650)	61	14	24
Xtrim-PET[55]	10	12	1.8	2.2 (400–700) 2.99 (250–650)	113.18 (250–650)	82.76	12.5	25.8
IRIS[32]	5.2	14	2.6	8 (250–750) 6.6 (350–750)	185 (250–750)	40	15.6	22.4
β-cubes[47]	5	12	NA	5.7 (435–588) 8[d] (385–640) 12.4 (255–765)	300 (435–588) 325[d] (385–640) 300[d] (255–765)	160 (435–588) 162[d] (385–640) 140[d] (255–765)	11.3 (435–588)	15.7 (435–588)
VECTor[39]	NA	NA	NA	0.31	NA	NA	NA	NA
MuPET[56]	3.4	14	600 ps	6.38 (350–650)	1100	354	12	28

Eplus-260[59]	2	NA	NA	1.8 (360–660)	NP	26.5[e]	NP	34.2[e]
MiniEXPLORER[60]	3.6	NA	609 ps	5[f] (425–650)	NP	1741[e]	NP	16.5[e]
MiniEXPLORER II[61]	2.7–2.9	11.7	409 ps	51.8 (kcps/MBq)[c] (430–1000)	NP	1712[e]	NP	19[e]

Abbreviations: ER, energy resolution; NA, not available; NECR, noise equivalent count rate; NP, not performed; SF, scatter fraction; TR, temporal resolution; TW, timing window.

[a] Energy window setting used for sensitivity and NECR evaluations are shown in parenthesis.
[b] LYSO-LYSO/LYSO-LGSO/LGSO-LGSO.
[c] Data were measured following NEMA NU 2-2012 standards.
[d] Approximated values estimated from the curves in the cited reference.
[e] Results were reported for monkey-like phantom.
[f] Data were measured following NEMA NU 2-2007 standards.
[g] Peak NECR value is not reached due to insufficient activity in the FOV.

Several scanners were designed specifically for NHP imaging. The Eplus-260 primate PET was recently constructed by the Institute of High Energy Physics, Chinese Academy of Sciences. This scanner used LYSO/PSPMT detection modules offering an extra-large bore (230 mm) and axial coverage (64 mm) allowing PET scanning of larger objects.[59] The reconstructed spatial resolution was measured to be 1.8 mm within the 50 mm TFOV with 1.8% sensitivity using a 360 to 660 keV energy window.

MiniEXPLORER I and II were developed by the EXPLORER Consortium in collaboration with Siemens Medical solutions (Knoxville, TN).[60,61] LSO/PMT detector modules of Siemens Biograph mCT clinical PET scanner model was redesigned to build MiniEXPLORER I total-body primate imager.[60] The scanner has an aperture of 435 mm and an AFOV of 475 mm, leading to 15% sensitivity and ~3 mm spatial resolution at the CFOV following NEMA NU 2-2012 standards [62] the second version of the scanner, MiniEXPLORER II was also adopted for veterinary applications and human brain imaging.

DESIGN CONSIDERATIONS AND PERFORMANCE CHARACTERIZATION OF PRECLINICAL PET SCANNERS
Detector Material and Conceptual Design Considerations

It has long been known that the emergence of LSO scintillators in 1992 revolutionized the PET imaging portfolio in various aspects.[63] MicroPET scanner series was the first enjoying the superior benefits of LSO arrays.[13] Among all types of scintillator materials used in PET scanners, L(Y)SO scintillators are still the materials of choice due to their outstanding characteristics in terms of density (7.4 g/cm^3), effective atomic number (Z = 66), light output (75%), and decay constant (40 ns).[7] However, the major drawback of these scintillators is the intrinsic radiation emitted from Lutetium-176 with 202 and 307 keV prompt gamma photons, which limits the minimum amount of the activity detectable by the scanner. This might be an issue in low-dose studies, such as cell tracking or gene expression research.[64] Moreover, lutetium background activity is not deemed critical in clinical imaging but could affect image quality, particularly in compact small bore scanners, such as miniaturized preclinical machines that implement wider energy windows due to lower injected activities. Although by increasing the lower level of energy discriminator (LLD) up to 350 keV one could eliminate single photons emitted from Lutetium background, the summed energy of single photons

could still cover the photopeak window and degrade the contrast of PET images. The contribution of these photons is dictated by the amount of lutetium used in the scanner design and system geometry. For instance, the intrinsic count rate is about 4 cps for VrPET,[65] 186 kcps for NanoPET/MR imaging,[29] and 145 kcps for Hyperion II^D insert.[66] Albeit these limitations, background photons could be used in daily quality control of the detectors, energy calibration, DOI extraction, PET-CT registration, and also time-of-flight (TOF) applications in clinical PET scanners.[67] Other scintillation materials, such as BGO, have been widely used in the early generation of preclinical PET scanners owing to its high atomic number (Z = 83) and photofraction of 41.5% at 511 keV, yielding higher detection capability in a more compact and costless design. YAP crystals were also used in early designs such as YAP-(S)PET and Tier-PET scanners.[19,68] Although YAP crystal presents better temporal properties, it was not considered a good candidate owing to its lower detection efficiency. Other scintillation materials such as LuYAP have been used in conjunction with LYSO in ClearPET phoswich detectors. LGSO and GSO crystals have also found interest in phoswich arrays, such as SuperArgus and LabPET models.

GSO scintillator has also been investigated in the APET scanner, the prototype version of Philips Mosaic-HP. However, after 6 months it was substituted by LSO owing to inferior properties of GSO, particularly in terms of light yield and density.[20,69] Performance comparison of APET(LSO) and APET(GSO) under the same testing conditions proved that scintillator choice affects different aspects of scanner performance. Because LSO crystal generates around 3.75 times more photons than GSO, better crystal identification and thus narrower FWHM and full-width at tenth-maximum were achieved for APET(LSO). Measurements using a ^{68}Ge line source have been shown as good as twice higher sensitivity and noise equivalent count rate (NECR) for APET(LSO).

As mentioned earlier, the chemical composition of the scintillator directly influences many aspects of system performance, such as detection efficiency, energy resolution, time resolution, and counting rate performance. These effects will be discussed in the following sections in more detail. The other key factor that should be taken into account when devising a small-animal scanner is the shape of the detector arrangements. Unlike clinical scanners, commonly adopting cylindrical geometries, various designs were proposed for small-animal PET scanners to push the limitations for spatial resolution and sensitivity, including stationary multipanel (VECTor, PETbox), rotating multihead (rPET-1, YAP(S)PET, VrPET), rotating ring (ClearPET, IRIS PET/CT), boxlike arrangement (G-series, PETbox4), and polygon or ringlike orientation, which are the most prevailing configurations for full-ring models. The multihead configuration could be used more efficiently in dual-purpose PET/SPECT acquisitions such as YAP(S)PECT and VECTor models, but such design suffers from low geometric efficiency and imaging artifacts regarding lower packing fraction. Further concerns that may arise with the multihead scheme is head misalignment, which hinders ultimate image quality as well as quantitative accuracy. According to simulation studies, the best design to maximize detection efficiency is boxlike configuration.[70] Scanners with polygon layout manifest a nonuniform pattern of resolution degradation across the transaxial FOV in contrast to ringlike cylinders owing to dead regions in polygon designs generated by arranging rectangular blocks around an annulus that negatively affects system efficiency and uniformity.[55,66,71]

The type of light sensor used to measure the scintillator output is as, if not more, important than scintillation crystals in determining overall scanner's performance. Among the many alternatives available, including PMTs, position-sensitive PMTs (PSPMTs), and multichannel PMTs (MC-PMTs), APDs, and SiPMs; are the default choices in PET devices intended for small-animal imaging.[72] The bulky size of conventional PMTs renders them unsuitable for one-to-one coupling, particularly in high-resolution scanners with small crystal arrays. However, PSPMTs composed of multiple anodes with individual outputs that share a common glass tube provide more accurate spatial information regarding their structure. Although most of the preclinical scanners are still based on PSPMTs, PET inserts benefit from superior advantages of MR imaging–compatible solid-state photosensors, such as APDs and SiPMs.[66,71,73,74] For the first time, APDs have been used on the Sherbrooke PET scanner and its successor, the LabPET. These photodiode detectors offer a multitude of advantages over PMTs, including small size, lower cost, and magnetic tolerance. The small dimensions of APDs in comparison to PMTs enable one-to-one coupling in high-performance scanners, which in turn improves spatial and energy resolution of the scanner. However, the downsides of APD photosensors are the small gain and inferior timing properties that make them less tempting in preclinical applications. The inherent limitations of APDs were addressed by the introduction of Geiger mode APDs or SiPMs. These assemblies are refined versions of APDs with fine microcell arrays, called single-photon avalanche diodes (SPADs) operating in the Geiger regime. SiPMs boast favorable advantages relative to conventional PMTs, such as comparable intrinsic gain, minimal dark noise, compactness, immunity to magnetic and electric fields, and also lower price. SiPMs are now available both in analog and digital formats. In an analog SiPM, signals from individual SAPD cells are summed up to determine timing and energy information. However, in digital mode, the signal is produced in each micro-SAPD with its time-stamp information. Digital SiPMs give clear improvements in energy and temporal resolutions and also provide lower temperature sensitivity as opposed to analog counterparts. Hyperion Π^D is the first preclinical model with digital SiPM readout electronics.[66]

In quest of submillimetric range resolution, the application of indirect room-temperature compound semiconductor detectors such as cadmium-telluride (CdTe) and CZT was also investigated.[7,75] Unlike scintillation-based detectors in which the spatial resolution is mainly limited by crystal element size, in semiconductor detectors, the intrinsic spatial resolution is determined by the fine pitch between adjacent electrodes. The fine structure imaging PET scanner developed at Tokyo university pioneered the use of CdTe detectors for high-resolution preclinical studies.[76] The system gantry was built out of 10 detection units around an annulus with 70 mm diameter and 26 mm axial coverage. Each detection unit consists of 2 detector layers of CdTe with a 0.6 mm offset to measure 3-dimensional (3D) position information. With such a design, the study found a 0.74 mm FWHM tangential resolution. Another ultra-high-resolution CZT-based PET scanner with 4-sided box geometry and selectable TFOV is under development at Stanford University.[75,77] The scanner provides 80 × 80 × 80 mm³ FOV by using CZT detectors with 40 × 40 × 5 mm³ dimensions in an edge-on configuration. These detectors are more compact in size and provide fine energy resolution (~3% at 511 keV) due to direct charge conversion process, superior packing fraction (~99%), and more importantly, ultrafine spatial resolution. Another factor reflecting the superiority of CZT over its scintillation counterpart is the capability of 3D event positioning to reduce the magnitude of the parallax error. There are however several technical concerns in using CZT in

PET, including poor timing resolution and lower atomic number.[7]

Spatial Resolution

Spatial resolution is the finest detail that can be resolved by a PET scanner, which is a function of several compounding factors. These include pixel pitch size, positron range, noncollinearity of annihilation photons, ring diameter, detector readout, coupling scheme, and image reconstruction algorithm. The spatial resolution of a PET system is primarily governed by the detector element size.[78] The conventional crystal element size in animal scanners is approximately less than 1.5 to 2 mm. Although this resolution meets the basic requirements for rat imaging, it is not sufficient for divulging fine details in the mice.[5] Ignoring the physical factors, the best achievable empirical spatial resolution equals to half the pitch size between adjacent detector elements. Therefore, the most straightforward approach to improve PET's spatial resolution without sacrificing detection capability is incorporating minuscule but lengthy crystal elements. The main limitations associated with such design are poor light collection efficiency and parallax error, which is more dominant in close geometries.[7] These issues lead to the use of relatively shorter crystals in animal scanners (10 ~ 13 mm) in comparison with those in clinical scanners. However, in current designs, such as PETbox prototypes and G-series, narrow crystals with 5 mm and 7.5 mm thicknesses were used taking advantage of the high absorption efficiency of BGO crystals, which ultimately preserves photon collection ability while minimizing parallax contribution in a close-packed layout. The other elegant advantage of box geometry is the equivalent propagation of the penetration effect across the system's FOV known as parallax error.[43]

Over the years, different innovative methods were investigated to alleviate parallax phenomena (**Fig. 2**), at least partly, by measuring the interaction point within each crystal element. The most conventional and practical one is using multilayer crystals to allocate each event to the actual interaction depth. Some commercial scanners, such as ClairvivoPET, and newly developed prototype models, such as MADPET4 and MRS-PET, are based on dual-layered offset arrays of LYSO/LYSO pairs.[53,71,74] Several investigators extended this approach to 4 layers and even 8 layers of detectors.[79,80] The initial investigations of 4-layered LSO detectors by single-side readout pattern specialized for small-animal jPET-RD proved the feasibility of the method.[79] The alternative depth encoding technique is incorporating phoswich

design compromised of multilayered crystals with different scintillation materials, such as (LYSO/LuYAP) in the ClearPET, (LYSO/LGSO) in LabPET series, (LYSO/GSO) in SuperArgus, and (LYSO/BGO) in GNEXT, where the DOI information is obtained from the differences in decay times between the layers. Because in the multilayered approach the accuracy of DOI assessment is directly determined by the number of detector layers and the thickness of each layer, the method is less effective in small-bore PET scanners.[27,53] Moreover, the multilayer paradigm bears several penalties, such as increasing the design complexity and electronic channels as well as out-of-FOV scattered photons, which is the main source of scattered radiation in preclinical setting. NEMA-based evaluation of preclinical PET scanners proved the increased contribution of scattered photons in multilayered systems.[6] Another popular technology to implement continuous DOI information is dual-end readout. In this case, two photosensors are placed at both ends of each crystal element. The ratio of the signal amplitude generated in each photosensor allows the determination of the depth of photon's impact. It has been shown that this technique facilitates a DOI resolution of ~2 mm using PSAPDs.[81] In a follow-up study, a dedicated brain mice prototype was developed based on tapered crystals read out from both ends using PSPADs.[82] For this design, a DOI resolution of ~1.5 mm was obtained by irradiating the crystals with a 1-mm width collimated beam. More recently, detector blocks with 0.5-mm LSO arrays with double-end SiPMs were fabricated to serve as building blocks of a high-resolution small-animal PET with DOI capability. With this configuration, a DOI accuracy of 1.84 mm FWHM was obtained.[83] A similar method was implemented in a new dual-ended PET insert with 48 detector blocks and AFOV of 106 mm. DOI resolution of 1.96 mm was measured for the insert composed of $1 \times 1 \times 20$ mm^3 LYSO crystals read out by SiPMs from each crystal end. Preliminary investigations of the PET insert indicated a uniform spatial resolution of 0.8 mm within the 50 mm of the scanner's TFOV with 15% sensitivity using an energy window of 250 to 750 keV.[83] The attenuation caused by the front photosensor, poor timing, and energy resolution, unavoidable gap regions between detection modules and twice more the number of photosensors are the major limitations of this readout technique. The most promising and cost-efficient solution seems to be continuous DOI encoding, which is feasible by means of monolithic crystal slabs. Monolithic crystals grasped attention in the market of dedicated scanners due to their excellent 3D positioning

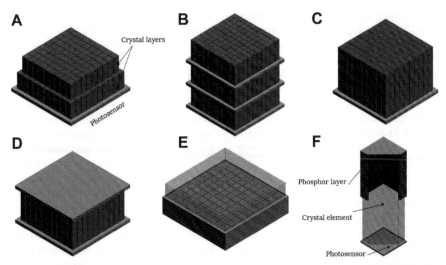

Fig. 2. Strategies for depth of interaction encoding. Dual-layered arrays with relative offset (*A*), Direct depth of interaction encoding using multiple crystal layers read out individually (*B*), Phoswich detectors compromised of multi-layered crystals with different scintillation materials (*C*), Dual-ended readout method (*D*), Monolithic crystal (*E*), phosphor-coating approach (*F*).

properties, easy and inexpensive production process, and high packing ratio.[34,47] The main concern of continuous crystals is the challenging calibration process to measure the hit position. Using a 5-layer DOI measurement, a DOI resolution of 1.6 mm was achieved for the β-cube scanner.[47] To extract the DOI information in the β-cube, a maximum likelihood algorithm was developed to achieve depth-dependent light spread function. DOI encoding in Albira detection slabs is based on the width of the light distribution, which becomes narrower as the interaction point gets closer to the photodetector. Another ongoing design using monolithic slabs is the DigiPET scanner tailored for rodent brain imaging.[84] The proposed design used LYSO slabs with $32 \times 32 \times 5$ mm³ dimensions optically assembled with digital SiPMs. The scanner has 4-sided box geometry generating $32 \times 32 \times 32$ mm³ FOV. For event positioning in DigiPET, a collimated 0.4-mm pencil beam was used. The variance of the light distribution following the irradiation of monolithic crystal with the pencil beam was used to extract DOI information. With such a design, a spatial resolution of 0.6 mm, DOI resolution of 1.6 mm, energy resolution of 23%, and coincidence time resolution of 529 ps were obtained. A different methodology enabling continuous DOI encoding is the phosphor-coating approach.[85] In this method, one face of the crystal is coated by a thin layer of phosphor material, which could absorb the scintillation light and re-emit depth-dependent phosphor light with some delay, whereas the other end of the crystal is coupled

to the photodetector. The light reaching the photodetector surface is a mixture of the scintillation light and delayed phosphor light. If a gamma photon strikes close to the photodetector, the amount of light received by the photosensor has a short decay time. However, if the photon hits the crystal far away from the photodetector, most of the photons detected by the photosensor are phosphor-emitted lights with long decay time.

Unlike polygon and ring orientations, the radial FWHM in dual-head scanners decreases toward the edges of the TFOV, which arises from the small number of detected events at the periphery of TFOV due to the absence of detector elements in these regions.[68] Therefore, the number of oblique line of responses (LORs) passing the center is more than in the edge regions, which consequently impairs the spatial resolution at the scanner's CFOV.

Spatial resolution blurring is affected not only by the radial distance from the center of the TFOV but also by the axial position of the object. Results from different studies indicated that the spatial resolution in the axial center is poorer than one-fourth offset due to a significant number of slanted LORs passing through the center. The effect is more pronounced for scanners with large AFOV.[18,53] As is the case with the radial resolution, deterioration of the axial spatial resolution is highly likely to occur in large axial spans as a consequence of DOI phenomena in the axial axis of the scanner. This nonuniformity is hampered by rebinning techniques before 2D reconstruction. As demonstrated on the Inveon-DPET scanner, the axial spatial resolution depends on the maximum ring difference,[18] increasing the MRD from 1 to 79 leads to 0.8 mm deterioration of axial resolution. By selecting small ring differences while incorporating a 2D reconstruction scheme or using full 3D reconstruction methods, one could achieve a more homogenous spatial resolution within the whole AFOV. Although the effect of noncollinearity is less significant in small bore preclinical scanners, the FWHM broadening due to positron range effect is directly related to the type of radiotracer injected to the animal body and may contribute to resolution degradation, particularly when this range is larger than the scanner's intrinsic resolution. Several studies investigated the impact of positron range effect in small-animal imaging. Disselhorst and colleagues[86] performed a set of experiments to assess the effect of positron range on image quality metrics by scanning the NEMA quality phantom filled with several positron emitters. It has conclusively been shown that the finite positron range limits the overall spatial resolution in the Inveon-DPET. Similar results were obtained for microPET focus through imaging line sources filled with ^{18}F, ^{19}N, and ^{68}Ga embedded in a cylindrical phantom filled with tissue-equivalent materials. The results recognized the deleterious effect of positron range, particularly in low-density materials and long-range positron emitters.[87] Remarkable improvements in quantitative values were recently reported for [^{68}Ga] DOTA-labeled scan of mice by implementing positron range correction in the small-animal ARGUS PET/CT scanner.[88] Lastly, for high-resolution PET scanners with smaller aperture size and miniature detector elements, positron range is the dominant factor in FWHM blurring, whereas, for large-scale detector rings, noncollinearity of annihilated photons becomes more prominent.[89]

Sensitivity

In PET imaging, the sensitivity refers to the minimum number of detected true events per unit of activity within the FOV. High-detection efficiency leads to a small but biologically more relevant amount of injected dose, rapid acquisition, lower motion artifacts, and hence higher visual quality of the resulting images. For the first-generation commercial PET scanners customized for murine studies, the sensitivity was less than ~5%, reaching about 18.1%, for the very latest generation (see **Table 3**). The overall sensitivity of a PET scanner is defined as a combination of geometric and intrinsic factors.[70] The geometric efficiency is determined with detector ring diameter as well as the axial length of the scanner, whereas the

intrinsic efficiency depends strongly on detector properties, packing fraction, and energy and time window settings. Scanners with a small radius and long axial FOV exhibit higher detection capability due to large solid angle coverage. State-of-the-art preclinical PET scanners have a wide range of ring diameters (50–250 mm) and axial FOV (45–151 mm) perfectly suitable for various applications. Decreasing the distance between the detectors and radioactive sources would increase the number of incident annihilation photons at the cost of increasing parallax-related errors. A different strategy would be to incorporate adjustable detector rings to fit the size of the scanned object as is the case with YAP(S)PET[19] and ClearPET.[21] Apart from the benefits, such designs come at the cost of additional mechanical complexity.

Increasing the number of axial rings to elongate the axial extension implies higher detection capability foremost but also facilitates whole-body imaging, a desirable feature for dynamic and gated studies. Furthermore, a long AFOV mitigates the nonuniformity problems associated with multibed reconstruction schemes. Most preclinical PET scanners have an axial FOV greater than 100 mm to cover a wide range of laboratory rodents in one session. Among the commercially available systems, the largest AFOV belongs to triple-ring Albira (148 mm), ClairvivoPET (151 mm), and Si78 (up to 149–200 mm).[37,53,90]

Aside from scanner geometry, several intrinsic factors compromise the number of detected annihilation events. Scintillation materials, such as BGO, with high stopping power and high effective atomic number increase the chance of photon absorption in each element by boosting the photoelectric absorption. Systems composed of BGO crystals provide higher peak efficiency even with shorter crystal elements less than 10 mm, compared to other systems with approximately equivalent axial coverage.[41,42,45] Increasing the thickness of detector elements would further enhance the possibility of photon absorption in each detector pixel but increases the positioning errors introduced by parallax, as explained earlier. The other determinant factor influencing system inherent sensitivity is the scanner packing, which is determined by the detector fill factor (active to the total area of the detector), interblock spacing, and inter-ring distance. The gap area between adjacent crystals occupied by reflective materials (to decrease intercrystal crosstalk) as well as dead zones between detection modules in polygon orientation would increase the number of undetected photons. Intermodular gaps not only decrease system sensitivity but also hinder image

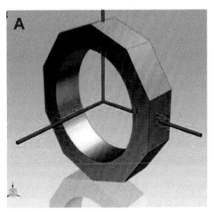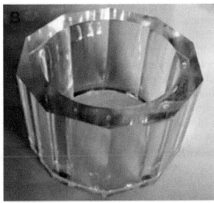

Fig. 3. Schematic view of a PET scanner based on single monolithic crystal ring (*A*) and manufactured monolithic LYSO tube (*B*). Reprinted from Gonzalez and colleagues[93] (The figure is licensed under Creative Commons Attribution 4.0 License).

quality by introducing starlike artifacts. The most conventional method to cover dead regions between adjacent modules consists increasing the number of transaxial detection blocks. This technique is reflected in G8 design by increasing the number of transaxial modules in contrast to its previous version (G4).[43] Moreover, using tapered shape crystals instead of conventional rectangular detection blocks yields further improvement in system sensitivity by filling the transaxial interblock gaps, as used in the X-PET subsystem of the FLEX Triumph model and the Albira scanner. This concept was previously investigated in Lab-PET systems through the use of trapezoid phoswich detectors, and also applied in newly developed scanners, such as the MuPET system. Monte Carlo simulations reported 60% enhancement in scanner sensitivity using tapered arrays instead of traditional cuboid models. Besides, experimental setups implied 11% degradation in spatial resolution when using tapered shaped crystals compared with rectangular crystals.[91] This effect is mainly attributed to increasing the crystal cross-section along the depth direction.[92]

A more elegant approach, called gapless PET was proposed more recently.[93] To build a gapless PET scanner, a monolithic PET tube is considered instead of individual detection blocks. The simulated scanner is made up of a monolithic LYSO tube (**Fig. 3**) with a cylindrical inner surface and a polygonal outer face to accommodate conventional pixelated SiPMs. Comparison of the proposed design with conventional polygonal multiblock PET (for the same geometry) indicated 20% reduction in production cost and 30% enhancement in system sensitivity and count rate capability of the scanner.[93] The same concept was also implemented by another group with different geometric parameters. The simulated scanner, called AnnPET, enables 10% sensitivity achieved using a single LYSO annulus with 50 mm inner ring diameter and 72 mm axial extension.[94] However, a miniaturized PET imager has been constructed recently using a monolithic cylinder with 48.5 mm inner diameter and 5 mm length. The performance characterization of the scanner, called LOR-PET, is not available at the time of writing.[95]

Another important factor that will compromise the imaging performance is the homogeneity of the sensitivity profile along the z-axis of the scanner, which is controlled by the number of rings in the axial direction. Single-ring scanners offer more uniform profiles with a peak at the center of the detection ring, which drops linearly toward the edges of the AFOV, whereas the sensitivity profile of multiblock scanners deviate from typical behavior as a consequence of axial gaps between adjacent rings.[33,66] Additionally, in the single-ring orientation, the lack of axial uniformity may arise from block misalignment across the AFOV. This inhomogeneity could be mitigated by using more accurate normalization methods.[96]

Moreover, the number of detected events is affected by acquisition parameters, such as energy window, timing window settings, scan duration, and injected amount of radiotracer. Wider windows yield a drastically higher amount of photons accepted during acquisition at the expense of a higher percentage of unwanted random and scattered photons. For the G8 scanner, increasing the LLD from 150 to 350 keV with a fixed upper-level-discriminator shows about an 8% reduction in the scanner's central sensitivity.[43] For the β-cube scanner, the sensitivity increased by 2.17-fold when using (255-765 keV) energy window instead of (435-588 keV).[47] Increasing the width of the timing window up to twice the system temporal resolution improves the system detection sensitivity, but further increases in the timing window seem not to have an additional effect on overall system sensitivity. Yang and colleagues[97] investigated the effect of timing window on the absolute sensitivity of the microPETII scanner with 3 ns coincidence timing resolution. Their study has shown small dependency of scanner sensitivity with respect to timing windows beyond 10 ns. These findings were later confirmed by Kim and colleagues.[17] Another attractive and novel strategy to increase system sensitivity is Compton PET concept, which uses the kinematics of Compton scattering to recover scattered photons concerning the direction of entry of photons.[98,99] Similar to true events, the recovered scattered photons could then be used within the reconstruction process to boost the signal-to-noise ratio further. This could be achieved through CZT detectors with high energy and positioning resolution. The animal bed and other assemblies within the FOV could also compromise the scanner's sensitivity. To decrease the adverse effects of attenuation and scattering arising from the animal holder, the fiber Carbon bed is considered in some scanners, such as the microPET R4, NanoScan PET/MR imaging, Inveon-DPET, and Xtrim-PET scanners.

Count-Rate Performance

The NECR is the most relevant metric indicating the system's ability to record true events relative to scattered and random coincidences. The overall counting performance of a PET device depends on a combination of factors, such as pulse pile-up, detector dead-time, signal resolving time, scintillator decay time, system sensitivity, object size, distribution of activity over the FOV, and acquisition parameters. To improve the signal-to-noise ratio and hence image quality, the injected activity should correspond to at least 90% to 95% the peak NECR of the scanner.

As a rule of thumb, higher detection efficiency leads to higher NECR but the relation is not trusted in all situations. For instance, some state-of-the-art scanners, such as PETbox4, G4, and G8 show high sensitivity but relatively low peak NECR, which is mainly due to undesirable temporal properties of BGO (300 ns decay time).[42–44] Crystals with short decay time, such as LSO, represents a more favorable count rate tolerance by reducing the chance of pile-up events. Further improvements in NECR could be achieved by incorporating electronic boards with lower noise and

shorter integration time. This issue is considered in MuPET design by developing special home-made pile-up event recovery channels in the FPGA board, which drastically ameliorates system counting behavior. The type of photodetector used to sense the scintillation light is of paramount importance in time resolution and detection throughput of the scanner. Systems with high temporal resolution peak at higher counting rate, such as the Inveon (1.22 ns, 1670 kcps),[100] MuPET (600 ps, 1100 kcps),[56] NanoPET (1–2 ns, 430 kcps),[30] NanoPET/MR imaging (1–2 ns, 406 kcps),[29] or fully digital systems, such as Hyperion Π^D (605 ps, 483 kcps).

Most preclinical scanners have adopted light sharing readout methods to decrease the number of electronic channels and signal processing complexity. Compared to one-to-one coupling, systems with block detector designs and light sharing electronics are more susceptible to increased pile-up events at a high flux rate, because a large number of crystals fires every photosensor. To exemplify this point, one could compare LabPET12 with individual pixel readout to other scanners with similar geometry such as ClearPET. With the same energy window, LabPET12 represented ~ 4 times better counting performance, which is partly ascribed to the individual readout scheme.[6]

As mentioned in the preceding section, systems with larger AFOV, small bore, and higher packing fraction saturate at higher NECR. The best examples to support this statement are microPET families. Increasing the packing fraction, extending the AFOV and improving readout electronics contribute to higher gain in NECR at low amount of activity, as achieved in the Inveon-DPET in comparison to its forerunners.[6,18] Moreover, the inverse effect of ring diameter on system count tolerance can be evidenced by comparing the Focus120 unit with Focus220 in which an increase in detector ring diameter up to 83% suggests 30% reduction in NECR. In LabPET scanners, a 50% increase in AFOV length results in a 30% improvement in peak NECR, at the expenses of only a 2% increase in the scatter fraction ratio. As expected, partial ring geometries present smaller NECR (<100 kcps) in comparison to more constrained designs.[6,21] A two-fold improvement in the number of detection modules in the VrPET scanner compared to rPET-1 version approximately doubles the NECR values.[28] Approximately similar improvements have been achieved for PETbox prototypes when shifting from dual-head model to 4-head box geometry.[41,42] In addition, lower NECR values were reported for PET/MR imaging inserts with small AFOV, such as MRS-PET

(61.9 kcps),[74] SimPET-S (42.4 kcps),[101] MADPET4 (29.0 kcps),[71] and the scanner reported by Stortz and colleagues[102] (20.8 kcps).

In addition to the abovementioned factors, other important parameters controlling the NECR properties of the scanner are the size of the object being imaged and the distribution of activity within the FOV. For larger objects, the NECR peaks more quickly. NEMA evaluation of preclinical scanners revealed that the peak NECR for a micelike phantom is higher than that of ratlike and monkeylike phantoms. This effect is mainly attributed to the increasing number of scattered and attenuated true events with increasing phantom diameter. The dependency of count rate characteristics on energy and time window settings was studied for several scanners. For the microFocus120 scanner, higher NECR and scatter ratio were achieved for wider energy and timing windows.[17] However, these variations are more pronounced for ratlike phantom compared with micelike phantom. Similar results were observed for the Trans-PET scanner. For micelike phantom, NECR values of 110 and 62 kcps were measured using 250 to 750 keV and 350 to 650 keV windows, respectively.[49] For the β-cube benchtop, 4% to 10% improvements in NECR were reported for (385-640 keV) energy window compared with (435-588 keV) settings.[47] Decreasing the LLD from 350 keV to 250 keV exhibits 2-fold enhancement in NECR magnitude measured in MADPET4.[71] In comparison, for the LabPET12, increasing the LLD from 100 to 200 keV improves the peak NECR of ratlike phantom from 141 to 179 kcps by limiting the scattered events. However, by further increasing the LLD (up to 350 keV), the NECR decreases to 90 kcps due to decreasing the number of true coincidences.[26] Reducing the width of the temporal window in the Mosaic-HP improves the scanner count performance without compromising detection sensitivity to true coincidence events.[69] Hence, the acquisition parameters should be adjusted according to the size of the object and scanner performance. For small objects, such as mice, one could benefit from wider energy windows to achieve higher sensitivity and NECR. However, for larger animals and multianimal imaging, highest NECR could be achieved through limiting energy and timing windows. From the NECR point of view, although the characteristics of preclinical scanners are different, almost all of them are adequate for the typical range of activity used in preclinical research (~30 MBq).

Energy and Temporal Resolution

The main parameter influencing the energy resolution is the number of light quanta collected from the scintillator, which in turn is driven by the scintillator light yield, crystal refraction index, doping material, crystal element size, the coupling material, the wavelength of the scintillator light, and the quantum efficiency of the photodetectors. Crystals with higher luminosity such as L(Y)SO exhibit better characteristics in terms of energy and timing resolution. To decrease the light loss and improve light collection efficiency, each scintillator element is enclosed by reflective materials. The other important factor is the refractive index of the crystalline composition. As the light guide between the scintillator and photosensor is conventionally made of glass, scintillators with lower refraction index, such as LSO and GSO (~1.5), show better light collection properties through minimizing the refracted photons that occur at the crystal/light guide interface. Using improved light guides in the Inveon-DPET scanner resulted in 8% improvement in energy resolution compared with first-generation models (P4, R4).[18,100] Similar results were also observed in the G8 scanner. Incorporating pixelated light guides in G8 instead of the 1 mm clear glass used in G4 suggested considerable improvements in energy resolution.[43] The quantum efficiency of the photosensor is also of paramount importance to achieve better energy and timing performance by decreasing the amount of statistical noise.[103] To date, breaking the barrier of 11% energy resolution and <1 ns becomes possible thanks to impressive properties of LSO/SiPM detectors, which are becoming the common theme in next-generation application-specific systems.[47,55,66] Besides the factors mentioned above, multiplexing readout and light sharing techniques hinder the energy and temporal precision. Using one-to-one coupling would help to promote energy and temporal characterization by decreasing the light loss at photodetector junction.[104] In a more recent study, a new strategy was developed to improve light collection efficiency while preserving spatial resolution and sensitivity of the detector blocks. In this new design, four layers of LYSO slabs were stacked together, such that each layer was optically separated from the adjacent layers and read out by SiPM arrays from 4 sides, results in energy and timing resolution of 10.38% and 348 ps, respectively.[99] The type of doping material is also another pertinent issue. Several studies investigated the types of doping materials to determine the optimum concentration of co-doping. It was verified that 0.5 mol % Yb-doped LSO: Ce crystals offer 2-fold lower afterglow compared with LSO:Ce crystals.[105] Another study reported that Li doping improves the light yield of LSO:Ce by ~20% while decreasing the scintillation decay time up to

42.1 ns.[106] There are also other parallel efforts in this context. It was demonstrated that 0.04% Ca co-doped LSO: Ce exhibits superior light output (35,000 photons/MeV) and shorter decay time (31 ns), rendering it the best choice for TOF-PET scanners.[107] In a further study, sub-100 ps time resolution was obtained for a $2 \times 2 \times 3$ mm^3 LSO:Ce co-doped 0.4% Ca.[108] energy and timing resolutions are significantly imposed by the detector element size.[104] As discussed earlier, the most prominent disadvantages associated with thin and long crystals are parallax error, decreased energy and timing resolutions. The former could be mitigated using DOI strategies, whereas the latter remains a challenge for low aspect ratio crystals used in high-resolution scanners. Several strategies were proposed to retain the energy resolution without the limiting design trade-offs present in low aspect ratio, such as side readout techniques. Moreover, through the emergence of indirect semiconductor detectors, superior energy resolution (~3% at 511 keV) is feasible. As mentioned earlier, high energy resolution allows efficient rejection of scattered events and thus improvement of image contrast.

Apart from the abovementioned factors, the temporal resolution of a PET scanner is mainly affected by all elements involved in the detection chain: the scintillation crystal, the photosensor, light guide, and other components of the processing electronics. Scintillators with short decay time coupled to photodetectors with fast temporal response (fast raising time, fast transition time, and high quantum efficiency) are the primary components affecting coincidence timing resolution.[109] Improved temporal resolution ensures efficient rejection of undesirable random coincidences, which adds background to emission data and hence counteracts the resulting image quality. It is worth noting that the advantages of improved energy and timing resolution will not be significant in rodent imaging due to the small fraction of scattered and random coincidences. Some of the recent designs specialized for moderate or large nonhuman primate animals, such as Hyperion Π^D, Eplus-260, and MiniEXPLORER I could benefit from improved timing resolution for TOF-PET reconstruction.[59,61,66] The TT-TOF project based on Silicon pixel sensors with 16 steplike modules is being developed.[110], which is expected ... is expected to achieve 30 ps time resolution using Silicon-Germanium (Si-Ge) amplifiers in the pixel sensor. As the temporal resolution continues to be improved, the impetus grows for unlocking TOF imaging in small-animal imaging that would not have been dreamt possible in the preclinical era.

SUMMARY AND FUTURE TRENDS

Because of the poor performance of clinical PET scanners for scanning small animals, a tremendous effort put into designing dedicated PET systems with finer spatial resolution, higher detection capabilities, minimum cost, and easy accessibility to fulfill the basic requirements of in vivo imaging to support longitudinal and noninvasive scanning of animal models with high statistical power. Since its emergence, several dedicated PET scanners with various design features and characteristics were developed in academic and corporate settings to meet preclinical researchers' higher-than-ever expectations. Some of these systems are still at the prototype stage for further evaluations, whereas some of them are commercially available and installed in research laboratories. Therefore, an updated overview of these dedicated small-animal PET scanners is provided emphasizing recent advances instrumentation. The identified limitations and challenges may help to predict future directions and depict a more realistic roadmap for this miniaturized and small-scale systems. To precisely translate and correlate the preclinical findings to clinical outcomes, around 0.5 mm spatial resolution is desired. Today, high-end state-of-the-art technologies approach submillimetric spatial resolution, breaking a barrier that could open the door to more specific applications and more accurate quantification by eliminating the partial volume issue. However, there are still ongoing efforts in this era to achieve more uniform volumetric resolution and consistent performance across the whole active volume of the scanner at a lower price. In this direction, cost-efficient monolithic slabs will continue to gain in popularity. The same can be expected for full digital SiPM photodetectors, which hold promises toward next-generation multimodality scanners, such as hybrid PET/MR imaging scanners. It should be mentioned that improved crystalline materials or more novel compositions and co-doping agents along with more advanced readout electronics may be available in the foreseeable future, which permits to incorporate TOF capability in state-of-the-art animal scanners. It is envisaged that more novel configurations, such as monolithic crystal rings, will foster a new era for high-performance scanners at a lower cost. However, the challenges of such designs are still not realized. It seems that direct semiconductor detectors, such as CZT, will continue to push themselves into commercial systems. In the light of these detectors, next-generation models will likely become available in a more concise fashion, particularly for more specialized tasks, such as dedicated brain imagers for awake and behaving mice, which is eminently desirable in neuroscience studies. It should be emphasized that in addition to hardware design, there is still much that needs to be done in terms of fast, accurate, and reliable image reconstruction techniques. Research efforts are still required to evaluate and optimize current reconstruction algorithms and tuning acquisition settings for a variety of applications. Increasing demands for kinetic modeling, as well as high throughput imaging, will highlight the less noticed but significant role of quantitative corrections in preclinical settings as well. Although much effort is geared toward developing highly efficient scanners for preclinical research, still there is ample room for further improvements to save cost, time, and improved noise-resolution tradeoffs.

ACKNOWLEDGMENTS

This work was supported through grant No. 36950 from Tehran University of Medical Sciences and Health Services, Iran and the Swiss National Science Foundation, Switzerland under grant SNRF 320030_176052.

REFERENCES

1. Cuccurullo V, D Di Stasio G, Schillirò ML, et al. Small-animal molecular imaging for preclinical cancer research: μPET and μSPECT. Curr Radiopharm 2016;9(2):102–13.
2. Epstein F, Catana C, Tsui B, et al. Small-animal molecular imaging methods. J Nucl Med 2010;51(0 1): 18S–32S.
3. Toyohara J, Ishiwata K. Animal tumor models for PET in drug development. Ann Nucl Med 2011; 25(10):717–31.
4. Phelps ME. Positron emission tomography provides molecular imaging of biological processes. Proc Natl Acad Sci USA 2000;97(16):9226–33.
5. Chatziioannou AF. PET scanners dedicated to molecular imaging of small animal models. Mol Imaging Biol 2002;4(1):47–63.
6. Goertzen AL, Bao Q, Bergeron M, et al. NEMA NU 4-2008 comparison of preclinical PET imaging systems. J Nucl Med 2012;53(8):1300–9.
7. Levin CS, Zaidi H. Current trends in preclinical PET system design. PET Clin 2007;2(2):125–60.
8. Tai YC, Laforest R. Instrumentation aspects of animal PET. Annu Rev Biomed Eng 2005;7:255–85.
9. Watanabe M, Uchida H, Okada H, et al. A high resolution PET for animal studies. IEEE Trans Med Imaging 1992;11(4):577–80.
10. Watanabe M, Okada H, Shimizu K, et al. A high resolution animal PET scanner using compact PS-PMT detectors. IEEE Trans Nucl Sci 1997;44(3): 1277–82.
11. Rajeswaran S, Bailey DL, Hume S, et al. 2D and 3D imaging of small animals and the human radial artery with a high resolution detector for PET. IEEE Trans Med Imaging 1992;11(3):386–91.
12. Bloomfield P, Rajeswaran S, Spinks T, et al. The design and physical characteristics of a small animal positron emission tomograph. Phys Med Biol 1995;40(6):1105.
13. Cherry SR, Shao Y, Silverman R, et al. MicroPET: a high resolution PET scanner for imaging small animals. IEEE Trans Nucl Sci 1997;44(3):1161–6.
14. Tai Y-C, Chatziioannou A, Siegel S, et al. Performance evaluation of the microPET P4: a PET system dedicated to animal imaging. Phys Med Biol 2001;46(7):1845.
15. Knoess C, Siegel S, Smith A, et al. Performance evaluation of the microPET R4 PET scanner for rodents. Eur J Nucl Med Mol Imaging 2003;30(5):737–47.
16. Tai Y-C, Ruangma A, Rowland D, et al. Performance evaluation of the microPET focus: a third-generation microPET scanner dedicated to animal imaging. J Nucl Med 2005;46(3):455–63.
17. Kim JS, Lee JS, Im KC, et al. Performance measurement of the microPET focus 120 scanner. J Nucl Med 2007;48(9):1527–35.
18. Kemp BJ, Hruska CB, McFarland AR, et al. NEMA NU 2-2007 performance measurements of the Siemens Inveon™ preclinical small animal PET system. Phys Med Biol 2009;54(8):2359.
19. Del Guerra A, Di Domenico G, Scandola M, et al. High spatial resolution small animal YAP-PET. Nucl Instrum Methods Phys Res A 1998;409(1–3):537–41.
20. Huisman MC, Reder S, Weber AW, et al. Performance evaluation of the Philips MOSAIC small animal PET scanner. Eur J Nucl Med Mol Imaging 2007;34(4):532–40.
21. Cañadas M, Embid M, Lage E, et al. NEMA NU 4-2008 performance measurements of two commercial small-animal PET scanners: ClearPET and rPET-1. IEEE Trans Nucl Sci 2010;58(1):58–65.
22. National Electrical Manufacturers Association. NEMA standards publication NU 4-2008: performance measurements of small animal positron emission tomographs. Rosslyn (VA): National Electrical Manufacturers Association; 2008. p. 1–23.
23. Prasad R, Ratib O, Zaidi H. Performance evaluation of the FLEX triumph X-PET scanner using the national electrical manufacturers association NU-4 standards. J Nucl Med 2010;51(10):1608–15.
24. Prasad R, Ratib O, Zaidi H. NEMA NU-04-based performance characteristics of the LabPET-8™ small animal PET scanner. Phys Med Biol 2011; 56(20):6649.
25. Bergeron M, Cadorette J, Beaudoin J-F, et al. Performance evaluation of the LabPET APD-based

digital PET scanner. IEEE Trans Nucl Sci 2009; 56(1):10–6.

26. Bergeron M, Cadorette J, Bureau-Oxton C, et al. Performance evaluation of the LabPET12, a large axial FOV APD-based digital PET scanner. IEEE Nucl Sci Symp Conf Rec (NSS/MIC) 2009;4017–21.

27. Wang Y, Seidel J, Tsui BM, et al. Performance evaluation of the GE healthcare eXplore VISTA dual-ring small-animal PET scanner. J Nucl Med 2006; 47(11):1891–900.

28. Lage E, Vaquero JJ, Sisniega A, et al. VrPET/CT: Development of a rotating multimodality scanner for small-animal imaging. IEEE Nucl Sci Symp Conf Rec 2008;4671–4.

29. Nagy K, Tóth M, Major P, et al. Performance evaluation of the small-animal nanoScan PET/MRI system. J Nucl Med 2013;54(10):1825–32.

30. Szanda I, Mackewn J, Patay G, et al. National Electrical Manufacturers Association NU-4 performance evaluation of the PET component of the NanoPET/CT preclinical PET/CT scanner. J Nucl Med 2011;52(11):1741–7.

31. Sarnyai Z, Nagy K, Patay G, et al. Performance evaluation of a high-resolution nonhuman primate PET/CT system. J Nucl Med 2019;60(12):1818–24.

32. Belcari N, Camarlinghi N, Ferretti S, et al. NEMA NU-4 performance evaluation of the IRIS PET/CT preclinical scanner. IEEE Trans Radiat Plasma Med Sci 2017;1(4):301–9.

33. Pajak MZ, Volgyes D, Pimlott SL, et al. NEMA NU4-2008 performance evaluation of Albira: a two-ring small-animal PET system using continuous LYSO crystals. Open Med J 2016;3(1):12–26.

34. Sánchez F, Orero A, Soriano A, et al. ALBIRA: a small animal PET/SPECT/CT imaging system. Med Phys 2013;40(5):051906.

35. Balcerzyk M, Kontaxakis G, Delgado M, et al. Initial performance evaluation of a high resolution Albira small animal positron emission tomography scanner with monolithic crystals and depth-of-interaction encoding from a user's perspective. Meas Sci Technol 2009;20(10):104011.

36. González AJ, Aguilar A, Conde P, et al. Next generation of the Albira small animal PET based on high density SiPM arrays. IEEE Nuclear Science Symposium and Medical Imaging Conference (NSS/MIC) 2015;1–4.

37. Bruker. True trimodal preclinical PET SPECT CT system. 2020. Available at: https://www.bruker.com/products/preclinical-imaging/nuclear-molecular-imaging/pet-spect-ct.html. Accessed March 20, 2020.

38. Walker MD, Goorden MC, Dinelle K, et al. Performance assessment of a preclinical PET scanner with pinhole collimation by comparison to a coincidence-based small-animal PET scanner. J Nucl Med 2014;55(8):1368–74.

39. Goorden MC, van der Have F, Kreuger R, et al. VECTor: a preclinical imaging system for simultaneous submillimeter SPECT and PET. J Nucl Med 2013;54(2):306–12.

40. MILabs. MILabs simultaneous sub-mm PET-SPECT opens new avenues for advanced research. 2020. Available at: https://www.milabs.com/vector/. Accessed March 20, 2020.

41. Zhang H, Bao Q, Vu NT, et al. Performance evaluation of PETbox: a low cost bench top preclinical PET scanner. Mol Imaging Biol 2011;13(5):949–61.

42. Gu Z, Taschereau R, Vu N, et al. NEMA NU-4 performance evaluation of PETbox4, a high sensitivity dedicated PET preclinical tomograph. Phys Med Biol 2013;58(11):3791.

43. Gu Z, Taschereau R, Vu NT, et al. Performance evaluation of G8, a high-sensitivity benchtop preclinical PET/CT tomograph. J Nucl Med 2019; 60(1):142–9.

44. Herrmann K, Dahlbom M, Nathanson D, et al. Evaluation of the Genisys4, a bench-top preclinical PET scanner. J Nucl Med 2013;54(7):1162–7.

45. Sofie. GNEXT PET/CT. 2020. Available at: https://sofie.com/a-hrefproductsproductsa. Accessed March 20, 2020.

46. Wei Q, Wang S, Ma T, et al. Performance evaluation of a compact PET/SPECT/CT tri-modality system for small animal imaging applications. Nucl Instrum Methods-Phys Res A 2015;786:147–54.

47. Krishnamoorthy S, Blankemeyer E, Mollet P, et al. Performance evaluation of the MOLECUBES β-CUBE—a high spatial resolution and high sensitivity small animal PET scanner utilizing monolithic LYSO scintillation detectors. Phys Med Biol 2018; 63(15):155013.

48. MOLECUBES. B-CUBE. 2020. Available at: http://www.molecubes.com/b-cube/. Accessed March 20, 2020.

49. Zhu J, Wang L, Kao C-M, et al. Performance evaluation of the trans-PET® BioCaliburn® SH system. Nucl Instrum Methods Phys Res A 2015;777:148–53.

50. Wang L, Zhu J, Liang X, et al. Performance evaluation of the Trans-PET® BioCaliburn® LH system: a large FOV small-animal PET system. Phys Med Biol 2014;60(1):137.

51. Teuho J, Han C, Riehakainen L, et al. NEMA NU 4-2008 and in vivo imaging performance of RAYCAN trans-PET/CT X5 small animal imaging system. Phys Med Biol 2019;64(11):115014.

52. RAYCAN. All-digital small animal PET. 2019. Available at: http://ray-can.com/en/. Accessed March 20, 2020.

53. Sato K, Shidahara M, Watabe H, et al. Performance evaluation of the small-animal PET scanner ClairvivoPET using NEMA NU 4-2008 standards. Phys Med Biol 2015;61(2):696.

54. Mizuta T, Kitamura K, Iwata H, et al. Performance evaluation of a high-sensitivity large-aperture small-animal PET scanner: ClairvivoPET. Ann Nucl Med 2008;22(5):447–55.

55. Amirrashedi M, Sarkar S, Ghafarian P, et al. NEMA NU-4 2008 performance evaluation of Xtrim-PET: a prototype SiPM-based preclinical scanner. Med Phys 2019;46(11):4816–25.

56. Wong W-H, Li H, Baghaei H, et al. Engineering and performance (NEMA and animal) of a lower-cost higher-resolution animal PET/CT scanner using photomultiplier-quadrant-sharing detectors. J Nucl Med 2012;53(11):1786–93.

57. SEDECAL. SuperArgus PET/CT. 2020. Available at: https://www.scintica.com/products/superargus-sed ecal-pet-ct-preclinical-systems/. Accessed March 20, 2020.

58. MRSolutions. Preclinical imaging systems. 2020. Available at: https://www.mrsolutions.com/products/imaging-systems/. Accessed March 20, 2020.

59. Pei C, Baotong F, Zhiming Z, et al. NEMA NU-4 performance evaluation of a non-human primate animal PET. Phys Med Biol 2019;64(10):105018.

60. Berg E, Zhang X, Bec J, et al. Development and evaluation of mini-EXPLORER: a long axial field-of-view PET scanner for nonhuman primate imaging. J Nucl Med 2018;59(6):993–8.

61. Lyu Y, Lv X, Liu W, et al. Mini EXPLORER II: a prototype high-sensitivity PET/CT scanner for companion animal whole body and human brain scanning. Phys Med Biol 2019;64:075004.

62. Nema NU. NU 2-2012 performance measurements of positron emission tomographs. Rosslyn (VA): National Electrical Manufacturers Association; 2012.

63. Melcher CL. Scintillation crystals for PET. J Nucl Med 2000;41(6):1051–5.

64. Goertzen AL, Suk JY, Thompson CJ. Imaging of weak-source distributions in LSO-based small-animal PET scanners. J Nucl Med 2007;48(10):1692–8.

65. Lage E, Vaquero J, Sisniega A, et al. Design and performance evaluation of a coplanar multimodality scanner for rodent imaging. Phys Med Biol 2009;54(18):5427.

66. Hallen P, Schug D, Weissler B, et al. PET performance evaluation of the small-animal Hyperion IID PET/MRI insert based on the NEMA NU-4 standard. Biomed Phys Eng Express 2018;4(6):065027.

67. Rothfuss H, Moor A, Young J, et al. Time alignment of time of flight positron emission tomography using the background activity of LSO. IEEE Nuclear Science Symposium and Medical Imaging Conference (NSS/MIC) 2013;1–3.

68. Weber S, Herzog H, Cremer M, et al. Evaluation of the TierPET system. IEEE Trans Nucl Sci 1999;46(4):1177–83.

69. Surti S, Karp JS, Perkins AE, et al. Imaging performance of A-PET: a small animal PET camera. IEEE Trans Med Imaging 2005;24(7):844–52.

70. Habte F, Foudray A, Olcott P, et al. Effects of system geometry and other physical factors on photon sensitivity of high-resolution positron emission tomography. Phys Med Biol 2007;52(13):3753.

71. Omidvari N, Cabello J, Topping G, et al. PET performance evaluation of MADPET4: a small animal PET insert for a 7 T MRI scanner. Phys Med Biol 2017;62(22):8671.

72. Lewellen TK. Recent developments in PET detector technology. Phys Med Biol 2008;53(17):R287.

73. Schug D, Lerche C, Weissler B, et al. Initial PET performance evaluation of a preclinical insert for PET/MRI with digital SiPM technology. Phys Med Biol 2016;61(7):2851.

74. Vrigneaud J-M, Mcgrath J, Courteau A, et al. Initial performance evaluation of a preclinical PET scanner available as a clip-on assembly in a sequential PET/MRI system. Phys Med Biol 2018;63(12):125007.

75. Gu Y, Matteson J, Skelton R, et al. Study of a high-resolution, 3D positioning cadmium zinc telluride detector for PET. Phys Med Biol 2011;56(6):1563.

76. Ishii K, Kikuchi Y, Matsuyama S, et al. First achievement of less than 1 mm FWHM resolution in practical semiconductor animal PET scanner. Nucl Instrum Methods Phys Res A 2007;576(2–3):435–40.

77. Abbaszadeh S, Levin CS. 3-D position sensitive CZT PET system: current status. IEEE Nuclear Science Symposium, Medical Imaging Conference and Room-Temperature Semiconductor Detector Workshop (NSS/MIC/RTSD) 2016;1–2.

78. Moses WW. Fundamental limits of spatial resolution in PET. Nucl Instrum Methods Phys Res A 2011;648:S236–40.

79. Tsuda T, Murayama H, Kitamura K, et al. Performance evaluation of a subset of a four-layer LSO detector for a small animal DOI PET scanner: jPET-RD. IEEE Trans Nucl Sci 2006;53(1):35–9.

80. Inadama N, Murayama H, Tsuda T, et al. Optimization of crystal arrangement on 8-layer DOI PET detector. IEEE Nucl Sci Symp Conf Rec 2006;5:3082–5.

81. Yang Y, Wu Y, Qi J, et al. A prototype PET scanner with DOI-encoding detectors. J Nucl Med 2008;49(7):1132–40.

82. Yang Y, Bec J, Zhou J, et al. A prototype high-resolution small-animal PET scanner dedicated to mouse brain imaging. J Nucl Med 2016;57(7):1130–5.

83. Kuang Z, Wang X, Fu X, et al. Dual-ended readout small animal PET detector by using 0.5 mm

pixelated LYSO crystal arrays and SiPMs. Nucl Instrum Methods Phys Res A 2019;917:1–8.

84. España S, Marcinkowski R, Keereman V, et al. DigiPET: sub-millimeter spatial resolution small-animal PET imaging using thin monolithic scintillators. Phys Med Biol 2014;59(13):3405.

85. Du H, Yang Y, Glodo J, et al. Continuous depth-of-interaction encoding using phosphor-coated scintillators. Phys Med Biol 2009;54(6):1757.

86. Disselhorst JA, Brom M, Laverman P, et al. Image-quality assessment for several positron emitters using the NEMA NU 4-2008 standards in the Siemens Inveon small-animal PET scanner. J Nucl Med 2010;51(4):610–7.

87. Alva-Sánchez H, Quintana-Bautista C, Martínez-Dávalos A, et al. Positron range in tissue-equivalent materials: experimental microPET studies. Phys Med Biol 2016;61(17):6307.

88. Cal-Gonzalez J, Vaquero JJ, Herraiz JL, et al. Improving PET quantification of small animal [68 Ga] DOTA-labeled PET/CT studies by using a CT-based positron range correction. Mol Imaging Biol 2018;20(4):584–93.

89. Levin CS, Hoffman EJ. Calculation of positron range and its effect on the fundamental limit of positron emission tomography system spatial resolution. Phys Med Biol 1999;44(3):781.

90. Spinks T, Karia D, Leach M, et al. Quantitative PET and SPECT performance characteristics of the Albira Trimodal pre-clinical tomograph. Phys Med Biol 2014;59(3):715.

91. St James S, Yang Y, Bowen SL, et al. Simulation study of spatial resolution and sensitivity for the tapered depth of interaction PET detectors for small animal imaging. Phys Med Biol 2009;55(2):N63.

92. Yang Y, James SS, Wu Y, et al. Tapered LSO arrays for small animal PET. Phys Med Biol 2010;56(1):139.

93. Gonzalez AJ, Berr SS, Cañizares G, et al. Feasibility study of a small animal PET insert based on a single LYSO monolithic tube. Front Med 2018;5:328.

94. Stolin AV, Martone PF, Jaliparthi G, et al. Preclinical positron emission tomography scanner based on a monolithic annulus of scintillator: initial design study. J Med Imaging (Bellingham) 2017;4(1):011007.

95. Xie S, Zhao Z, Yang M, et al. LOR-PET: a novel PET camera constructed with a monolithic scintillator ring. IEEE Nuclear Science Symposium and Medical Imaging Conference (NSS/MIC) 2017;1–3.

96. Badawi RD, Marsden P. Developments in component-based normalization for 3D PET. Phys Med Biol 1999;44(2):571.

97. Yang Y, Tai Y-C, Siegel S, et al. Optimization and performance evaluation of the microPET II scanner for in vivo small-animal imaging. Phys Med Biol 2004;49(12):2527.

98. Yoon C, Lee W, Lee T. Simulation for CZT Compton PET (Maximization of the efficiency for PET using Compton event). Nucl Instrum Methods Phys Res A 2011;652(1):713–6.

99. Peng P, Judenhofer MS, Cherry SR. Compton PET: a layered structure PET detector with high performance. Phys Med Biol 2019;64(10):10LT01.

100. Magota K, Kubo N, Kuge Y, et al. Performance characterization of the Inveon preclinical small-animal PET/SPECT/CT system for multimodality imaging. Eur J Nucl Med Mol Imaging 2011;38(4):742–52.

101. Ko GB, Yoon HS, Kim KY, et al. Simultaneous multiparametric PET/MRI with silicon photomultiplier PET and ultra-high-field MRI for small-animal imaging. J Nucl Med 2016;57(8):1309–15.

102. Stortz G, Thiessen JD, Bishop D, et al. Performance of a PET insert for high-resolution small-animal PET/MRI at 7 tesla. J Nucl Med 2018;59(3):536–42.

103. Surti S, Karp JS. Advances in time-of-flight PET. Phys Med 2016;32(1):12–22.

104. Cates JW, Levin CS. Advances in coincidence time resolution for PET. Phys Med Biol 2016;61(6):2255.

105. Starzhinskiy N, Sidletskiy OT, Tamulaitis G, et al. Improving of LSO (Ce) scintillator properties by co-doping. IEEE Trans Nucl Sci 2013;60(2):1427–31.

106. Wu Y, Tian M, Peng J, et al. On the role of Li+ co-doping in simultaneous improvement of light yield, decay time, and afterglow of Lu2SiO5: Ce3+ scintillation detectors. Phys Status Solidi Rapid Res Lett 2019;13(2):1800472.

107. Spurrier M, Szupryczynski P, Rothfuss H, et al. The effect of co-doping on the growth stability and scintillation properties of lutetium oxyorthosilicate. J Cryst Growth 2008;310(7–9):2110–4.

108. Nemallapudi MV, Gundacker S, Lecoq P, et al. Sub-100 ps coincidence time resolution for positron emission tomography with LSO: Ce codoped with Ca. Phys Med Biol 2015;60(12):4635.

109. Lecoq P, Auffray E, Brunner S, et al. Factors influencing time resolution of scintillators and ways to improve them. IEEE Trans Nucl Sci 2010;57(5):2411–6.

110. Bandi Y, Benoit M, Cadoux F, et al. The TT-PET project: a thin TOF-PET scanner based on fast novel silicon pixel detectors. J Instrum 2018;13(01):C01007.

111. Mediso medical imaging systems. nanoScan SPECT/CT/PET. 2016. Available at: http://www.mediso.com/products.php?fid52,11&pid590. Accessed March 20, 2020.

Reinventing Molecular Imaging with Total-Body PET, Part I
Technical Revolution in Evolution

Babak Saboury, MD, MPH[a,b,c,]*, Michael A. Morris, MD, MS[a,b],
Faraz Farhadi, BS[a], Moozhan Nikpanah, MD[a], Thomas J. Werner, MS[c],
Elizabeth C. Jones, MD, MPH, MBA[a], Abass Alavi, MD[c]

KEYWORDS

• Total-body PET • Molecular imaging • Radiophenomics • Parametric PET • Systems biology

KEY POINTS

- TB-PET provides 40-fold improvement to signal-to-noise ratio (SNR) over conventional PET because of novel scanner geometry.
- SNR has two parts, physiologic SNR and biologic SNR.
- TB-PET SNR gains are used to reduce patient radiation dose, perform more delayed imaging, perform faster imaging, or to perform whole-body dynamic imaging.

INTRODUCTION

Around 350 years after Vesalius' masterpiece Roentgen discovered the x-ray. Vesalius' work was focused on attentive description of human structure and anatomy. *De humani corporis fabrica* revolutionized medicine by putting more importance on "observation and scientific description" than commentaries on and hermeneutics of the writings of Greek fathers. The same happened after discovery of this "new way of observation" by "x-ray vision."

About 80 years after Vesalius, William Harvey published *De motu cordis*, and for the first time showed how to observe experimental measurement of physiologic function. By a strange coincidence, about 80 years after Roentgen's discovery, the first molecular and physiologic imaging using ^{18}F-fluorodeoxyglucose (FDG) and the rectilinear scanner set the course toward PET.[1–3] Molecular imaging awakened clinicians to noninvasive imaging of disease pathophysiology.[4]

PET devices have evolved with more efficient detectors and faster electronics. However, the major limitation of current clinical PET devices is that most of the patient's body is out of view of the scanner while the informative signal emits from throughout the body constantly. As a consequence more than 80% of flux with potential diagnostic information is lost while scanning the patient. This loss of information is detrimental to patient care. In addition to that wastefulness, the signal detection efficacy of the remaining 20% of the body inside the field of view (FOV) is suboptimal and only 3% to 5% of the coincident photons within the FOV that escape from the body without being scattered or attenuated are detected. It is estimated that the efficiency of the scanners could

Sources of Funding: None.
Declaration of conflict of interest: None.
[a] Department of Radiology and Imaging Sciences, Clinical Center, National Institutes of Health, 9000 Rockville Pike, Bethesda, MD 20892, USA; [b] Department of Computer Science and Electrical Engineering, University of Maryland, Baltimore County, Baltimore, MD, USA; [c] Department of Radiology, Hospital of the University of Pennsylvania, 3400 Spruce St, Philadelphia, PA 19104, USA
* Corresponding author. 9000 Rockville Pike, Bethesda, MD 20892.
E-mail address: babak.saboury@nih.gov

PET Clin 15 (2020) 427–438
https://doi.org/10.1016/j.cpet.2020.06.012
1556-8598/20/Published by Elsevier Inc.

be increased 100 times in an ideal situation.[5] Based on that potential, the Explorer Consortium was conceived to team up scientists from the University of Pennsylvania and University of California, Davis with support and funding from the National Institutes of Health to pursue the goal of creating a total-body PET (TB-PET).[6] Almost 15-years after the first conceptualization by Cherry and Badawi, the first TB-PET-computed tomography (CT) scanner (uEXPLORER) obtained Food and Drug Administration (FDA) clearance and became commercially available in the United States in February 2019.[7]

TB-PET is not just an elongated PET scanner. Numerous improvements in PET technology over the years make possible the new TB-PET geometry, which captures coincidence photons occurring within the patient's body even when emitted at wide oblique angles.[5,8,9] Increase in axial FOV to 194 cm by assembling eight detector rings[7] provides the opportunity to increase acceptance angle up to $57°$[7] and having more than 90×10^9 lines-of-response.[7,10,11] Using more than half a million crystal-elements in detector modules of this device improves the time-resolution to 430 ps with an exceptional coincidence time window of 4.5 ns.[7] The PennPET prototype has demonstrated improved time-resolution to less than 250 ps.[5] TB-PET registers more counts per unit of radioactivity in the body (kcps/MBq) over the entire axial length of the detector array simultaneously, without the need for individual bed positions.[7]

Overall TB-PET effective sensitivity increase is a combination of two factors: increased efficiency of coincident photon detection, and reduction in bed positions caused by increased axial FOV. The PennPET prototype (three ring; 64-cm axial FOV) was reported to have sensitivity approximately nine times the sensitivity of a single-ring conventional PET (**Fig. 1**).[12] Computer simulations predicted an overall approximate 40-times effective sensitivity increase for a 200-cm FOV compared with the conventional 20-cm FOV using a cylindrical phantom approximating the size of an adult human.[5,13–15] To estimate the effect size of the coincident photon detection improvement in TB-PET, a simulation study showed four- to five-fold increase in signal from a point-source or a small organ (eg, heart or liver)[5] (**Fig. 2**).[15] To better understand the impact of the second component, only one single bed position is needed to acquire the imaging volume of the entire body, compared with conventional PET requiring five to six bed positions (**Fig. 3**).[7,12,16]

TB-PET is still a technology on the rise with currently only one FDA-approved device in the world and few prototype systems in development. One of the proposed limitations in implementation and wide clinical application of the total-body approach to PET imaging has been the price of the scanner. This may be in part due to substantial increase in the amount of detector material needed to build the total body scanner with such geometric coverage, which results in increased manufacturing cost. To mitigate this aspect of manufacturing expense, alternative cost-saving designs have been proposed and investigated, including spacing the detector ring to expand the same number of detector elements over a longer axial dimension.

Zein and colleagues[17] investigated this method by using sparse ring detector configuration, in which two or more spaced out PET gantries are used to increase the axial FOV. Authors demonstrated comparable image quality between PET systems with extended and compact detector rings.

When discussing from the economic standpoint, it is important to differentiate the price tag of the scanner from manufacturing cost. To the best of our knowledge there is no scientific evidence evaluating the actual manufacturing cost associated with full-length FOV. Although the number of detectors inside the scanner increase 10-fold, this only implies a 10-fold increase in detector cost, not the total production cost. Inferring the manufacturing cost from the market price tag is not a reliable method in economics and econometrics. The current market price of TB-PET manufacturing with complete geometric coverage is substantially more than a conventional PET system. A fact that should be considered is that these current estimated costs are not the manufacturing cost of a commercialized unit but more related to the lack of a production line and research and development efforts invested in production of a new technology. TB-PET is yet to take the path from an invention to innovation before one can comment on the cost-effectiveness of this technology.

An innovative new commercial medical imaging device may enter the market with high initial market price point.[18] In the case of TB-PET this price point may be acceptable due to increases in efficiency, quality of patient care, significant radiation dose reduction. The "first do no harm" principle holds that it is the ethical duty of clinicians to ensure that avoidance of potential risks to the patient is paramount in

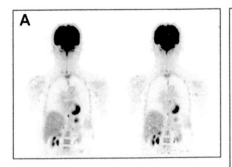

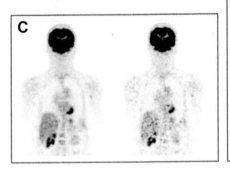

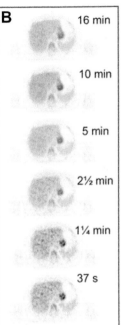

Fig. 1. Early PennPET prototype with 64-cm axial FOV. Imaging was performed after administration of ^{18}F-FDG PET for various acquisition durations and at different time points to assess image quality. (*A*) Coronal ^{18}F-FDG PET images 1.5 hours following injection with 16-minute acquisition (*left*) versus 2-minute acquisition (*right*). (*B*) Axial images through the liver with 16-minute acquisition down to 37-second acquisition. (*C*) Coronal images acquired 0.75 hours after injection for 16 minutes (*left*) and 2 minutes (*right*). (This research was originally published in Pantel AR, Viswanath V, Daube-Witherspoon ME, et al. PennPET Explorer: Human Imaging on a Whole-Body Imager. J Nucl Med. 2020;61(1):144-151.)

determining the clinical benefits of an imaging modality.[19]

TECHNICAL ADVANTAGES

In this section we describe the technical principles and advantages that this new technology will bring about to PET imaging in a manner relevant to clinicians.

Increased effective sensitivity allows the clinician to select among several strategies to improve clinical capabilities using TB-PET. These strategies are all related to the signal-to-noise ratio (SNR) equation (see **Fig. 2**, Eq. 1).[5] It should be appreciated that SNR has two types: physical SNR (SNR_{phys}) and biologic SNR (SNR_{bio}).

We begin by discussing some advantages provided by increasing the SNR_{phys} (see **Fig. 2**, Eq. 2). When using TB-PET with the same current clinical parameters, imaging is obtained with higher SNR_{phys}. Increased SNR_{phys} means the detection power of imaging is increased. The PennPET prototype was able to achieve brain voxel resolution of $1 \times 1 \times 1$ mm^3 with a 20-minute scan.[12] Taking advantage of improved contrast resolution can allow the molecular imaging clinician to see that which was previously unseeable (see **Fig. 2**, Eq. 3).

The increased effective sensitivity of TB-PET also allows the system to tolerate lower radiotracer activity or decreased scan time while maintaining an equivalent SNR. TB-PET affords new unique capabilities, such as dose reduction, delayed imaging, and better temporal resolution (**Fig. 4**, Eq. 1).

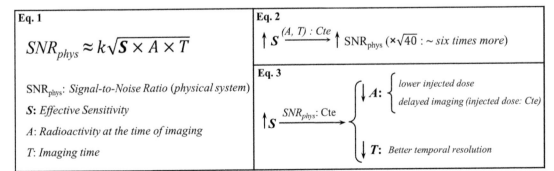

Eq. 1

$$SNR_{phys} \approx k\sqrt{S \times A \times T}$$

SNR_{phys}: *Signal-to-Noise Ratio (physical system)*

S: *Effective Sensitivity*

A: *Radioactivity at the time of imaging*

T: *Imaging time*

Eq. 2

$$\uparrow S \xrightarrow{(A,\ T)\ :\ Cte} \uparrow SNR_{phys}\ (\times\sqrt{40}\ :\ \sim six\ times\ more)$$

Eq. 3

$$\uparrow S \xrightarrow{SNR_{phys}:\ Cte} \begin{cases} \downarrow A: \begin{cases} lower\ injected\ dose \\ delayed\ imaging\ (injected\ dose:\ Cte) \end{cases} \\ \downarrow T: Better\ temporal\ resolution \end{cases}$$

Fig. 2. In a PET image, signal-to-noise ratio (SNR) is proportional to the effective sensitivity of the scanner (S), injected activity (A), and imaging time (T).

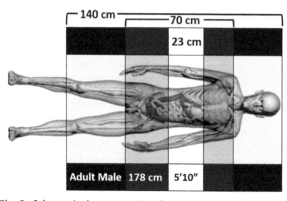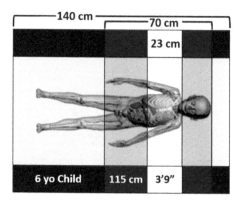

Fig. 3. Schematic demonstrating the expected coverage of the average adult by conventional PET FOV (~23 cm) compared with simulated TB-PET FOV (~70 cm and ~140 cm) as simulated by the XCAT digital phantoms (Segars and colleagues 2010, Kainz and colleagues 2019). (Originally published in Viswanath, V., Daube-Witherspoon, M.E., Schmall, J.P., Surti, S., Werner, M.E., Muehllehner, G., Geagan, M.J., Perkins, A.E., Karp, J.S., 2017. DEVELOPMENT OF PET FOR TOTAL-BODY IMAGING. Acta Phys. Pol. B 48, 1555–1566.)

Lower Dose

The amount of radiation dose in PET imaging is predominantly determined by the amount of radiotracer used in an examination. To maintain diagnostic quality and cope with the low sensitivity of current PET scanners, the SNR is increased by using a higher amount of radiotracer to increase the number of detected decay events. Sensitivity gains of TB-PET, largely because of its broad geometric coverage, allows reduction of the injected activity by a factor of 40 (see **Fig. 4**, Eq. 2). This significant reduction in patient administered radiotracer dose in TB-PET occurs while keeping SNR_{phys} equal to conventional whole-body PET. Many factors have contributed to reduced radiation exposure by PET/CT imaging in the past two decades. An example is improved CT scanner technology and reconstruction methods, which have provided lower dose attenuation correction for CT scanning. Another example is three-dimensional acquisition and time-of-flight

PET, which have improved SNR and somewhat reduced necessary radiotracer dosages. These improvements, although important, have contributed minimally to dose reduction compared with TB-PET. The FDA-approved 194-cm TB-PET was reported to be capable of allowing imaging with 25 MBq (0.7 mCi) ^{18}F-FDG or less (**Fig. 5**).[7] It has been postulated that the ^{18}F-FDG injected dose could potentially be reduced to 9.25 MBq (250 µCi) with similar or even better SNR than conventional PET because of reduced dead time and random fraction at these lower activities.[5] TB-PET has the potential to decrease radiation exposure by an order of magnitude.

The dose reduction strategy could make immuno-PET a clinical reality. A challenge with Zr-89 agents is the high radiation dose per scan because of the long half-life of Zr-89 (78.41 hours) and the high gamma emission (77%; 909 keV). A typical 37-MBq (1 mCi) imaging dose of Zr-89 can expose the patient to 20 to 50 mSv. With TB-PET total radiation dose for immuno-PET

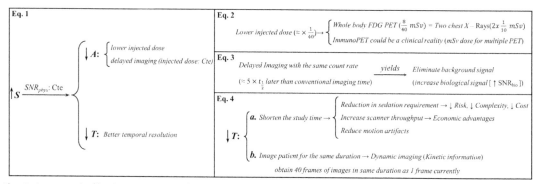

Fig. 4. Improved effective sensitivity of the TB-PET scanner can provide advantages in several areas.

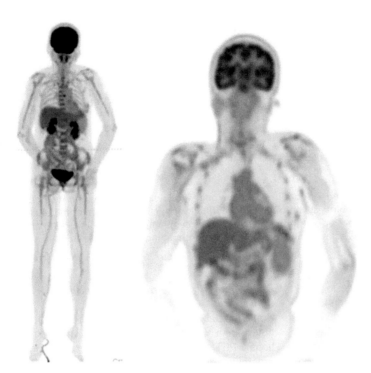

Fig. 5. Total-body maximum intensity projection (*left*) and coronal view of the upper body (*right*) of a patient who was injected with 25 MBq into a vein in the right lower leg and scanned for 10 minutes after 52.5 minutes of uptake time. (Originally published in JNM. Badawi RD et al. First Human Imaging Studies with the EXPLORER Total-Body PET Scanner. J Nucl Med 2019;60:299-303. © SNMMI.)

examinations could be reduced to sub-mSv, less than low-dose chest CT.

Radiotracer delivery to more remote locations or use of radiotracers with a shorter half-life are ancillary benefits of the low-dose capabilities of TB-PET. These effects could broaden the range of commercially available radiotracers.

Delayed Imaging

The time interval between injection of radiotracer and initiation of imaging serves two purposes: accumulation of radiotracer in the location of interest over time based on tracer pharmacokinetics (signal)[20–22] while washing out the off-target activity from the background (noise) (see **Fig. 4**, Eq. 3).[23] By increasing the time interval, these two processes contribute to an increase in SNR_{bio}.[20,24] This paradigm demonstrated clinical utility for atherosclerosis detection and quantification[25] and brain imaging.[24]

Although many studies suggest a potential benefit of more delayed imaging, conventional PET scanners are prone to error and suboptimal function if the imaged activity is lower than expected. Use of TB-PET-improved effective sensitivity helps to overcome this technologic limitation by maintaining SNR at lower radiotracer activities present during delayed imaging. The FDA-approved TB-PET/CT demonstrated the ability to acquire diagnostic quality imaging up to 10 hours after ^{18}F-FDG administration[7] (**Fig. 6**).[12] Similarly, the results from the PennPET prototype suggested improved SNR in lymph nodes (**Fig. 7**)[12] and the liver.[12]

This gained SNR_{bio} is particularly beneficial for antibody-based radiotracers, where the nonspecific background activity is the major reason for failure during the past 20 years. It is reported, for instance, that Zr-89 can be imaged for up to 30 days because of the increased sensitivity afforded by TB-PET.[26,27]

Better Temporal Resolution

Contrary to other clinical imaging systems, such as CT or MR imaging, temporal resolution in PET is not limited by any physical or electronic processes, such as gantry rotation or pulse sequences. This simultaneous acquisition of all the emitted data makes PET a remarkable modality for in vivo tracking of biomedical processes. However, this intrinsic temporal resolution is limited by counting statistics of detected decay events.[28] By covering the total human body, TB-PET allows for PET studies to start with the same amount of administered activity and increase the counts per second. This approach allows the required coincidence photon counts to be obtained faster per unit of space (increased temporal resolution). This technical advantage could be used in two ways: by shortening study time, or by obtaining more

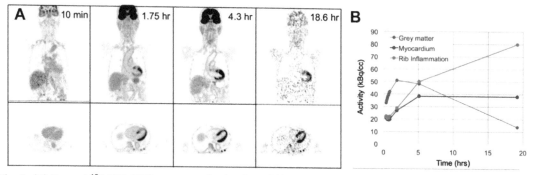

Fig. 6. (*A*) Coronal ^{18}F-FDG PET images acquired at four different time points following injection (as noted in the frame) and axial images of the same time points as the frames above. (*B*) Plot of activity at the midtime of each scan in the gray matter (*blue*), myocardium (*red*), and rib inflammation (*green*). (Originally published in Pantel AR, Viswanath V, Daube-Witherspoon ME, et al. PennPET Explorer: Human Imaging on a Whole-Body Imager. J Nucl Med. 2020;61(1):144-151.)

frames during the same acquisition time in conventional PET to extract kinetic information (see **Fig. 4**, Eq. 4); this high temporal resolution would create opportunities for studying rapidly changing phenomena (eg, fast pharmacokinetics), and motion-frozen imaging of organs prone to motion artifacts. In one study, Zhang and colleagues[28] took advantage of the high temporal resolution of TB-PET, combined with dynamic image reconstruction, to perform ultrahigh-resolution (100 ms) dynamic imaging capturing the fast dynamics of initial radiotracer distribution (**Fig. 8**). This ability to perform fast functional imaging with total-body coverage is a capability that has not yet existed in any other imaging modality.

Faster imaging: ease of use and motion diminution

Conventional PET requires at least 10 to 20 minutes for a whole-body examination. In conventional PET, motion artifacts typical of quiet breathing are ubiquitous in the lower lungs and upper abdomen. Motion and partial volume effects can often make small structures, such as the adrenal glands, difficult to resolve. It is reported that TB-PET can achieve an increased voxel resolution of $1.2 \times 1.2 \times 1.45$ mm^3 to resolve the smaller structures in the brain while maintaining image quality without motion correction (see **Fig. 4**, Eq. 4a).[7]

Increased temporal resolution can translate into other practical clinical benefits. TB-PET is

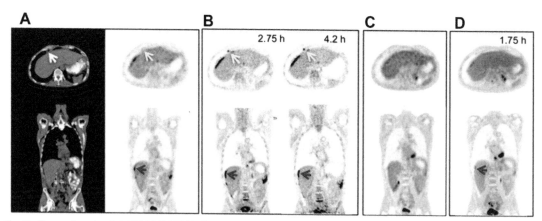

Fig. 7. Coronal and axial 18F-FDG PET/CT images in a patient with metastatic colon cancer with perihepatic disease (*red arrows*) and epinephric lymph node involvement (*yellow and white arrows*) shown using (*A*) the standard clinical PET protocol, (*B*) 2.75-hour and 4-hour delayed protocols for 10-minute acquisitions on the PennPET, (*C*) Follow-up standard clinical PET scan at 3 months, and (*D*) 1.75-hour delayed protocol for 20-minute acquisition on PennPET that showed improvement in perihepatic disease and epiphrenic lymph node. (Originally published in Pantel AR, Viswanath V, Daube-Witherspoon ME, et al. PennPET Explorer: Human Imaging on a Whole-Body Imager. J Nucl Med. 2020;61(1):144–151.)

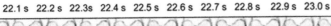
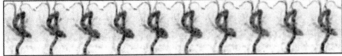
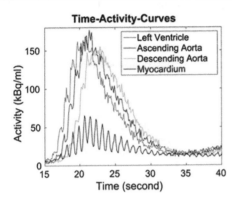

Fig. 8. (*Top*) Maximum intensity projection images reconstructed from a dynamic PET acquisition of 10 consecutive frames starting at 22 seconds postinjection. (*Bottom*) Dynamic time activity curves generated from 100-m frames. (Originally published in Zhang, X., Cherry, S.R., Xie, Z., Shi, H., Badawi, R.D. and Qi, J., 2020. Subsecond total-body imaging using ultrasensitive positron emission tomography. Proceedings of the National Academy of Sciences, 117(5), pp.2265-2267.)

reported to provide similar image quality with a 30-second acquisition in many patients and debatably down to 18.75 seconds in a single bed position.[7] At this speed of whole-body acquisition, the authors suggest TB-PET be performed in a single-breath-hold in many patients.[5,29] Patients with difficulty tolerating longer scan times (eg, those of conventional PET and MR imaging) or with difficulty remaining still may tolerate TB-PET with appropriate coaching without the need for sedation or anesthesia. The faster scan time could also allow much higher throughput in a department or outpatient molecular imaging center, helping to justify the increased cost over conventional PET. It is projected that the entire scan time could be decreased to less than 5 minutes including positioning, allowing 15-minute patient blocks to be used for up to 40 examinations per 10-hour working day similar to CT.[5]

Whole-body dynamic imaging: extension of dual-time-point imaging paradigm

PET tracer biodistribution is a dynamic process impacted by underlying biochemical, physiologic, and pharmacologic processes in vivo. In the current clinical practice, information acquired over a single time period or frame at late time points is reconstructed to create images for diagnosis. This static approach to a dynamic process and its corresponding quantification measure of metabolic activity, known as standardized uptake value (SUV), is a time-dependent method that may not accurately capture these processes.[30]

Dynamic PET imaging seeks to collect a series of frames of data over a given time interval to address SUV limitations.[31] These data are analyzed at the region of interest level, which reduces statistical noise over the voxel level by sampling the time activity curve over a given volume. Data can also be used during image reconstruction for quantification of physiologic parameters, a method known as parametric PET imaging. Parametric PET imaging can potentially reveal useful information about tissue physiologic and molecular profile (radiophenomics).[30]

In conventional PET imaging, two major acquisition methods have been developed to achieve dynamic PET imaging. Single bed position was introduced to scan a limited axial FOV over a sequence of time frames enabling acquisition of useful tracer kinetic parameters. To include more than one organ in the dynamic study, one needs to acquire data from an extended portion of the body. To gain this goal, multibed-position dynamic PET methodologies have been investigated. However, this approach introduces significant challenges because this method requires multiple whole-body passes within the same time, resulting in short acquisition time frames per bed position, hence low SNR.[31,32]

To reconstruct and generate images from dynamic information and to address challenges associated with modeling of tracer kinetic information different strategies have been developed. Some of the more often used methods include the streamlined graphical analysis developed by Patlak and colleagues[33] (Patlak plot), spectral analysis that is based on the decomposition of the tissue response after radiotracer injection, and complex full compartmental modeling methods that are more informative but also more sensitive to statistical noise.[30]

The gained temporal resolution in TB-PET could also be invested in the context of dynamic imaging. In the current PET scanners the dead time that occurs at high activities and high random event rates prevent the acquisition of high-SNR images in short time periods. Therefore, the ability to perform high-resolution, dynamic imaging studies with tracer kinetic modeling is limited because the short time frame datasets are always noisy. The high efficiency of TB-PET can provide the opportunity for high SNR dynamic imaging, allowing for real-time functional imaging of biochemical, molecular, and physiologic processes with total-body coverage (see **Fig. 4**, Eq. 4b).[5]

Sokoloff and colleagues[34,35] developed a meticulous complex compartmental model to measure the metabolic rate of glucose consumption. Sokoloff's model was used on autoradiographs of the rat brain after administration of ^{14}C-deoxyglucose (^{14}C-DG) and extensively validated. Around the same time, FDG was

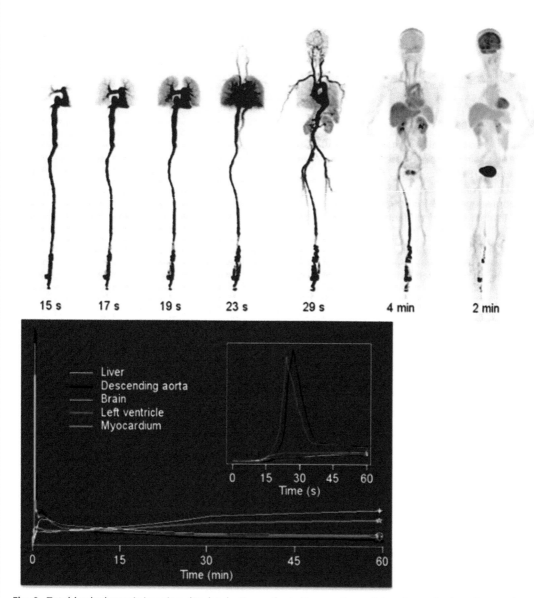

Fig. 9. Total-body dynamic imaging. (*Top*) Selections of rotating maximum intensity projections from a dynamic scan of a patient. Frame duration is 1 second, except for the two left-most images, which have frame durations of 1 minute. (*Bottom*) Time–activity curves for selected anatomic regions. (*Bottom inset*) Time–activity curves for first minute of acquisition. (Originally published in JNM. Badawi RD et al. First Human Imaging Studies with the EXPLORER Total-Body PET Scanner. J Nucl Med 2019;60:299-303. © SNMMI.)

administered for the first time to two normal human volunteers by Abass Alavi in August 1976 at the University of Pennsylvania. From the dawn of clinical FDG imaging, extensive efforts were made to use that complex compartmental model for accurate measurement of glucose metabolic rate (MR_{gluc}); however, those complex compartmental models were never adopted in the clinical setting because of impracticality of requirements (multiple arterial sampling) and assumption-dependency of the calculations. Subsequently, many attempts were made to simplify measurement of MR_{gluc}.

One of those approaches was developed by Patlak and coworkers.[33,36] Patlak's method elegantly simplified the process, with less dependency on model assumptions, and calculated MR_{gluc} based on dynamic FDG PET imaging (termed "Patlak plot"). Patlak's model has proven valuable in PET research and clinical use. However, this approach also required use of PET table time for a long duration and it remained clinically and financially impractical for routine use. In an attempt to mitigate the limitation of PET scanner access, Hustinx and colleagues[37] developed the concept of dual-time-point (DTP) imaging as a clinically feasible data acquisition schema with almost equal accuracy of the MR_{gluc} measurement. This equivalency was elegantly described and validated by van den Hoff and colleagues[38]; they showed an analytical relationship between the Patlak-derived K_m ($K_m \sim MR_{gluc}$) and DTP-derived K_s as shown in the following equation:

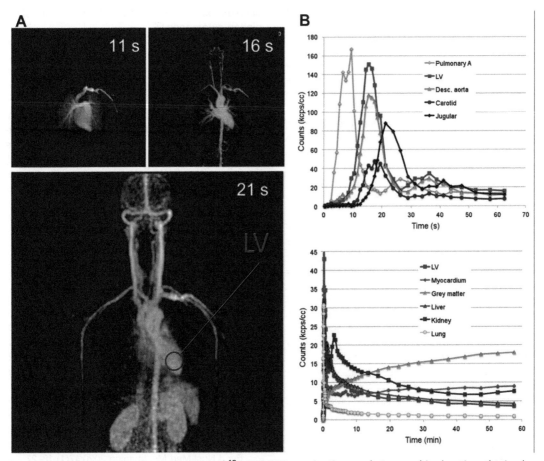

Fig. 10. (*A*) Maximum intensity projections of ^{18}F-FDG PET examination, each 1 second in duration obtained on the PennPET TB-PET prototype. (*B*) Blood input function time activity curves over the first hour for major organs following injection of radiotracer. LV, left ventricle. (Originally published in Pantel, Austin R., Varsha Viswanath, Margaret E. Daube-Witherspoon, Jacob G. Dubroff, Gerd Muehllehner, Michael J. Parma, Daniel A. Pryma, Erin K. Schubert, David A. Mankoff, and Joel S. Karp. 2020. "PennPET Explorer: Human Imaging on a Whole-Body Imager." Journal of Nuclear Medicine: Official Publication, Society of Nuclear Medicine 61 (1): 144–51.)

$$\begin{cases} K_s = \dfrac{1}{\sqrt{A}} \times \dfrac{B}{\Delta t} \\[2mm] A = C_{second-time-point}^{aorta} \times C_{first-time-point}^{aorta} \\[2mm] B = C_{second-time-point}^{lesion} - C_{first-time-point}^{lesion} \\[2mm] \Delta t = \text{time interval between two points} \end{cases}$$

The story of FDG and the resilient ways that researchers moved ahead to keep the dream of better quantification alive should be the roadmap for all the new tracers and modalities. There is a dire need for the same comprehensive yet practical quantification methods for newly approved tracers, such as ^{68}Ga-DOTA-TATE. The astonishing confusion around the SUV_{max} measurement of neuroendocrine tumors is addressed by use of this roadmap. Even in the current clinical setting DTP-PET can enlighten the clinical confusion of ^{68}Ga-DOTA-TATE activity measurements.[39] Indeed, similar principles apply to all receptor-based radiotracers. Prostate-specific membrane antigen (PSMA) PET imaging should also be informed by this history and try to move toward more feasible quantification.[40] DTP imaging should not be a luxury in the ivory towers of academia; it is a needed procedure for day-to-day clinical practice. Molecular imaging physicians should strive for demonstrating the clinical utility of reliable, well-defined quantification techniques, such as DTP-PET, to foster CPT code development to support practical clinical implementation.

Implementing DTP FDG PET as a clinically feasible equivalent to the Patlak method opened the door of kinetic information extraction to routine clinical practice, particularly in the realm of tumor biology characterization and inflammation versus neoplasia differentiation. The next step in the odyssey of MR_{gluc} measurement is harnessing the temporal resolution of TB-PET. DTP-based MR_{gluc} quantification with TB-PET will be more efficient and more robust (multiple-time-point approach). Compared with conventional whole-body PET, the temporal resolution capabilities of TB-PET for dynamic quantification are almost magical.

The combination of increased temporal resolution, although having the entire body in the FOV, creates the opportunity for a new paradigm of whole-body dynamic PET imaging. The FDA-approved 194-cm TB-PET scanner will provide whole-body coverage for most of the population (average human height range, 142.2–185.6 cm worldwide). The sensitivity is higher in the central part of the FOV and decreases toward the edges of the scanner.[41] With TB-PET, region-specific time activity curves of the entire body are acquired simultaneously for the first time (**Fig. 9**).[7] Pharmacokinetics of a radiotracer are dynamically assessed for a systems biology approach to disease. Studying tracer physiology in various vital or pathologic organs and tissues simultaneously over time will lead to a better understanding of systemic disease processes and treatments (**Fig. 10**).[12]

SUMMARY

TB-PET is a technical revolution in evolution with a huge potential to address some limitations of the conventional PET scanners. This advancement could be considered as an innovation that could change the landscape of medical imaging in the coming years. In the "image wisely" era, by public awareness about radiation exposure where gradual advancement in dose reduction is applauded, a 4000% reduction in patient radiation dose exposure is a new stage in the concept of radiation awareness.[42]

With the traditional approach to PET imaging for a given dose of radiation received by the patient a significant proportion of valuable data is lost, hence exhausting diagnostic opportunities and reducing the informative value of this clinical examination compared with its invasive burden. With the patient already having paid the fixed radiation price by receiving a certain tracer dose at the time of injection, it is our ethical duty to collect all the information that can be used for patient care. This trend is the inevitable destiny of medical imaging; it is up to the medical community to align with all the scanner manufacturers to move toward this goal sooner, rather than later.

REFERENCES

1. Alavi A, Reivich M. Guest editorial: the conception of FDG-PET imaging. Semin Nucl Med 2002;32(1):2–5.
2. Ido T, Wan C-N, Casella V, et al. Labeled 2-deoxy-D-glucose analogs. 18F-labeled 2-deoxy-2-fluoro-D-glucose, 2-deoxy-2-fluoro-D-mannose and 14C-2-deoxy-2-fluoro-D-glucose. J Labelled Comp Radiopharm 1978;14(2):175–83.
3. Alavi A, Hess S, Werner TJ, et al. An update on the unparalleled impact of FDG-PET imaging on the day-to-day practice of medicine with emphasis on management of infectious/inflammatory disorders. Eur J Nucl Med Mol Imaging 2020;47(1):18–27.
4. Hess S, Blomberg BA, Zhu HJ, et al. The pivotal role of FDG-PET/CT in modern medicine. Acad Radiol 2014;21(2):232–49.
5. Cherry SR, Jones T, Karp JS, et al. Total-body PET: maximizing sensitivity to create new opportunities

for clinical research and patient care. J Nucl Med 2018;59(1):3–12.

6. Cherry SR, Badawi RD, Karp JS, et al. Total-body imaging: transforming the role of positron emission tomography. Sci Transl Med 2017;9(381). https://doi.org/10.1126/scitranslmed.aaf6169.

7. Badawi RD, Shi H, Hu P, et al. First human imaging studies with the EXPLORER total-body PET scanner. J Nucl Med 2019;60(3):299–303.

8. Segars WP, Sturgeon G, Mendonca S, et al. 4D XCAT phantom for multimodality imaging research. Med Phys 2010;37(9):4902–15.

9. Kainz W, Neufeld E, Bolch WE, et al. Advances in computational human phantoms and their applications in biomedical engineering: a topical review. IEEE Trans Radiat Plasma Med Sci 2019;3(1):1–23.

10. Berg E, Zhang X, Bec J, et al. Development and evaluation of mini-EXPLORER: a long axial field-of-view PET scanner for nonhuman primate imaging. J Nucl Med 2018;59(6):993–8.

11. Lv Y, Lv X, Liu W, et al. Mini EXPLORER II: a prototype high-sensitivity PET/CT scanner for companion animal whole body and human brain scanning. Phys Med Biol 2019;64(7):075004.

12. Pantel AR, Viswanath V, Daube-Witherspoon ME, et al. PennPET explorer: human imaging on a whole-body imager. J Nucl Med 2020;61(1):144–51.

13. Poon JK. The performance limits of long axial field of view PET scanners. Davis (CA): University of California; 2013.

14. Poon JK, Dahlbom ML, Moses WW, et al. Optimal whole-body PET scanner configurations for different volumes of LSO scintillator: a simulation study. Phys Med Biol 2012;57(13):4077–94.

15. Surti S, Pantel AR, Karp JS. Total Body PET: Why, How, What for? IEEE Transactions on Radiation and Plasma Medical Sciences 2020;4(3):283–92. Available at: https://ieeexplore.ieee.org/abstract/document/9056798/casa_token5NTPSPgSONToAAAAA:zifFWCuiZyM0xSEYlo9QNC_EdO0iThLYJwMV_Scs5qtYpvcfPAFAGQy1tkPLTamVsaRjkqosAQ.

16. Viswanath V, Daube-Witherspoon ME, Schmall JP, et al. Development of PET for total-body imaging. Acta Phys Pol B Proc Suppl 2017;48(10):1555–66.

17. Zein SA, Karakatsanis NA, Issa M, et al. Physical performance of a long axial field-of-view PET scanner prototype with sparse rings configuration: a Monte Carlo simulation study. Med Phys 2020;47(4):1949–57.

18. Smith-Bindman R, Miglioretti DL, Larson EB. Rising use of diagnostic medical imaging in a large integrated health system. Health Aff 2008;27(6):1491–502.

19. Gerber TC, Gibbons RJ. Weighing the risks and benefits of cardiac imaging with ionizing radiation. JACC Cardiovasc Imaging 2010;3(5):528–35.

20. Basu S, Kung J, Houseni M, et al. Temporal profile of fluorodeoxyglucose uptake in malignant lesions and normal organs over extended time periods in patients with lung carcinoma: implications for its utilization in assessing malignant lesions. Q J Nucl Med Mol Imaging 2009;53(1):9.

21. Pauwels EK, Ribeiro MJ, Stoot JH, et al. FDG accumulation and tumor biology. Nucl Med Biol 1998;25(4):317–22.

22. Zhuang H, Pourdehnad M, Lambright ES, et al. Dual time point 18F-FDG PET imaging for differentiating malignant from inflammatory processes. J Nucl Med 2001;42(9):1412–7.

23. Cheng G, Alavi A, Lim E, et al. Dynamic changes of FDG uptake and clearance in normal tissues. Mol Imaging Biol 2013;15(3):345–52.

24. Houshmand S, Salavati A, Hess S, et al. An update on novel quantitative techniques in the context of evolving whole-body PET imaging. PET Clin 2015;10(1):45–58.

25. Kwiecinski J, Berman DS, Lee S-E, et al. Three-hour delayed imaging improves assessment of coronary 18F-sodium fluoride PET. J Nucl Med 2019;60(4):530–5.

26. Rosenkrans ZT, Cai W. Total-body PET imaging for up to 30 days after injection of Zr-89-labeled antibodies. J Nucl Med 2020;61(3):451–2.

27. Berg E, Gill H, Marik J, et al. Total-body PET and highly stable chelators together enable meaningful 89Zr-antibody PET studies up to 30 days after injection. J Nucl Med 2020;61(3):453–60.

28. Zhang X, Cherry SR, Xie Z, et al. Subsecond total-body imaging using ultrasensitive positron emission tomography. Proc Natl Acad Sci U S A 2020;117(5):2265–7.

29. Nehmeh SA, Erdi YE, Meirelles GSP, et al. Deep-inspiration breath-hold PET/CT of the thorax. J Nucl Med 2007;48(1):22–6.

30. Bentourkia M, 'hamed, Zaidi H. Tracer kinetic modeling in PET. PET Clin 2007;2(2):267–77.

31. Karakatsanis NA, Lodge MA, Tahari AK, et al. Dynamic whole-body PET parametric imaging: I. Concept, acquisition protocol optimization and clinical application. Phys Med Biol 2013;58(20):7391–418.

32. Karakatsanis NA, Casey ME, Lodge MA, et al. Whole-body direct 4D parametric PET imaging employing nested generalized Patlak expectation–maximization reconstruction. Phys Med Biol 2016;61(15):5456.

33. Patlak CS, Blasberg RG, Fenstermacher JD. Graphical evaluation of blood-to-brain transfer constants from multiple-time uptake data. J Cereb Blood Flow Metab 1983;3(1):1–7.

34. Sokoloff L. [1-14C]-2-deoxy-d-glucose method for measuring local cerebral glucose utilization. Mathematical analysis and determination of the "lumped"

constants. Neurosci Res Program Bull 1976;14(4): 466–8.

35. Sokoloff L, Reivich M, Kennedy C, et al. The [14C] deoxyglucose method for the measurement of local cerebral glucose utilization: theory, procedure, and normal values in the conscious and anesthetized albino rat. J Neurochem 1977;28(5):897–916.

36. Patlak CS, Blasberg RG. Graphical evaluation of blood-to-brain transfer constants from multiple-time uptake data. Generalizations. J Cereb Blood Flow Metab 1985;5(4):584–90.

37. Hustinx R, Smith RJ, Benard F, et al. Dual time point fluorine-18 fluorodeoxyglucose positron emission tomography: a potential method to differentiate malignancy from inflammation and normal tissue in the head and neck. Eur J Nucl Med 1999;26(10): 1345–8.

38. van den Hoff J, Hofheinz F, Oehme L, et al. Dual time point based quantification of metabolic uptake rates in 18F-FDG PET. EJNMMI Res 2013;3(1):16.

39. Farhadi F, Saboury B, Jones E. How to interpret and report 68Ga-DOTA-TATE PET/CT standard uptake value (SUV) measurement? Pearls and pitfalls. J Nucl Med 2019;60(supplement 1):1150.

40. Basu S, Kwee TC, Torigian D, et al. Suboptimal and inadequate quantification: an alarming crisis in medical applications of PET. Eur J Nucl Med Mol Imaging 2011;38(7):1381.

41. Cherry SR. The 2006 Henry N. Wagner Lecture: of Mice and men (and Positrons)—Advances in PET imaging technology. J Nucl Med 2006;47(11): 1735–45.

42. Mayo-Smith WW, Morin RL. Image wisely: the beginning, current status, and future opportunities. J Am Coll Radiol 2017;14(3):442–3.

Prospects and Clinical Perspectives of Total-Body PET Imaging Using Plastic Scintillators

Paweł Moskal, PhD*, Ewa Ł. Stępień, PhD*

KEYWORDS

- J-PET • PET imaging • Total-body PET imaging • Multitracer imaging • Positronium imaging
- ^{82}Rb-chloride • ^{44}Sc-PSMA • Plastic scintillators

KEY POINTS

- Total-body PET opens a new diagnostic paradigm with prospects for personalized disease treatment, yet the high cost of the current crystal-based PET technology limits dissemination of total-body PET in hospitals and even in the research clinics.
- The J-PET tomography system is based on axially arranged low-cost plastic scintillator strips. It constitutes a realistic cost-effective solution of a total-body PET for broad clinical applications.
- High sensitivity of total-body J-PET and triggerless data acquisition enable multiphoton imaging, opening possibilities for multitracer and positronium imaging, thus promising quantitative enhancement of specificity in cancer and inflammatory diseases assessment.
- An example of dual tracer analysis, becoming possible with total-body J-PET system, could be a concurrent application of Food and Drug Administration–approved ^{82}Rb-Chloride and [^{18}F]FDG, allowing simultaneous assessment of myocardium metabolic rate and perfusion of the cardiovascular system.

INTRODUCTION

As modern medicine advances toward personalized treatment of patients, it requires highly specific and sensitive tests to diagnose disease. The advent of total-body PET (TB-PET) systems[1–6] opens new perspectives for the precision medicine enabling detection of pathologies on a molecular level in the whole patient body simultaneously, before they lead to the functional or structural abnormalities.[7,8] TB-PET imaging creates a new paradigm for precision medicine, yet not fully exploited, enabling simultaneous imaging of metabolism rate in close and distant organs, reducing drastically the whole-body scan time or the dose delivered by the radiopharmaceutical agent (by a factor of approximately 40 with respect to typical current clinical PET systems).[3] Introduction of

TB-PETs extends the PET application to diagnosis of a wider group of patients (eg, children and pregnant women) and systemic diseases, as for example, autoimmune diseases, cardiovascular diseases, or active rheumatoid diseases[8–10] by simultaneous multiorgan kinetic modeling, currently not possible with the ~25 cm axial filed-of-view scanners.[11,12] Kinetic model-based parametric imaging may also deliver additional complementary diagnostic information to that available from standard static standardized uptake value (SUV) images.[13–15]

However, introduction of the TB-PET scanners in the common clinical practice encounters challenges of the high cost, estimated to approximately $10 million or more for a single TB-PET system built based on the current technology

Marian Smoluchowski Institute of Physics, Jagiellonian University, ul. S. Lojasiewicza 11, Kraków 30-348, Poland
* Corresponding authors.
E-mail addresses: p.moskal@uj.edu.pl (P.M.); e.stepien@uj.edu.pl (E.Ł.S.)

PET Clin 15 (2020) 439–452
https://doi.org/10.1016/j.cpet.2020.06.009
1556-8598/20/© 2020 The Authors. Published by Elsevier Inc. This is an open access article under the CC BY-NC-ND license (http://creativecommons.org/licenses/by-nc-nd/4.0/).

using crystal scintillators.[4] High price is a serious barrier factor in using this device not only in hospital facilities but even in medical research clinics.

Therefore, there is a need for new technical solution that would enable to substantially decrease the cost of the extended axial field-of-view (AFOV) PET, where approximately half of the cost is in scintillators, and the other half of the costs is in silicon photomultipliers (SiPM) and electronics.[16]

The ongoing investigations aiming at cost reduction focuses on the possibilities of (1) scintillator thickness reduction[17]; (2) sparse detector configurations[18,19]; and (3) application of BGO crystals[20,21] with Cherenkov light readout for the improved timing properties.[22–25]

The reduction of detector thickness decreases the sensitivity approximately as a square of the reduction thickness coefficient, whereas the cost of scintillators decreases only linearly without reducing the costs of electronics. Similarly, in the sparse configuration, the sensitivity drops as square of the decrease of the number of detector components.[18] An application of BGO crystals may reduce costs of the scintillators by a factor 2 to 3[16]; however, at the same time the costs may increase due to the increased requirements and complications for the of readout electronics needed for taking advantage of both scintillation and Cherenkov light.

Therefore, it is claimed that only a spectacular decrease in the price, while maintaining the key parameters such as total-body dynamic/kinetic imaging, will accelerate the dissemination process of the TB-PET imaging.[26] In general it is also important to decrease the costs of the whole diagnostic process, which includes not only PET imaging enabling detection of the presence of diseased tissues based on SUV, but also histologic assessments of tissues requiring biopsies for distinguishing among the inflammatory, infected, and cancerous tissues and for evaluating the grade of cancer malignancy.

Therefore, the effective translation of TB-PET for wide use in clinics, in view of the precision diagnosis tailored to the individual patient, requires significant decrease of costs of the TB-PET construction with respect to the pioneering EXPLORER PET technology and an increase of specificity in cancer and inflammatory diseases assessment.

In this article, we discuss the principle of operation of the new Jagiellonian-PET (J-PET) tomography system developed at the Jagiellonian University, Cracow, Poland, based on axially arranged low-cost plastic scintillator strips, as contrasted with the current PET scanners with radially arranged expensive crystal blocks. J-PET enables cost-effective construction of PET with long AFOV, up to 2.5 m and more, which would enable high sensitivity imaging of the whole human body, with high and uniform sensitivity over the whole patient from the brain to the feet. Imaging with such a large AFOV would open new perspective for diagnosis of diseases affecting the body and brain simultaneously. J-PET may be constructed as a modular, light and portable TB-PET, enabling reconfiguration of the tomographic volume, which may help to extend PET diagnosis further by including patients who cannot be examined with the standard PET due to factors such as obesity or claustrophobia.

Further on, we discuss the properties of the economic total-body J-PET (TB-J-PET), and its prospects for performing both the simultaneous multitracer imaging and *positronium imaging*. The newly proposed *positronium imaging* is being developed based on properties of positronium atoms produced in the intramolecular voids in the patient's cells during the routine PET diagnosis,[27–30] and it is promising for enhancing the specificity of cancer and inflammatory diseases assessment in TB-PET diagnostics.

PROSPECTS FOR TOTAL-BODY PET IMAGING WITH PLASTIC SCINTILLATORS

The J-PET tomography scanner is constructed from plastic scintillator strips read out at both ends by matrices of SiPM. Schematic view of the axial cross-section of the scanner is shown in **Fig. 1**, whereas the left panel of **Fig. 2** presents a perspective view. The position and time of the interaction of annihilation photons is determined by measurement of the times of scintillation light signals arrivals to the edges of the scintillators.[31] Light attenuation by plastic scintillators is by more than 1 order of magnitude lower than in the crystal scintillators, and that enables effective light transport even in strips of a few meters' length (for example, attenuation length for BC-408 plastic scintillator amounts to 380 cm compared with approximately 21 cm to 40 cm for the LYSO crystal).[32–34] The signals from SiPMs are probed in the voltage domain with the time accuracy of approximately 20 ps by newly developed

---

[a]The Netherlands has the tallest people in the world, where the average height of men is 1.83 m (https://adc.bmj.com/content/90/8/807).

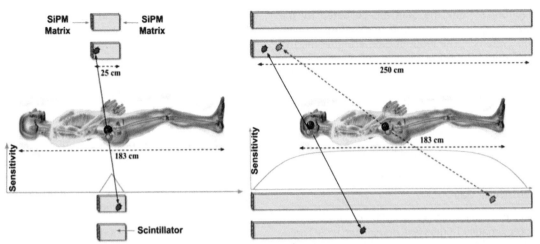

Fig. 1. Schematic view of the axial cross section of the J-PET tomograph composed of the 2 detection layers. Left and right panels illustrate the cases of J-PET with 25 cm and 250 cm AFOV and the 183-cm-tall patient.[a] The single detection module consists of a scintillator strip read out by two SiPM matrices. The cross section of the plastics strips designed for the TB-J-PET is 6 mm × 30 mm. Here it is presented not to scale. Solid and dashed arrows indicate exemplary lines of response (LOR) originating from e⁺e⁻ annihilation. The interaction distance from the center of the scintillator is determined by the difference in times the two signals reach both ends of the scintillator strip. The position along the LOR is determined from time difference measured between two strips. In practice, more advanced methods of hit-time and hit-position were developed, which take advantage of the variation of the signal shape as a function of the hit-position.[39,40] Superimposed charts indicate the sensitivity (in arbitrary units) along the AFOV. It was calculated using the formula described in reference.[29] The presented sensitivity includes also the attenuation of annihilation photons in the patient. The attenuation in the patient flattens the sensitivity inside the long AFOV scanner. The value of sensitivity is given in arbitrary units, however the values in the left and right figures are shown in the same scale.

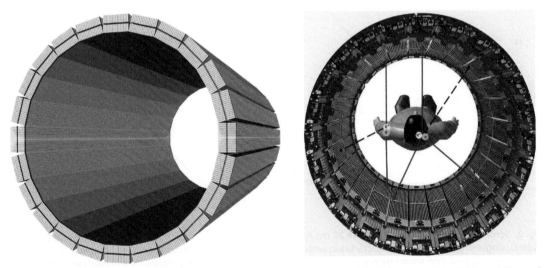

Fig. 2. (*Left*) Perspective view of the design of two-layer TB-J-PET scanner. Each layer consists of 24 modules each including 16 scintillator strips with cross-section of 6 mm × 30 mm. (*Right*) Photograph of the single-layer (with 50 cm AFOV) modular J-PET prototype with superimposed representations of electron-positron annihilation in the patient's body for 2 and 3 photon events (*red solid arrows*) and the associated prompt gamma rays (*blue dashed arrows*) emitted by the β⁺γ radionuclide such as for example, ⁴⁴Sc or ⁸²Rb. The single-layer J-PET prototype with AFOV = 50 cm weighs only approximately 60 kg. It consists of 24 modules each built from plastic scintillator strips (*black*) read out at both ends by SiPMs equipped with the dedicated front-end and digitizing electronics visible in the foreground.[35,36]

electronics[35] and the data are collected by the novel triggerless and reconfigurable data acquisition system.[36] The readout data are streamed to the Central Controller Module and then to a permanent storage.[36] For data processing and simulations, a dedicated software framework was developed.[37] The hit-position and hit-time are reconstructed by the dedicated reconstruction methods based on the compressing sensing theory[38] and the library of synchronized model signals.[39]

Sensitivity Gain

Plastic scintillators (1.02–1.06 g/cm³)[32,41] are approximately 7 times less dense than LYSO crystals (7.0–7.4 g/cm³)[42] and hence less effective for the registration of annihilation photons. However, the axial arrangement of plastic strips with the SiPM readout at the ends provides compensation for the lower registration efficiency by application of multilayer geometry with concentric detector layers,[43] as is visualized in **Figs. 1** and **2** (left). The overall imaging sensitivity depends on the geometric acceptance of the detector, efficiency of the registration of annihilation photons, efficiency of the selection of events contributing to

the PET image formation, and on the attenuation of photons in the imaged object/patient. Annihilation photons emitted at small angles to the cylinder axis (dashed LOR in **Fig. 1**, right) are strongly attenuated in the patient body and effectively the sensitivity for registration and selection of image forming events saturates at approximately 50 cm from the tomograph edges, as indicated by the blue line in the right panel of **Fig. 1**, instead of growing almost linearly toward the detector center as is in the case of short AFOV systems, as indicated in the left panel of **Fig. 1**. The solid and dashed lines in **Fig. 1** indicate examples of a moderately and very oblique lines-of-response, respectively.

To quantitatively estimate the gain in the scanner sensitivity with the extension of the AFOV and to compare the sensitivity gains between the crystal and plastic based scanners, we performed calculations under the assumption that the compared scanners are in the form of a cylinder with the diameter of 80 cm and thickness of 1.81 cm (LYSO) and 6 cm (2 layers of plastic scintillators with 3-cm thickness each). In the left panel of **Fig. 3** we present obtained results taking into account attenuation of photons in the body

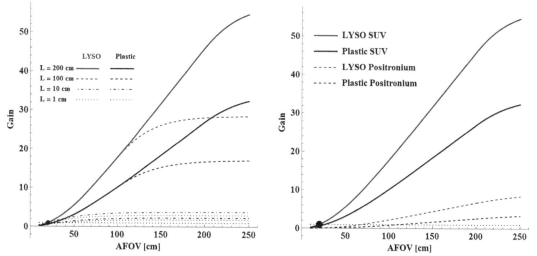

Fig. 3. Sensitivity gain with respect to the 20 cm AFOV LYSO PET (indicated with *blue*) for a small lesion (L = 1 cm object), single organ (L = 10 cm object), brain with torso (L = 100 cm long object) and the total body (200 cm long object). Blue dotted line shows gain equal to unity. Sensitivity includes the probability of registration and selection of image forming events as well as attenuation of photons in the body (water phantom with 20 cm diameter and 200 cm long). Results as a function of the axial length for LYSO (1.81 cm thick) and plastic (two 3-cm-thick layers) PET detectors are shown. The meaning of line types is explained in the legends. The red and black colors indicate results for the LYSO and plastic scintillators, respectively. (*Left*) Results of sensitivity gain for the standard 2γ annihilation photons imaging. (*Right*) The sensitivity for the standard 2γ imaging of the SUV is compared to the sensitivity of the triple-coincidence 2γ + prompt *positronium* imaging.[27–29] In the right panel only the results obtained for the total-body imaging (for source of L = 200 cm) are shown. Calculations were performed assuming energy of the prompt gamma of 1157 keV as emitted by the ⁴⁴Sc isotope.[44]

as well as the changes of interaction probability as a function of the angle under which the photon is entering the detector. The attenuation was estimated approximating the body with a water phantom of 20 cm diameter and 200 cm long.

For the whole-body scan (estimated for the 200-cm-long object) the sensitivity for the 200 cm AFOV scanner, with respect to the 20 cm AFOV PET, is enhanced by a factor of approximately 46 for the LYSO based and by a factor of approximately 27 for the plastic based TB-J-PET scanner, respectively. The gain for brain plus torso imaging (approximated by a 100-cm-long object) saturates for the AFOV of approximately 150 cm, and increases by a factor of approximately 28 for the LYSO PET and by a factor of 15 for the plastic PET. In case of the single organ or a lesion (short 10 cm or 1 cm objects) the gain is already saturated for systems with 70 cm AFOV and reaches values of approximately 3.8 and 2.3 (for the 10-cm object) and 3.0 and 1.8 (for the 1 cm object) for LYSO and plastic PET, respectively.

National Electrical Manufacturers Association Characteristics: Spatial Resolution, Noise Equivalent Count Rate, Sensitivity and Scatter Fraction

The spatial resolution, sensitivity, scatter fraction and noise equivalent count rate (NECR) for the J-PET were estimated[45] using GATE simulation software,[46] following the National Electrical Manufacturers Association (NEMA) NU 2 to 2012 standards.

For a strip length of 100 cm with cross-section of 4 mm × 20 mm and an additional layer of wavelength shifter as the readout,[47] the point spread function (PSF) in the center of the scanner is equal to 3 mm (radial, tangential) and 6 mm (axial). For the double layer geometry, the NECR peak of 300 kcps is reached at 40 kBq/mL activity concentration and the sensitivity at the center amounts to 14.9 cps/kBq. Whereas for the TB-J-PET with AFOV of 200 cm and a scintillators with cross-section of 6 mm × 30 mm, the PSF is estimated to 4.9 mm (radial, tangential) and 7 mm (axial), the NECR peak of 600 kcps is reached at 25 kBq/mL activity concentration, and the sensitivity at the center amounts to 38 cps/kBq. The scatter fraction is estimated to approximately 35%. These values can be compared with PSF of 4 mm and 3 mm, the NECR of 1435 kcps and 1000 kcps, sensitivity at the center of 191.5 cps/kBq and 55 cps/kBq and scatter fraction of 35.8% and 32% for uEXPLORER[16] and Penn PET EXPLORER,[2] respectively.

Multiphoton Imaging

High sensitivity of TB-PET scanners opens opportunities for application in PET scans of events with the emission of 3 or more photons. The triggerless data acquisition system of the J-PET tomograph[36] enables detection of all events including multiphoton annihilations and prompt gammas, not restricted to the standard double annihilation photons coincidences as it is in the current PET scanners. Triggerless mode opens the possibility for flexible selection of events at the software level.[37] This may include selection of double, triple and in general multicoincidence events. In particular it enables registration and identification of 2 ($e^+e^- \rightarrow 2\gamma$) and 3 photon ($e^+e^- \rightarrow 3\gamma$) annihilations, as well as prompt gamma emitted in case of some isotopes referred to as $\beta^+\gamma$ emitters, such as for example, ^{10}C, ^{14}O, ^{22}Na, ^{34}Cl, ^{44}Sc, ^{48}V, ^{52}Mn, ^{55}Co, ^{60}Cu, ^{66}Ga, ^{69}Ge, ^{72}As, ^{76}Br, ^{82}Rb, ^{86}Y, ^{94}Tc, ^{110}In, ^{124}I.[44] Some examples of multiphoton events are shown pictorially in the right panel of **Fig. 2**. After emission of positron the $\beta^+\gamma$ emitters change into the daughter nucleus in an excited state. The daughter nucleus subsequently de-excites through emission of 1 or several gamma quanta. For example, in the case of Scandium the reaction chain is as follows: ^{44}Sc $\rightarrow$ ^{44}Ca* e^+ v $\rightarrow$ ^{44}Ca γ e^+ v, where v denotes neutrino that escapes from the body undetected.

In the current PET imaging procedures, prompt gammas and $e^+e^- \rightarrow 3\gamma$ annihilations constitute a source of unwanted background. In the body a fraction of 3γ annihilation events constitutes approximately 0.5% only[28]; however, prompt gamma may accompany almost each annihilation as it is in the case of for example, ^{44}Sc radionuclide.[44] However, these multiphoton coincidences may be useful for diagnosis.[28] Capability of J-PET to register and identify the signals from prompt gammas and from 2γ and 3γ annihilations allows for tagging the events originating from various isotopes. This information enables classification of registered events according to the radiotracer, and hence enables diagnosis with 2 or more tracers simultaneously during single PET examination.[48] Therefore, in case of the $\beta^+\gamma$ emitters, an additional prompt gamma may be used not only for improving the spatial resolution by combining 2γ PET with the various types of Compton cameras for the registration of the prompt gamma as discussed, for example, in Refs.[49–53] but it may also be used for the simultaneous multitracer imaging[48] and for the newly developed positronium lifetime imaging, which is a promising approach for the in vivo assessment of tissue pathology.[27–29]

Example of Multitracer Imaging Applications with Total-Body Jagiellonian-PET

Despite potential advantage in PET imaging, especially in TB-PET, and broad accessibility of suitable tracers, the β-emitters application is still limited, and to date only a few clinical trials have been conducted. The summary of published results of the preclinical and clinical studies is presented in **Table 1**. Among the previously listed 18 isotopes, only one is approved by the Food and Drug Administration (FDA) (^{82}Rb) and only 2 (^{44}Sc and ^{124}I) are clinically applied and few of them were tested preclinically.[54]

The trivalent β-emitters as ^{44}Sc, ^{66}Ga, and monovalent ^{124}I are especially promising because they

i. Can be delivered by the same class of chelators or carries as their commonly used analogues (isotopes): DOTA,[61] IMP,[58] PIB,[71] NOTA,[62] PSMA-617[67]

ii. Can be attached to tracers approved in clinical trials: PSMA-617,[68,74] Herceptin (trastuzumab),[70] cetuximab[75]

iii. Can recognize the same targets: EGFR[58] HER2 ^{44}Sc-DOTA-ZHER2:342,[72–] CAIX,[55,56] Integrin $\alpha_V\beta_3$,[59] PSMA,[69] SST2R[64]

iv. Can be used in dual analysis with 2 radiotracers "pairs": ^{124}I-trastuzumab/^{18}F-FDG[70]

This unique feature of the aforementioned radionuclides over the standard 2γ radionuclides, which emit additional prompt γ (eg, ^{44}Sc, ^{66}Ga, ^{82}Rb, ^{124}I) provides another rationale for the application of the TB-PET concept.

These radiotracers can be used in the TB-PET simultaneously and complementarily with for example, FDG to shorten the time between dosing of a radiopharmaceutical and a PET scan, which would reduce a diagnostic window, optimize the uptake and clearance of each radiotracer and minimize the risk of radiopharmaceuticals decay.

Table 1
Summary of ^{44}Sc, ^{66}Ga and ^{124}I labeled tracers proposed for PET cancer imaging

Cell/Tissue Molecular Characteristics	Targets	Tracers (Preclinical and Clinical Studies)
Mutations or genome instability	CAIX mutEGFR (de2-7)	^{124}I-cG250[a,55–57] ^{124}I-IMP-R4-ch806[58]
Inducing angiogenesis	Integrin $\alpha_V\beta_3$	^{66}Ga-DOTA-E−[c(RGDfK)]$_2$[59] ^{44}Sc-DOTA-RGD[60] ^{44}Sc-DOTA/NODAGA-RGD[61]
	CD105	^{66}Ga-NOTA-GO-TRC105[62]
Activating motility and mobility	Integrin $\alpha_V\beta_3$	^{66}Ga-DOTA-E−[c(RGDfK)]$_2$[59] 44Sc-DOTA-RGD[60] ^{44}Sc-DOTA/NODAGA-RGD[61]
	CD44v6	^{124}I-cMAb U36[63]
Expressing specific surface antigens	SSTR2 PSMA	^{44}Sc-DOTATOC[a,64,65] ^{124}I-J591[66] ^{66}Ga-PSMA-617[67]] ^{44g}Sc-PSMA-617[68,69,a]
	HER2	^{124}I-trastuzumab[70,a] ^{124}I-PIB-ZHER2:342[71] ^{44}Sc-DOTA-ZHER2:342[72]
	CEA	^{124}I anti-CEA mAbs (cT84.66)[73]

Abbreviations: CAIX, carbonic anhydrase IX, enzyme expressed in the cell membrane of clear cell renal carcinoma; CD105, endoglin, surface glycoprotein identified as angiogenesis regulator; CD44v6, type I transmembrane glycoprotein, which promotes cell adhesion and binds vascular endothelial growth factor (VEGF); CEA, Carcinoembryonic antigen; cG250, chimeric antiCAIX monoclonal antibody, girentuximab; cRGDfK, cyclo(Arg-Gly-Asp-Phe-Lys) peptide, motif specific for integrin binding; DOTA, 1,4,7,10-Tetraazacyclododecane- N,N′,N′′,N′′′- tetraacetic acid, bifunctional chelator also known as tetraxeten; DOTATATE, compound containing 3-tyrosine-octreotate and DOTA; DOTATOC, compound containing 1-phenyloalanine-3-tyrosine-octreotide and DOTA; EGFR, epidermal growth factor receptor; GO, graphen oxide; HER2, herceptin 2 receptor, receptor tyrosine-protein kinase erbB-2, also known as CD340, binding herceptin (trastuzumab); IMP-R4, MCC-Lys(MCC)-Lys(X)-d-Tyr-d-Lys(X)-OH peptide, bifunctional chelator; J591, humanized anti-PSMA monoclonal antibody; NOTA, 1,4,7-triazacyclononane-1,4,7-triacetic acid, chelator; PIB, p-iodobenzoate; PSMA, prostate-specific membrane antigen; SSTR2, somatostatin receptor type 2; TRC105, chimeric anti-CD105 monoclonal antibody; ZHER2, affibody molecule of a small (6–7 kDa) protein based on the Z domain (58 a.a.) derived from *staphylococcal* protein A
ᵃ Clinical trials.

The golden example of a dual tracer analysis application that became possible with TB-PET, is the FDA-approved [82]Rb-Chloride, which when applied concurrently with [^{18}F] fludeoxyglucose (FDG) would enable simultaneous assessment of metabolic rate and perfusion, mainly in the cardiovascular system.[54,76] This would allow to assess coronary arteries' occlusion and myocardium necrotic zone, as a perfusion (oxygen supply) and viability (oxygen consumption) synchronized tests.

Another example worth clinical trials, becoming possible with TB-PET, could be an early diagnostics of neuroendocrine and HER2-positive tumors via simultaneous applications of radiopharmaceuticals labeled with 2 different radionuclides, [44]Sc and ^{18}F, allowing for monitoring of the cancer receptor system (eg, using [44]Sc-DOTATE) end its metabolic activity (eg, using [^{18}F]FDG) at the same time.

Positronium Imaging

One of the examples of multiphoton imaging is the recently proposed positronium mean lifetime tomography,[27–30] which can deliver information complementary to the currently used SUV-based parameters.[77] During the PET imaging, a positron emitted by the radionuclide annihilates with the electron in the patient's body, directly or via formation of the metastable positronium atom. In the human body, positronium atoms are formed in up to approximately 40% of cases of positron-electron annihilations.[78,79] Positronium is an atom built from an electron and a positron (anti-electron). It is not stable but annihilates with emission of photons. In a quarter of the cases it appears as a short-lived (125 ps) para-positronium and in three-quarters of cases as ortho-positronium with mean lifetime in the vacuum of 142 ns. In the tissue ortho-positronium mean lifetime strongly depends on the size of intramolecular voids (free volumes between atoms), whereas its formation probability depends on the voids concentration (**Fig. 4**). In the body, the mean lifetime of ortho-positronium varies from approximately 1.8 ns in pure water to approximately 4 ns in human skin.[80] Moreover, both formation probability and mean lifetime depend on the concentration of the bio-fluids and bio-active molecules[81,82] and the mean lifetime can be established in the human body with the precision of approximately 20 ps.[29]

There are investigations demonstrating differences between normal and cancerous cells with changes of the positronium lifetime during dynamic processes undergoing in model and living biological systems.[79–81,85–95] Therefore, positronium may be used as a sensor of the surrounding tissue environment, and imaging of its properties inside the patient body may serve as additional diagnostic indicator. In general, positronium imaging can be defined as a method for the position-sensitive reconstruction of positronium properties (such as mean lifetime, formation probability, and 3γ/2γ rate ratio) within the imaged object.[27–30] Imaging of positronium lifetime and its formation probability requires applications of isotopes emitting prompt gamma, while 3γ/2γ rate ratio is accessible with all kinds of β+ emitters.[96]

In case of the mean lifetime positronium image, registration of the prompt gamma is used to determine the time of the emission of the positron (which is within tens of picoseconds equal to the time of the formation of the positronium atom) and the registration of annihilation photons is used for the determination of the position and time of the positronium annihilation.[28,29] The most effective way of the positronium mean lifetime image reconstruction is based on the registration of annihilations of ortho-positronium into 2 photons, which may occur in the tissue due to the pick-off[84] and conversion processes[82,97,98] and that is approximately 70 times more frequent than annihilation into 3 photons.[28,29] In this case, the back-to-back photons are used to reconstruct the decay time and decay position of ortho-positronium atom on an event-by-event basis. Reconstruction of the time difference distribution between annihilation and the emission of the positron enables to determine the positronium's mean lifetime for each image voxel.[29]

Time resolution of positronium imaging depends predominantly on the statistics of events reconstructed in the image voxel whereas the spatial resolution depends mainly on the PET time resolution.[29] Current clinical time of flight (TOF)-PETs[12] achieve down to 210 ps and small laboratory type detectors reach CRT of even 30 ps equivalent to position resolution of 4.5 mm along the line of response.[99] Therefore, with the continuous improvement of the time resolution[25,100] it may become feasible in not so distant future to reconstruct positronium image directly as a density distribution of annihilation points.[29,30] Resent simulation studies[29] indicate that the PSF of positronium image equals to approximately 5 mm (radial and axial) for CRT = 50 ps. In comparison, for the CRT of approximately 500 ps, as presently achieved by the uEXPLORER TB-PET, the PSF of positronium image would equal to 30 mm (radial) and 7 mm (axial).[29]

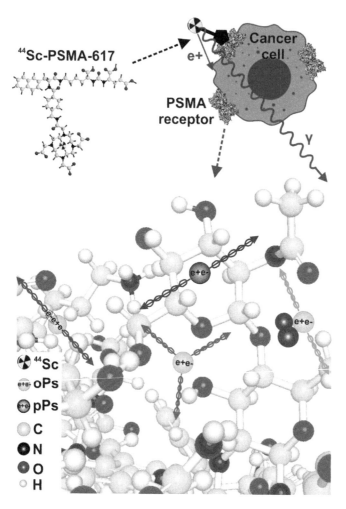

Fig. 4. Pictorial representation of the basic processes involved in the "positronium tomography" using the example of examination of the prostate cancer. The PSMA-617 ligand) labeled with radionuclide ^{44}Sc attaches to the PSMA receptors highly expressed in prostate epithelial cells.[83] ^{44}Sc isotope emits positron (e$^+$) and prompt gamma (γ) via following process: ^{44}Sc $\rightarrow$ ^{44}Ca* e$^+$ v $\rightarrow$ ^{44}Ca γ e$^+$ v.[44] Positron interacting with electrons may form positronium atoms (indicated as oPs or pPs) inside cell molecules including intermolecular voids in PSMA receptors as indicated in the lower part of the sketch. Prompt gamma may be detected in the tomograph to give the signal approximately the time of positronium formation. Arrows indicate photons originating from the annihilation of para- and ortho-positronium inside free space between atoms (*magenta* and *orange arrows*), respectively. Black arrows indicate annihilation of ortho-positronium through the interaction with the electron from the surrounding molecule[84] and green arrows illustrate photons from the conversion of ortho-into para-positronium via interaction with the oxygen molecule[82] and subsequent decay of para-positronium to 2γ.[27]

As an example of the possible application we use here the diagnosis of the prostate cancer. Prostate-specific membrane antigen (PSMA), (which is commonly used as a target for prostate cancer imaging and treatment) is a nonsoluble type 2 integral membrane protein with carboxypeptidase activity.[101] PSMA is overexpressed in prostate cancer cells, correlates to prostate-specific antigen blood levels and reflects tumor aggressiveness diagnosed both in tissue biopsies and in prostate cancer imaging.[102,103] In patients having castration-resistant prostate cancer metastasis, there is an unmet need to apply imaging-guided prostate cancer therapy based on total-body scanning and real-time theranostics.[104] For this purpose [44Sc]Sc-PSMA-617 for PET imaging is the most suitable radiotracer[68] (see **Fig. 4**). Application of [44Sc]Sc-PSMA-617 with TB-PET would enable an enhancement of accurate diagnostics by simultaneous reconstruction of the positronium image.

Sensitivity of Multitracer and Positronium Imaging with Total-Body PET Scanners

Multitracer imaging and mean lifetime positronium imaging requires registration of triple coincidences with 2 photons from e$^+$e$^-$ (Ps) $\rightarrow$ 2γ annihilation and prompt gamma emitted by the $\beta^+\gamma$ isotope as for example, ^{44}Sc. Registration of the prompt gamma enables a determination of the time of the formation of positronium, and registration of the correlated annihilation photons (2 or 3) allows for the determination of the position and time of the positronium annihilation.[28,29,105,106] However, the requirement of the registration and identification of the prompt gamma, in addition to the 2 back-to-back annihilation photons, decreases significantly the imaging sensitivity with respect to the standard PET 2γ imaging. Right panel of **Fig. 3** shows sensitivity gain calculated with respect to the standard 2γ metabolic imaging with the 20 cm axial-length LYSO detector indicated with the blue dot. The figure compares results (dashed lines) for the sensitivity gain as a function of the AFOV for multitracer and positronium imaging (2γ+*prompt gamma*) with respect to the sensitivity gain for the standard SUV imaging (solid lines). Results presented in the right panel of **Fig. 3** were obtained for Scandium isotope as a $\beta^+\gamma$ emitter, which is decaying via the following reaction chain: $^{44}Sc \rightarrow {}^{44}Ca^* e^+ v \rightarrow {}^{44}Ca \; \gamma \; e^+ \; v$. Scandium was chosen as an example because it is one of the most promising $\beta^+\gamma$ isotopes for medical applications due to (1) its convenient half-lifetime (3.9 h), (2) emission of only single prompt 1157 keV gamma with high probability (99%), (3) short average time of prompt gamma deexcitation (1.6 ps), (4) chemical affinity enabling labeling of for example, DTPA and DOTA-peptides which may be attached for example, to trastuzumab-herceptin or PSMA tracers, respectively, and (5) it possesses therapeutic partners (^{47}Sc and ^{177}Lu) emitting low-energy electrons thus enabling theranostic approach.[44,107–109]

Fig. 3 indicates that for the current standard PET systems with 20 cm AFOV the (2γ+*prompt gamma*) sensitivity is by more than order of magnitude smaller with respect to the standard 2γ SUV imaging. However, with the increase of the AFOV the sensitivity gain of positronium and multitracer imaging increases strongly, and for the TB-PET scanner, with AFOV of 200 cm, it exceeds the sensitivities of the standard 2γ metabolic imaging with the PET scanners with AFOV = 20 cm by a factor of approximately 7.5 in case of LYSO TB-PET and by a factor of approximately 2.5 in case of the plastic TB-J-PET scanner.

SUMMARY AND PROSPECTS

The advent of TB-PET systems opens new possibilities for the personalized medicine. Increase of the AFOV to cover the total-body and the increase of whole-body scan's sensitivity by a factor of approximately 40 enables simultaneous dynamic imaging of all the organs, for the wider group of patients and diagnosis of systemic diseases.[16] Recently uEXPLORER, the first TB-PET, demonstrated kinetic and parametric imaging of all tissues in the human body simultaneously.[1,4,5]

These new imaging capabilities deliver significant quantitative improvements in diagnostic, prognostic and theranostic assessments of various oncological, cardiological, and neurologic diseases.[26] However, the extremely high cost of the uEXPLORER prevents its dissemination in hospitals and even in the research clinics. Therefore, the widespread use of TB-PET systems in a wide

clinical practice will be possible only after a drastic reduction in the production cost of such tomographs.

In this article, we have opined that the reduction of crystal thickness or exchange of the LYSO by BGO crystals will not lead to a significant enough reduction of production costs, and as a solution for the economic TB-PET we described the concept of the TB-J-PET system using axially arranged long strips of plastic scintillators with readout at the edges, instead of the typical detectors built form radially arranged blocks of heavy scintillator crystals.

Although the sensitivity increase expected for the TB-PET built from plastic scintillators is by approximately a factor of 2 lower with respect to the TB-PET built from crystals, it is still significant with respect to the current 20-cm to 25-cm-long LYSO PET systems: factor of 27 for total-body imaging and factor of approximately 2 for single organ imaging. Yet, the mechanical robustness of plastics with respect to crystals enable to make the plastic total-body scanner lightweight, modular and portable. A photograph of the 24-module prototype of such a scanner with 50 cm AFOV is shown in the right panel of **Fig. 2**. Modularity enables construction of PET with imaging chamber adjustable to the size of the patient, which could be of advantage in case of imaging of for example, obese or claustrophobic patients. Plastic TB-PET is a cost-effective solution for the long axial FOV PET scanner. Total cost of components of the plastic TB-PET is approximately 5 times less with respect to the crystal-based TB-PET systems. Cost of crystal scintillators constitutes approximately 50% of the total costs of the TB-PET scanner.[16] Plastic scintillators are more than an order of magnitude less expensive than LYSO crystals. Electronics and SiPMs constitute another ~50% of the costs of the crystal TB-PET, and in case of plastic PET with axially arranged scintillator strips these costs are significantly reduced because the readout is placed mainly at the ends of the cylindrical detector compared with the coverage of the full cylinder surface in case of the crystal PET detectors. Thus in case of plastic TB-PET, the cost of electronics are proportional to the trans-axial cross-section of the detector, whereas in case of crystal TB-PET they are proportional to the area of the detection cylinder. Overall the plastic TB-J-PET may be more than factor of 5 less expensive than the crystal-based TB-PET, making it a realistic cost-effective solution for the broad clinical applications.

High sensitivity and long AFOV of TB-PET opens new possibilities for diagnosis beyond the static

SUV index, improving diagnostic assessment specificity by access to kinetic and parametric imaging of all organs of the patient, simultaneously.[13,14] Then we presented examples of further diagnostic benefits of TB-PET system that arise from the possibility of effective multiphoton imaging opening prospects for the multitracer and positronium imaging and thus giving perspectives for the further quantitative increase of the diagnosis specificity. In the current PET imaging the prompt gamma emitted by $\beta^+\gamma$ isotopes as for example, ^{44}Sc constitutes a source of background. However, high sensitivity, triggerless data acquisition[36] and dedicated data selection algorithms[28,29,37,105,106,110,111] available at J-PET enable efficient registration of triple coincidences (see **Fig. 3**) corresponding to events with 2 back-to-back annihilation photons and prompt gamma. The additional information carried out by prompt gamma may be used for (1) disentanglement of images from different radiopharmaceuticals in case of simultaneous multitracer imaging,[48] and for (2) determination of the positronium mean lifetime image.[29]

Assessing of tumor status using multiple PET tracers has great potential for personalized oncology.[112] In clinical practice multitracer imaging may decrease significantly the time needed for the sequential imaging with more than 1 radiopharmaceutical that currently needs to be long between subsequent scans because of the long (many hours) biological decay time needed for cleaning up a tracer from the organism. Imaging with 2 different tracers at once is currently impractical with standard 2γ PET though it could enhance significantly the diagnostic possibilities (for example, by an early diagnostics of neuroendocrine and HER2 positive tumors) by delivering information of the tumor location (eg, from ^{18}F labeled radiopharmaceuticals) and simultaneously independent information of the tumor type (cancer receptor system) by use of for example, ^{44}Sc-DOTATATE radiopharmaceuticals, where DOTATATE possesses high binding affinity for the somatostatin receptors enhancing diagnostics quality of neuroendocrine cancers.[64] The scope of applications of radiopharmaceuticals labeled with Scandium (^{43}Sc, ^{44}Sc) is growing, particularly for oncologic imaging purposes.[64,113–116] Clinical trials with ^{44}Sc may be enhanced by the application of TB-J-PET which in addition to SUV and kinetic parametric images would deliver positronium lifetime image and may enable simultaneous double-tracer imaging. Finally it is worth stressing that a golden example of dual tracer analysis, becoming possible with TB-J-PET, could be a concurrent application of FDA-approved ^{82}Rb-Chloride and [^{18}F]FDG, allowing simultaneous assessment of myocardium metabolic rate and perfusion of the cardiovascular system.

ACKNOWLEDGMENTS

Authors are thankful to Prof. Stan Majewski and Dr Aleksander Gajos for reading and correcting the article, to Prof. Steven Bass and Prof. Jan Stanek for the perusal of the article and useful comments, and to Jyoti Chhokar, Dr Agnieszka Kamińska, Dr Daria Kisielewska, Pawel Kowalski, Szymon Parzych, and Shivani and Monika Szczepanek for the help in the preparation of the figures and calculations. The authors acknowledge support by the Foundation for Polish Science through the TEAM PIOR.04.04.00-00-4204/17 programme and by the Polish Ministry for Science and Higher Education through grant no. 7150/E-338/SPUB/2017/1.

REFERENCES

1. Badawi RD, Shi H, Hu P, et al. First human imaging studies with the EXPLORER total-body PET scanner. J Nucl Med 2019;60(3):299–303.
2. Karp JS, Viswanath V, Geagan MJ, et al. PennPET explorer: design and preliminary performance of a whole-body imager. J Nucl Med 2020;61(1):136–43.
3. Cherry SR, Badawi RD, Karp JS, et al. Total-body imaging: transforming the role of positron emission tomography. Sci Transl Med 2017;9(381):eaaf6169.
4. Cherry SR, Jones T, Karp JS, et al. Total-body PET: maximizing sensitivity to create new opportunities for clinical research and patient care. J Nucl Med 2018;59(1):3–12.
5. Zhang X, Xie Z, Berg E, et al. Total-body dynamic reconstruction and parametric imaging on the uEXPLORER. J Nucl Med 2020;61(2):285–91.
6. Surti S, Viswanath V, Daube-Witherspoom ME, et al. Benefit of improved performance with state-of-the art digital PET/CT for lesion detection in oncology. J Nucl Med 2020;120:242305.
7. Schmall JP, Karp JS, Alavi A. The potential role of total body PET imaging in assessment of atherosclerosis. PET Clin 2019;14(2):245–50.
8. McKenney-Drake ML, Moghbel MC, Paydary K, et al. 18F-NaF and 18F-FDG as molecular probes in the evaluation of atherosclerosis. Eur J Nucl Med Mol Imaging 2018;45(12):2190–200.
9. Nakajima R, Abe K, Sakai S. IgG4-related diseases; whole-body FDG-PET/CT may be easier to evaluate rare lesions. J Nucl Med 2017;58(suppl. 1):943.
10. Yamashita H, Kubota K, Mimori A. Clinical value of whole-body PET/CT in patients with active rheumatic diseases. Arthritis Res Ther 2014;16(5):423.

11. Grant AM, Deller TW, Khalighi MM, et al. NEMA NU 2-2012 performance studies for the SiPM-based ToF-PET component of the GE SIGNA PET/MR system. J Med Phys 2016;43(5):2334.

12. van Sluis J, de Jong J, Schaar J, et al. Performance characteristics of the digital biograph vision PET/CT system. J Nucl Med 2019;60(7):1031–6.

13. Zhang X, Xie Z, Berg E, et al. Total-body parametric imaging using kernel and direct reconstruction on the uEXPLORER. J Nucl Med 2019;60(suppl. 1):456.

14. Deng Z, Hu D, Ding Y, et al. A comparison of image quality with uMI780 and the first total-body uEXPLORER scanner. J Nucl Med 2019;60(suppl. 1):381.

15. Houshmand S, Salavati A, Hess S, et al. An update on novel quantitative techniques in the context of evolving whole-body PET imaging. PET Clin 2015; 10(1):45–58.

16. Vandenberghe S, Moskal P, Karp J. State of the art in total body PET. EJNMMI Phys 2020;7(1):35.

17. Surti S, Werner M, Karp J. Study of PET scanner designs using clinical metrics to optimize the scanner axial FOV and crystal thickness. Phys Med Biol 2013;58(12):3995–4012.

18. Zhang J, Knopp MI, Knopp MV. Sparse detector configuration in SiPM digital photon counting PET: a feasibility study. Mol Imaging Biol 2019;21(3): 447–53.

19. Zein SA, Karakatsanis NA, Issa M, et al. Physical performance of a long axial field-of-view PET scanner prototype with sparse rings configuration: a Monte Carlo simulation study. Med Phys 2020; 47(4):1949–57.

20. Zhang Y, Wong WH. System design studies for a low-cost high-resolution BGO PET with 1-meter axial field of view. J Nucl Med 2017;58(suppl.1):221.

21. Gonzalez-Montoro A, Sanchez F, Majewski S, et al. Highly improved operation of monolithic BGO-PET blocks. J Instrum 2017;12:C11027.

22. Brunner S, Schaart D. BGO as a hybrid scintillator/Cherenkov radiator for cost-effective time-of-flight PET. Phys Med Biol 2017;62(11):4421–39.

23. Kwon SI, Roncali E, Gola A, et al. Dual-ended readout of bismuth germanate to improve timing resolution in time-of-flight PET. Phys Med Biol 2019;64(10):105007.

24. Cates JW, Levin CS. Electronics method to advance the coincidence time resolution with bismuth germanate. Phys Med Biol 2019;64(17): 175016.

25. Gundacker S, Martinez Turtos R, Kratochwil N, et al. Experimental time resolution limits of modern SiPMs and TOF-PET detectors exploring different scintillators and Cherenkov emission. Phys Med Biol 2020;65(2):025001.

26. Majewski S. Imaging is Believing: The Future of Human Total Body Molecular Imaging Starts Now IL NUOVO CIMENTO 43 C (2020) 8, 3-5 September 2019, Accademia degli Zelanti e dei Dafnici, Acireale, Catania, Italy Proceedings of the FATA2019: FAst Timing Applications for nuclear physics and medical imaging.

27. Moskal P, Jasińska B, Stępień EŁ, et al. Positronium in medicine and biology. Nat Rev Phys 2019;1: 527–9.

28. Moskal P, Kisielewska D, Curceanu C, et al. Feasibility study of the positronium imaging with the J-PET tomograph. Phys Med Biol 2019;64(5): 055017.

29. Moskal P, Kisielewska D, Shopa R, et al. Performance assessment of the 2γ positronium imaging with the total-body PET scanners. EJNMMI Phys 2020;7(1):44.

30. Moskal P. Positronium Imaging. 2019 IEEE Nuclear Science Symposium and Medical Imaging Conference, Convention Centre, Manchester, UK, 26 October- 2nd of November, 2019 (NSS/MIC) https://doi.org/10.1109/NSS/MIC42101.2019.9059856.

31. Moskal P, Niedźwiecki Sz, Bednarski T, et al. Test of a single module of the J-PET scanner based on plastic scintillators. Nucl Instrum Methods Phys Res A 2014;764:317–21.

32. Saint Gobain. Available at: https://www.crystals.saint-gobain.com/. Accessed date: April 25, 2020.

33. Vilardi I, Braem A, Chesi E, et al. Optimization of the effective light attenuation length of YAP:Ce and LYSO:Ce crystals for a novel geometrical PET concept. Nucl Instrum Methods Phys Res A 2006;564:506–14.

34. Mao R, Zhang L, Zhu Y R. Optical and scintillation properties of inorganic scintillators in high energy physics. IEEE Trans Nucl Sci 2008;55(4):2425–31.

35. Pałka M, Strzempek P, Korcyl G, et al. Multichannel FPGA based MVT system for high precision time (20 ps RMS) and charge measurement. J Instrum 2017;12:P08001.

36. Korcyl G, Białas P, Curceanu C, et al. Evaluation of single-chip, real-time tomographic data processing on FPGA SoC devices. IEEE Trans Med Imaging 2018;37(11):2526–35.

37. Krzemień W, Gajos A, Gruntowski A, et al. Analysis framework for the J-PET scanner. Acta Phys Pol A 2015;127:1491–4.

38. Raczyński L, Moskal P, Kowalski P, et al. Compressive sensing of signals generated in plastic scintillators in a novel J-PET instrument. Nucl Instrum Methods Phys Res A 2015;786:105–12.

39. Moskal P, Zoń N, Bednarski T, et al. A novel method for the line-of-response and time-of-flight reconstruction in TOF-PET detectors based on a library of synchronized model signals. Nucl Instrum Methods Phys Res A 2015;775:54–62.

40. Raczyński L, Moskal P, Kowalski P, et al. Novel method for hit-positon reconstruction using voltage

signals in plastic scintillators and its application to the Positron Emission Tomography. Nucl Instrum Methods Phys Res A 2014;764:186–92.

41. Eljen technology, Physical Constants of plastic scintillators. Available at: https://eljentechnology. com/images/technical_library/Physical_Constants_ Plastic.pdf. Accessed date: April 25, 2020.

42. Mao R, Chen Wu C, Dai LE, et al. Crystal growth and scintillation properties of LSO and LYSO crystals. J Cryst Growth 2013;368:97–100.

43. Moskal P, Rundel O, Alfs D, et al. Time resolution of the plastic scintillator strips with matrix photomultiplier readout for J-PET tomograph. Phys Med Biol 2016;61(5):2025–47.

44. Sitarz M, Cussonneau JP, Matulewicz T, et al. Radionuclide candidates for $\beta+\gamma$ coincidence PET: an overview. Appl Radiat Isot 2020;155: 108898.

45. Kowalski K, Wiślicki W, Shopa RY, et al. Estimating the NEMA characteristics of the J-PET tomograph using the GATE package. Phys Med Biol 2018; 63(16):165008.

46. Jan S, Benoit D, Becheva E, et al. GATE v6: a major enhancement of the GATE simulation platform enabling modelling of CT and radiotherapy. Phys Med Biol 2011;56(4):881–901.

47. Smyrski J, Alfs D, Bednarski T, et al. Measurement of gamma quantum interaction point in plastic scintillator with WLS strips. Nucl Instrum Methods Phys Res A 2017;851:39–42.

48. Gajos A, Kamińska D, Moskal P, et al. Method for reconstructing multi-tracer metabolic and morphometric images and tomography system for multi-tracer metabolic and morphometric imaging. Patent Number: US 10339676. Official Gazette of the United States Patent and Trademark Office Patents; 2019.

49. Grignon C, Barbet J, Bardie M, et al. Nuclear medical imaging using $\beta + \gamma$ coincidences from 44Sc radio-nuclide with liquid Xenon as detection medium. Nucl Instrum Methods Phys Res A 2007; 571:42–5.

50. Donnard J, Chen W-T, Cussonneau J-P, et al. Compton imaging with liquid Xenon and 44Sc: recent progress toward 3 gamma imaging. Nucl Med Rev 2012;15(supp.C):64–7.

51. Lang C, Habs D, Parodi K, et al. Sub-millimeter nuclear medical imaging with high sensitivity in positron emission tomography using $\beta + \gamma$ coincidences. J Instrum 2014;9:P01008.

52. Oger T, Chen W-T, Cussonneau J-P, et al. A liquid xenon TPC for a medical imaging Compton telescope. Nucl Instrum Methods Phys Res A 2012; 695:125–8.

53. Thirolf PG, Lang C, Parodi K. Perspectives for highly-sensitive PET-based medical imaging using $\beta+\gamma$ coincidences. Acta Phys Pol A 2015;127:1441–4.

54. U.S. Food and Drug Administration. Available at: https://www.fda.gov/home   https://www.cardinal health.com/content/dam/corp/web/documents/factsheet/cardinal-health-fda-approved-radiopharma ceuticals.pdf. Accessed date: April 25, 2020.

55. Cheal SM, Punzalan B, Doran MG, et al. Pairwise comparison of 89Zr- and 124I-labeled cG250 based on positron emission tomography imaging and nonlinear immunokinetic modeling: in vivo carbonic anhydrase IX receptor binding and internalization in mouse xenografts of clear-cell renal cell carcinoma. Eur J Nucl Med Mol Imaging 2014; 41(5):985–94.

56. Larson SM, Motzer RJ, Pandit-Taskar N, et al. 124I-cG250 PET scan for early detection of response to sunitinib in patients (Pts) with metastatic clear cell renal cell carcinoma (MccRCC). J Clin Oncol 2012;30(0):362.

57. Khandani A, Wallen E, Rathmell K, et al. 124I-cG250 PET in clear cell renal cell carcinoma (ccRCC). J Nucl Med 2014;55(supp.1):1348.

58. Lee FT, O'Keefe GJ, Gan HK, et al. Immuno-PET quantitation of de2-7 epidermal growth factor receptor expression in glioma using 124I-IMP-R4-labeled antibody ch806. J Nucl Med 2010;51: 967–72.

59. Lopez-Rodriguez V, Gaspar-Carcamo RE, Pedraza-Lopez M, et al. Preparation and preclinical evaluation of (66)Ga-DOTA-E(c(RGDfK))2 as a potential theranostic radiopharmaceutical. Nucl Med Biol 2015;42(2):109–14.

60. Hernandez R, Valdovinos H, Chakravarty R, et al. 44Sc-labeled cyclic RGD peptide for PET imaging of integrin $\alpha v\beta 3$. J Nucl Med 2014;55(supp.1):6.

61. Domnanich KA, Müller C, Farkas R, et al. 44Sc for labeling of DOTA- and NODAGA-functionalized peptides: preclinical in vitro and in vivo investigations. EJNMMI Radiopharm Chem 2017;1(1):8 [published correction: 2018;3:13].

62. Hong H, Zhang Y, Engle JW, et al. In vivo targeting and positron emission tomography imaging of tumor vasculature with 66Ga-labeled nano-graphene. Biomaterials 2012;339160:4147–56.

63. Fortin MA, Salnikov AV, Nestor M, et al. Immuno-PET of undifferentiated thyroid carcinoma with radioiodine-labelled antibody cMAb U36: application to antibody tumour uptake studies. Eur J Nucl Med Mol Imaging 2007;34(9):1376–87.

64. Singh A, van der Meulen NP, Müller C, et al. First-in-human PET/CT imaging of metastatic neuroendocrine neoplasms with cyclotron-produced 44Sc-DOTATOC: a proof-of-concept study. Cancer Biother Radiopharm 2017;32(4):124–32.

65. Rösch F, Baum RP. Generator-based PET radiopharmaceuticals for molecular imaging of tumours: on the way to theranostics. Dalton Trans 2011; 40(23):6104–11.

66. Fung EK, Cheal SM, Fareedy SB, et al. Targeting of radiolabeled J591 antibody to PSMA-expressing tumors: optimization of imaging and therapy based on non-linear compartmental modeling. EJNMMI Res 2016;6(1):7.

67. Amor-Coarasa A, Kelly JM, Ponnala S, et al. 66Ga: a Novelty or a valuable preclinical screening tool for the design of targeted radiopharmaceuticals? Molecules 2018;23(10):2575.

68. Eppard E, de la Fuente A, Benešová M, et al. Clinical translation and first in-human use of [44Sc]Sc-PSMA-617 for PET imaging of metastasized castrate-resistant prostate cancer. Theranostics 2017;7(18):4359–69.

69. Khawar A, Eppard E, Sinnes JP, et al. [44Sc]Sc-PSMA-617 Biodistribution and dosimetry in patients with metastatic castration-resistant prostate carcinoma. Clin Nucl Med 2018;43(5):323–30.

70. Guo X, Zhou N, Chen Z, et al. Construction of 124I-trastuzumab for noninvasive PET imaging of HER2 expression: from patient-derived xenograft models to gastric cancer patients. Gastric Cancer 2020. https://doi.org/10.1007/s10120-019-01035-6.

71. Orlova A, Wållberg H, Stone-Elander S, et al. On the selection of a tracer for PET imaging of HER2-expressing tumors: direct comparison of a 124I-labeled affibody molecule and trastuzumab in a murine xenograft model. J Nucl Med 2009; 50930:417–25.

72. Honarvar H, Müller C, Cohrs S, et al. Evaluation of the first 44Sc-labeled Affibody molecule for imaging of HER2-expressing tumors. Nucl Med Biol 2017;45:15–21.

73. Bading JR, Hörling M, Williams LE, et al. Quantitative serial imaging of an 124I anti-CEA monoclonal antibody in tumor-bearing mice. Cancer Biother Radiopharm 2008;23(4):399–409.

74. Ruigrok EAM, van Weerden WM, Nonnekens J, et al. The future of PSMA-targeted radionuclide therapy: an overview of recent preclinical research. Pharmaceutics 2019;11(11):560.

75. Sihver W, Pietzsch J, Krause M, et al. Radiolabeled cetuximab conjugates for EGFR targeted cancer diagnostics and therapy. Pharmaceuticals (Basel) 2014;7(3):311–38.

76. Dibble EH, Yoo DC. Precision medicine and PET/Computed tomography in cardiovascular Disorders. PET Clin 2017;12:459–73.

77. Conti M, Bendriem B. The new opportunities for high time resolution clinical TOF PET. Clin Transl Imaging 2019;7:139–47.

78. Harpen MD. Positronium: review of symmetry, conserved quantities and decay for the radiological physicist. Med Phys 2004;31(1):57-61.

79. Jasińska B, Zgardzińska B, Chołubek G, et al. Human tissues investigation using PALS Technique. Acta Phys Pol B 2017;48:1737–47.

80. Chen H, Van Horn J, Ching Jean Y. Applications of positron annihilation spectroscopy to life science. Defect and Diffusion Forum 2012;331:275–93.

81. Jasińska B, Zgardzińska B, Chołubek G, et al. Human tissue investigations using PALS technique - free radicals influence. Acta Phys Pol A 2017;132:1556–9.

82. Stepanov PV, Selim FA, Stepanov SV, et al. Interaction of positronium with dissolved oxygen in liquids. Phys Chem Chem Phys 2020;22:5123–31.

83. Rahbar K, Afshar-Oromieh A, Jadvar H, et al. PSMA theranostics: current status and future directions. Mol Imaging 2018;17:1–9.

84. Garwin RL. Thermalization of positrons in metals. Phys Rev 1953;91:1571–2.

85. Kilburn D, Townrow S, Meunier V, et al. Organization and mobility of water in amorphous and crystalline trehalose. Nat Mater 2006;5:632-5.

86. Jean YC, Li Y, Liu G, et al. Applications of slow positrons to cancer research: search for selectivity of positron annihilation to skin cancer. Appl Surf Sci 2006;252:3166–71.

87. Jean Y, Chen H, Liu G, et al. Life science research using positron annihilation spectroscopy: UV-irradiated mouse skin Radiat. Phys Chem 2007;76:70–5.

88. Liu G, Chen H, Chakka L, et al. Applications of positron annihilation to dermatology and skin cancer. Phys Status Solidi C 2007;4:3912–5.

89. Liu G, Chen H, Chakka L, et al. Further search for selectivity of positron annihilation in the skin and cancerous systems. Appl Surf Sci 2008;255:115–8.

90. Yas RM, Al-Mshhdani AH, Elias MM, et al. Detection of line shape parameters in normal and abnormal biological tissues. Iraqi J Phys 2012;10:77–82.

91. Axpe E, Lopez-Euba T, Castellanos-Rubio A, et al. Detection of atomic scale changes in the free volume void size of three-dimensional colorectal cancer cell culture using positron annihilation lifetime spectroscopy. PLoS One 2014;9:1–5.

92. Pietrzak R, Borbulak S, Szatanik R. Influence of neoplastic therapy on the investigated blood using positron annihilation lifetime spectroscopy. Nukleonika 2013;58:199–202.

93. Kubicz E, Jasińska B, Zgardzińska B, et al. Studies of unicellular micro-organisms Saccharomyces cerevisiae by means of positron annihilation lifetime spectroscopy. Nukleonika 2015;60:749–53.

94. Kubicz E. Potential for biomedical applications of positron annihilation lifetime spectroscopy (PALS). AIP Conf Proc 2019;2182:050004.

95. Bura Z, Dulski K, Kubicz E, et al. Studies of the ortho-Positronium lifetime for cancer diagnostic. Acta Phys Pol B 2020;51:377.

96. Jasińska B, Moskal P. A new PET diagnostic indicator based on the ratio of 3γ/2γ positron annihilation. Acta Phys Pol B 2017;48:1577.

97. Consolati G, Quasso F. Positronium–oxygen interactions in polytrimethylsilylpropine membranes. Appl Phys 1998;B66:371–6.

98. Zgardzińska B, Białko W, Jasińska B. Ortho-para spin conversion of Ps by paramagnetic O2 dissolved inorganic compounds. Nukleonika 2015; 60(4):801–4.

99. Ota R, Nakajima K, Ogawa I, et al. Coincidence time resolution of 30 ps FWHM using a pair of Cherenkov-radiator integrated MCPPMTs. Phys Med Biol 2019;64(7):07LT01.

100. Lecoq P. Pushing the limits in time-of-flight pet imaging. IEEE Trans Rad Plasma Med Sci 2017;1: 473–85.

101. Silver DA, Pellicer I, Fair WR, et al. Prostate-specific membrane antigen expression in normal and malignant human tissues. Clin Cancer Res 1997; 3(1):81–5.

102. Bravaccini S, Puccetti M, Bocchini M, et al. PSMA expression: a potential ally for the pathologist in prostate cancer diagnosis. Sci Rep 2018;8(1): 4254.

103. Pereira Mestre R, Treglia G, Ferrari M, et al. Correlation between PSA kinetics and PSMA-PET in prostate cancer restaging: a meta-analysis. Eur J Clin Invest 2019;49(3):e13063.

104. Michalski K, Mix M, Meyer PT, et al. Determination of whole-body tumour burden on [68Ga]PSMA-11 PET/CT for response assessment of [177Lu]PSMA-617 radioligand therapy: a retrospective analysis of serum PSA level and imaging derived parameters before and after two cycles of therapy. Nuklearmedizin 2019;58(6):443–50.

105. Gajos A, Kamińska D, Czerwiński E, et al. Trilateration-based reconstruction of ortho-positronium decays into three photons with the J-PET detector. Nucl Instrum Methods Phys Res A 2016;819:54–9.

106. Kamińska D, Gajos A, Czerwiński E, et al. A feasibility study of ortho-positronium decays measurement with the J-PET scanner based on plastic scintillators. Eur Phys J C Part Fields 2016;76:445.

107. Müller C, Bunka M, Haller S, et al. Promising prospects for 44Sc-/47Sc-based theragnostics: application of 47Sc for radionuclide tumor therapy in mice. J Nucl Med 2014;55(10):1658–64.

108. Umbricht CA, Benesova M, Schmid RM, et al. 44Sc-PSMA-617 for radiotheragnostics in tandem with 177Lu-PSMA-617-preclinical investigations in comparison with 68Ga-PSMA-11 and 68Ga-PSMA-617. EJNMMI Res 2017;7(1):9.

109. Müller C, Domnanich KA, Umbricht CA, et al. Scandium and terbium radionuclides for radiotheranostics: current state of development towards clinical application. Br J Radiol 2018;91:20180074.

110. Dulski K, Curceanu C, Czerwiński E, et al. Commissioning of the J-PET detector in view of the positron annihilation lifetime spectroscopy. Hyperfine Interact 2018;239:40.

111. Dulski K, Zgardzińska B, Białas P, et al. Analysis procedure of the positronium lifetime spectra for the J-PET detector. Acta Phys Pol A 2017;132: 1637–40.

112. Kadrmas DJ, Hoffman JM. Methodology for quantitative rapid multi-tracer PET tumor characterizations. Theranostics 2013;3(10):757–73.

113. Hofman MS, Kong G, Neels OC, et al. High management impact of Ga-68 dotatate (gatate) PET/CT for imaging neuroendocrine and other somatostatin expressing tumours. J Med Imaging Radiat Oncol 2012;56(1):40–7.

114. Krajewski S, Cydzik I, Abbas K, et al. Cyclotron production of 44Sc for clinical application. Radiochim Acta 2013;101:333–8.

115. Huclier-Markai S, Kerdjoudj R, Alliot C, et al. Optimization of reaction conditions for the radiolabeling of DOTA and DOTA-peptide with 44m/44Sc and experimental evidence of the feasibility of an in vivo PET generator. Nucl Med Biol 2014; 41(Suppl):e36–43.

116. Walczak R, Krajewski S, Szkliniarz K, et al. Cyclotron production of 43Sc for PET imaging. EJNMMI Phys 2015;2:33.

New Challenges for PET Image Reconstruction for Total-Body Imaging

Nikos Efthimiou, PhD[a,b,*]

KEYWORDS

- Long axial field-of-view • Positron emission tomography • Image reconstruction • Quantification
- Dynamic acquisition • Parametric imaging • Data processing

KEY POINTS

- The presentation of the first human-size long axial field-of-view PET scanner removed many of the well-established limitations of traditional PET imaging.
- For quantitative PET imaging to be achieved, the typical PET corrections need to be applied but to some extent their relative importance has shifted.
- The combination of high sensitivity and advance regularization has demonstrated dynamic PET imaging and parametric maps that do not suffer from past limitations.
- The high data throughput requires new data processing and storage methods.
- Geometries with gaps can provide a cost-efficient alternative but in the cost of more complex detector modeling.

INTRODUCTION

Approximately 5 years ago, the National Institutes of Health–funded EXPLORER Consortium was formed to design and develop the first Total Body PET (TBP) scanner for clinical usage.[1] The idea was not new,[2] but the cost of the technology outweighed the benefits for many years to come.[3]

In this article, we present some of the major challenges, primarily in software, that had to be overcome to obtain the quantified TBP images that we have today. If one starts this journey from the hardware capacity to acquire and process the phenomenon amount for data looks long, from the software point of view it is shorter. Most of our methodologies were transferred from typical PET scanners.

Currently three Long PET scanners have presented; at University of Pennsylvania (Philadelphia, PA)(PennPET EXPLORER)[4], a long PET scanner developed at Krakow, Poland(J-PET)[5] and that designed at University of California, Davis (Davis, CA), and now commercialized under United Imaging.

These 3 scanners also represent 3 different *schools of thought*. The EXPLORER is a scanner of high sensitivity–high spatial resolution. The PennPET currently is being extended to 1.4 m (6 rings) and has a clear focus on the temporal benefits. Last, the J-PET has taken a very different approach with the use of plastic scintillators. It is mostly focused on nonclinical applications.[6]

Then, as the LAFOV gained traction, many old and new ideas for gap arrangements resurfaced, trying to achieve some of the benefits of the LAFOV with a more manageable cost.

For the reconstruction of quantitative static images, fast dynamic images, and low noise parametric maps, various challenges had to be addressed. Many of the preexisting correction

[a] PET Research Centre, Faculty of Health Sciences, University of Hull, Hull, UK; [b] Department of Radiology, Perelman School of Medicine, University of Pennsylvania, 156B John Morgan Building, 3620 Hamilton Walk, Philadelphia, PA 19104-6055, USA
* Department of Radiology, Perelman School of Medicine, University of Pennsylvania, 156B John Morgan Building, 3620 Hamilton Walk, Philadelphia, PA 19104-6055.
E-mail address: efthymin@pennmedicine.upenn.edu

methods, reconstruction algorithms, and techniques were translated directly to the LAFOV scanners. However, in the transition, their relative importance has shifted.[7,8] Please note that the amount of detail released by each of the 2 main groups is not the same, and over the years their methods were expanded and developed.

QUANTITATIVE IMAGE RECONSTRUCTION AND CORRECTIONS

The accuracy of PET images can be affected by a range of physical interactions among the emitted gamma photons, the matter, the detectors, the electronics response, acquisition modes, the software used for the various corrections, and finally the image reconstruction.[9]

Apart from the J-PET project,[10] statistically based iterative image reconstruction algorithms are used with LAFOV scanners. Iterative algorithms can achieve good image quality by using accurate statistical and physical models of the PET imaging process.

In this section, we highlight some key differences in the various data correction techniques between the LAFOV and typical PET scanners, with primary focus on their differential importance compared with typical PET scanners.

At this point, the axial acceptance angle (aa) should be introduced to the reader. That is, the maximum azimuthal angle that a line-of-response (LOR) can take. This can be given in terms of angle, ring difference, or maximum segment number.[11] It is used to moderate undesirable effects (heavily attenuated LORs, high number of multiple scattering, and extremely high input of data). Fig. 1 demonstrates simulated sensitivity profiles from a 2-m-long PET scanner for 2 acceptance angles. The simulations were performed using GATE Monte Carlo simulation toolkit.[12] As expected, the central axial positions are mostly affected.

Scattered Events and Correction

The possibility of increased Compton scattering and especially the ratio between multiple over single scattered photons was one of the earliest concerns in the design and development of LAFOV PET scanners. The main concern was that the Single Scatter Simulation (SSS),[13,14] arguably one of the most commonly used estimation methods, would not be able to account for the increase in multiple scattered events.

Initial simulation studies had shown that the Scatter Fraction (SF) depends on axial size of the scanner.[7] Without restrictions on the aa, it can increase from 28% to 52% with a clear remark on the possibility of higher multiples.[15] On the other

hand, simulations of the PennPET scanner demonstrated stable SF with respect to the size of the axial FOV.[8,16,17] It has been shown that the calculation of SFs of LAFOV scanners needs different-sized phantoms to be comparable with typical PET scanners.[18]

In most initial studies, scatter estimation was performed with an optimized version of time-of-flight (TOF) single scatter estimation.[7,8,19,20] As it is known that the distribution of the scattered photons is smooth, the procedure was performed on a heavily coarser grid. For example, the PENN-PET has reported the down-sampling to 36 detectors per ring and rings of 11 cm.

Since the publication of those initial studies, an extended version of SSS, which accounts for TOF and double scattering, has been presented.[21,22] However, the latest EXPLORER papers use a Monte Carlo–based method.[15,23] The advantage of the use of Monte Carlo simulations is a potentially more accurate scanner model and more complete physics on the expense of simulation time.[24]

Random Events and Correction

Random or accidental coincidences may occur when 2 photons from different but nearly simultaneous annihilations are detected accidently as a single coincidence event.

The EXPLORER random estimation is performed using the method presented by Knoll (2000).[15,25] PENN-PET just reports that the randoms are estimated from delayed convert to a sinogram, downsample and smooth, and include in image reconstruction model.

However, we should highlight the importance of the variable coincidence window that both groups use. Without it, the tradeoff between randoms and coincidence acceptance would not be acceptable. The 2 groups have adopted different approaches, but both are optimized to reject random coincidences. The EXPLORER has a coincidence window that extends with the distance of the 2 rings (4.5 ns to 6 ns) and the PENN-PET uses the intersection of the LOR with the phantom.

Parallax Error

The importance of parallax error was one highlighted by many researchers in early publications.[7,26,27] In brief, due to the high obliqueness of the LORs between distant rings, the axial spatial resolution can get significantly degraded. The effect depends on the depth of absorption and leads to inaccuracy in the determination of the correct ring. The parallax error can be significantly

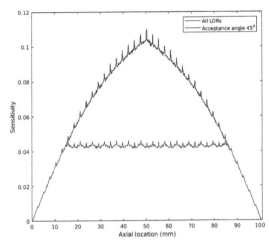

Fig. 1. Sensitivity profiles for all LORs and with a limiting acceptance angle of 45°, on a 2-m-long PET scanner, simulated with the GATE Monte Carlo toolbox.

suppressed by the use of a smaller acceptance angle. However, that also reduces the peak sensitivity.

Therefore, Point Spread Function (PSF) correction becomes critical.[15] For the calculation of teh PSF kernels point sources on distances equal to the voxel size, placed along the z axis, have been simulated. The following simulation toolkits have been used in various papers: GATE Monte Carlo simulation toolkit,[12] SimSET,[28] and EGS4.

Other methods, for the correction of the parallax error, that can be potential incorporated in TBP scanners in the future include the broader family of Depth-of-Interaction encoding schemes. However, the issues with these methods is they increase the number of LORs, proportional to the square of the number of depth-of-interaction bins.[29]

Detector Calibration

Detector calibration is a crucial procedure that ensures uniform detector response (efficiencies and geometry). In early simulation studies, the EXPLORER team reported the calculation of the normalization factors with a uniform cylinder[15]; however, their methodology in the physical scanner and other important procedures like energy and timing calibration have not been published.

Similarly, the UPenn team uses a thin steel and carbon fiber tube mounted on the gantry. The tube source is rotated slowly for approximately 1 hour and an integer number of ro-tations.[30] In addition, it has been reported that they follow a procedure similar to that of the Philips Digital Photon Counting tile sensors.[4] In brief, first the photon detection efficiency and timing digital con-version are calibrated, followed by energy, timing and offset values, per module.

MOTION CORRECTION

In all the LAFOV papers published to this date, motion correction is probably the correction that has been discussed the least.

In brief, 2 types of patient motion have been identified, the voluntary and the involuntary. The first originates from movements the patient makes out of discomfort (maybe due to a prolonged acquisition) and the involuntary, which includes the heartbeat and respiration.[31]

Patient motion can lead to a wide range of significant artifacts, from the misalignment between the attenuation map and the emission data,[32] to increased blurring in the images.[33] In typical PET scanners, researchers have tried various methods to extract a surrogate signal for the motion.[34] This is a huge list that includes devices such as pressure sensors attached to the patient, spirometers, to infrared or 3D cameras that track specific markers,[35,36] motion-compensated image reconstruction,[37] and deformation fields extracted with the use of MR imaging.

With a first glance, few of the options mentioned previously look optimized for LAFOV PET scanners, as their inner bore is very long for any external devices to have a good view of the patient. However, as it has been discussed, because of the short scanning duration (few minutes) the patient might not feel the need to reposition their body. In addition, for this short duration, the patient might be able to be coached to use controlled breathing, successfully. Moreover, it has been discussed that in sub-second dynamic scans the motion artifacts are not significant.

However, there is the possibility for another method that originates from radiotherapy but has not gained much traction in PET imaging: the use of a 4-dimensional (4D) computed tomography (CT) acquisition to extract the breathing motion model of the patient.[38] This method uses standard repeated fast helical acquisitions in combination with a simultaneous breathing surrogate measurement, and deformable image registration to extract the breathing pattern of a patient, as discussed in the article, unless that patient suffers from a respiratory issue. The modeled breathing pattern is likely to remain constant. Moreover, this model accounts to some extent for the cardiac cycle.

IMAGE RECONSTRUCTION ALGORITHMS

Typically, both groups use the Listmode (LM) Ordered Subsets-Expectation Maximization (OSEM) with TOF information, as the baseline reconstruction algorithm. However, EXPLORER has repeatedly reported use of Kernel Expectation Maximization (KEM).[39–42] PennPET makes use of blob basis functions for smoother images.[43] Typically, PennPET has reported the use of 25 subsets with 4 or 5 iterations.[44,45]

As has been pointed out, due to the extremely high sensitivity under typical acquisition settings, OSEM can provide images with good noise properties. **Fig. 2** demonstrates simulations of the XCAT anthropomorphic phantom[46] using PET geometries with different lengths. The simulated data were reconstructed using OSEM as implemented in STIR image reconstruction toolkit.[47] The aa was set to 40°. The background noise in the region of the liver, in terms of Coefficient of Variation (CoV) for the cases in **Fig. 2** are shown on **Fig. 3**. However, the background noise can be further reduced using Penalized Image Reconstruction.[48] Although the Fair penalty has demonstrated twofold noise reduction, the KEM is the one that has been used for the most challenging and impressive cases.

In brief, the Kernel method originates from the artificial intelligence applications and was originally proposed for use in synergistic applications and anatomic priors.[39] However, in this case, the kernel method is used to model PET imaging intensities as a function of feature points obtained from prior knowledge. The prior knowledge comes from low-noise PET images from long acquisitions. As will be presented in a later paragraph, this is a very powerful method in the case of short dynamic scans, which are smoothed using kernels calculated by the PET images from the total acquisition.

The KEM reconstruction has been compared with OSEM in dynamic imaging and the results showed that the image quality for short temporal frames was greatly improved.[22] In the same study, the benefits of the KEM were also discussed for the generation of parametric maps, showing improved contrast-versus-noise tradeoff.

Moreover, KEM has allowed the acquisition of sub-second dynamic frames. On such short time frames (100 ms) the total number of true events was reported as less than 1×10^6.[49] Comparison with OSEM showed a threefold improvement in root mean square error.

PennPET, on the other hand, has been designed to be able to process 100 10^6 singles per second and per ring, which in combination with the much better timing resolution can potentially simplify the reconstruction problem. This leads to very interesting future comparison between the 2 implementations.

DYNAMIC IMAGING

Arguably one of the early highlights of the LAFOV was the first human dynamic scan.[23] The scan demonstrated a 1-hour dynamic scan immediately after the intravenous injection. It was the first time that we were able to see the radiotracer propagating through the body with such clarity.

A dynamic acquisition captures over time the spatiotemporal distribution of the radiotracer. In typical PET scanners of 15 to 25 cm, most dynamic PET scans are performed for a single or multiple bed positions, each one capturing a small part of the human body, at a time. Commonly, 2 types of bed motion have been proposed and adopted, the classic step-and-shoot and the continuous bed motion. The order of the bed positions depends on the protocol.

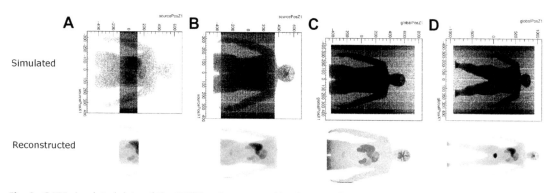

Fig. 2. GATE simulated data of the XCAT anthropomorphic phantom for 4 PET geometries: (*A*) 1, (*B*) 3, (*C*) 5, and (*D*) 8 blk rings. Each ring is approximately 233 mm. The data were reconstructed using OSEM with 12 subsets after 2 iterations. The acceptance angle was 40°.

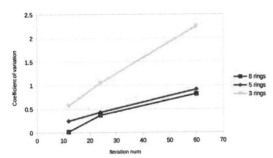

Fig. 3. CoV at the region of the liver for scanner with different axial coverage. The simulation in all cases was of 10 seconds, only true events were reconstructed.

However, LAFOV PET scanners naturally overcome this limitation, as dynamic data can be concurrently acquired from distant locations in the body, removing the temporal sampling issue. Furthermore, as the acquisition is not anymore divided in bed positions, there is an increase in the sensitivity.

Typical PET scanners require a minimum number of accumulated events, and thus acquisition time to achieve an acceptable signal-to-noise ratio. When this time is longer than the transients of the radiotracer kinetics in the tissue, the relevant dynamic information will be lost.[50]

The powerful combination of the high-sensitivity, single-bed position, and advanced image reconstruction allowed for the first sub-second dynamic PET study.[49] High temporal resolution PET is useful for studying blood flow, transit times, and fast radiotracer dynamics. The reported results showed time-activity-curves of the propagation of the radiotracer through the myocardium, with temporal resolution of 100 ms.

As of this date, the PENN-PET scanner is not complete with all the detector block rings. Therefore, in the only published study, patients were scanned for 1 hour with a dynamic protocol followed by delayed scans.[44] Having that said, the scanner was able to capture the time-activity curves for blood input function and major organs roughly with 1 second frames for first couple of minutes, eventually increasing to 300 seconds at tail of the hour.

TOTAL BODY PET SCANNERS AND PARAMETRIC IMAGING

In parametric imaging, physiologic parameters are extracted by PET dynamic acquisitions and kinetic modeling. A long-standing limitation in parametric imaging was the need for complex multibed acquisition to scan the full patient body.[51,52] This led to

long acquisition durations, large time gaps between the bed positions, increased motion artifacts, and so forth.

However, increased LAFOV axial coverage enables kinetic analysis of lesions beyond a typical axial FOV and ensures the inclusion of large vascular structures for input functions. Scan time of just a few minutes results in less movement and removal of the need for arterial blood sampling. Overall, the improvements lead to a significant reduction in administered dose.

Another common issue that parametric imaging with typical PET scanners had, was that the parametric maps were produced from generally noisy dynamic images. As discussed in the previous paragraph, even in sub-second dynamic acquisitions LAFOV scanners can produce images with good noise properties, even with the usage of a standard OSEM.

To this day, a systematic presentation of the TBP capabilities in parametric imaging has not been presented. One study by Zhang and colleagues[23] showed that due to the very high sensitivity, OSEM was capable of producing high-quality Patlak images. However, the use of KEM algorithm provided superior results in terms of both contrast and noise. Furthermore, if was shown that TB allows image-derived arterial input function to be determined from the aorta, which is not always feasible with typical PET scanners. Unfortunately, the effect of spill-in and spill-out counts in the carotid artery was not discussed in the paper.

DATA PROCESSING

The amount of data that the LAFOV scanners collect is staggering, both in the number of LORs in the dataspace and the potential singles rate. Reportedly, in a dynamic acquisition, the prompts count rate peaked at 27.9×10^6 events, a few orders of magnitude larger than for a typical PET scanner.

This requires both larger storage (we refer to the short-term H/Y buffers and the longer term HDDs in the PCs) and more powerful central processing unit and graphic processing unit (GPU).[53] Although, units of high parallelization and scalability (eg, clusters) are used, still, the requirement for reduction (or compression) of the data space is necessary and a common practice. As an example in the EXPLORER scanner crystal grouping is performed.

Then the data are sorted into coincidences in the hardware acquisition units, using a predefined axial acceptance angle. This design decision does help with the data storage, but in the long

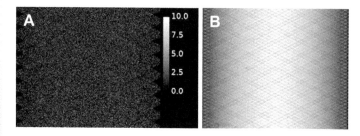

Fig. 4. (*A*) A single viewgram from the simulation of the generation of the normalization factors for a 2-m-long PET scanner. The datasets contained 2 billion events, yet the maximum value was 10 events. (*B*) Normalization factors generated using STIR with the application of rotational and translational symmetries.

term it prohibits the re-processing of the dataset under different settings, as the singles have been lost.

On the other hand, the PennPET collects singles that are then sorted in coincidences in software. This allows the minimization of the deadtime and allows for re-processing under different settings. It has been stated that the maximum aa will be less that the maximum, due to concerns of increased attenuation and reduction of the random/trues ratio. It has reported an aa of ± 40°,[11] but to the author's understanding the value has not been fixed.

Fig. 4A demonstrates a single viewgram of simulated data for the calculation of the normalization factors of a 2-m-long scanner. In total, in the dataset 10 billion events were included. The simulation process lasted 1 week on a cluster with 300 concurrent parallel processes and the maximum value in the viewgram is 10 events. For the generation of good-quality normalization factors, a utility in STIR, which uses a maximum-likelihood method and considers multiple symmetries (**Fig. 4**B), was used.[54,55]

The calculation of the System Response Matrix (SRM) is often associated with high computational cost and huge storage requirements. Both teams have used factorized arrays and the high sparsity, which can significantly reduce the storage requirements.[53]

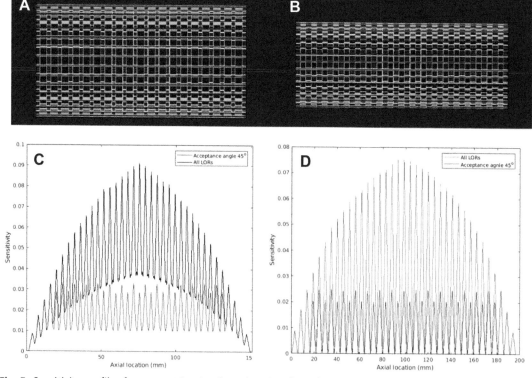

Fig. 5. Sensitivity profiles for geometries that introduced with uniformly distributed gaps for the elongation of the axial FOV. The number of detectors remained the same. (*A-B*) Geometries with evenly distributed gaps (chess-board); (*C-D*) corresponding sensitivity profiles for different acceptance angles.

In addition, even with Listmode reconstruction, the calculation of most correction factors must be performed in a projection space, which grows exponentially with the axial size of the scanner. Furthermore, the calculation of the sensitivity image includes a full BackProjection of all the LORs and the associated corrections. Moreover, in several papers to reduce the calculations, PSF kernels have been considered to be shift invariant. The time benefits of the LM reconstruction can be shown only after the initial calculations are finished.

The size of the reconstructed images has not been the same in every paper and the 2 projects. Matrices from the early 475 × 475 × 1355 with 1.425-mm voxel size for the EXPLORER to 2 × 2 × 2 mm^3 voxels or 4 × 4 × 2 mm^3 (the size of the matrix depended on the number of rings at the study) for PennPET. With the high sensitivity, the possibility to choose voxel size according to the number of detected events is open.

GAPS AND COST MANAGEMENT

The high sampling redundancy of fully 3D LAFOV PET together with its high cost has resurged the interest for the possibility of detector gaps.[56] Depending on the implementation, the gaps can have very different effects.[57]

Simulation studies have shown that a uniform spread of the gaps with a continuous bed motion is a viable alternative in the cost reduction.[58] In addition the presence of chess-board gaps can be effective in managing the loss of sensitivity[59] and provide better image quality compared with shorter full geometries.[60] In **Fig. 5**, the effect of uniform distributed gaps, for the elongation of the geometry, on the sensitivity profiles, is demonstrated. In addition, the effect of the acceptance angle is shown.

One more interesting design approach has been that of multiplex OpenPET, which can extend and contract axially, increasing the sampling in the region of interest.[61]

The aforementioned designs share the increased complexity in the calculation of the SRM and the relative corrections. For example, detector scattering can lead to significant LOR mispositioning that is hard to model. In addition, for moving parts, the calculation of geometric efficiencies must be repeated.

DISCLOSURE

The authors have nothing to disclose.

REFERENCES

1. Surti S, Pantel AR, Karp JS. Total body PET: why, how, what for? IEEE Trans Radiat Plasma Med Sci 2020;4(3):283–92.
2. Cherry SR, Dahlbom M, Hoffman EJ. High sensitivity, total body PET scanning using 3D data acquisition and reconstruction. IEEE Trans Nucl Sci 1992; 39(4):1088–92.
3. Jones T. Total body PET imaging from mice to humans. Front Phys 2020;8. https://doi.org/10.3389/fphy.2020.00077.
4. Karp JS, Viswanath V, Geagan MJ, et al. PennPET explorer: Design and preliminary performance of a whole-body imager. J Nucl Med 2020;61(1):136–43. https://doi.org/10.2967/jnumed.119.229997.
5. Niedzwiecki S, Bialas P, Curceanu C, et al. J-PET: a new technology for the whole-body PET imaging 2017. https://doi.org/10.5506/APhysPolB.48.1567.
6. Moskal P. Positronium Imaging, in 2019 IEEE Nuclear Science Symposium and Medical Imaging Conference (NSS/MIC), 2019, https://doi.org/10.1109/nss/mic42101.2019.9059856.
7. Zhang X, Badawi R, Cherry S, et al. Theoretical study of the benefit of long axial field-of-view PET on region of interest quantification. Phys Med Biol 2018;63. https://doi.org/10.1088/1361-6560/aac815.
8. Viswanath V, et al. GATE simulations to study extended axial FOVs for the PennPET Explorer scanner, in 2017 IEEE Nuclear Science Symposium and Medical Imaging Conference (NSS/MIC), 2017, https://doi.org/10.1109/nssmic.2017.8532747.
9. Zaidi H, Karakatsanis N. Towards enhanced PET quantification in clinical oncology. Br J Radiol 2018;91(1081):20170508.
10. Kowalski P, Wislicki W, Shopa RY, et al. Estimating the NEMA characteristics of the J-PET tomograph using the GATE package. Phys Med Biol 2018; 63(16). https://doi.org/10.1088/1361-6560/aad29b.
11. Vandenberghe S, Moskal P, Karp JS. State of the art in total body PET. EJNMMI Phys 2020;7(1):35.
12. Jan S, Santin G, Strul D, et al. GATE: a simulation toolkit for PET and SPECT. Phys Med Biol 2004; 49(19):4543–61.
13. Ollinger JM. Model-based scatter correction for fully 3D PET. Phys Med Biol 1996;41(1):153–76.
14. Watson CC, Newport D, Casey ME. A Single Scatter Simulation Technique for Scatter Correction in 3D PET 1996. p. 255–68. https://doi.org/10.1007/978-94-015-8749-5_18.
15. Zhang X, Zhou J, Cherry SR, et al. Quantitative image reconstruction for total-body PET imaging using the 2-meter long EXPLORER scanner. Phys Med Biol 2017;62(6):2465–85.
16. Viswanath V, et al. Development of PET for total-body imaging, Acta Phys Pol: 48(10).

17. Zein SA, Karakatsanis NA, Issa M, et al. Physical performance of a long axial field-of-view PET scanner prototype with sparse rings configuration: a Monte Carlo simulation study. Med Phys 2020; 47(4):1949–57.

18. Ghabrial A, Franklin D, and Zaidi H, Characterization of the scatter component in large axial field-of-view PET scanners: a Monte Carlo simulation study, in 2018 IEEE Nuclear Science Symposium and Medical Imaging Conference Proceedings (NSS/MIC), 2018, https://doi.org/10.1109/nssmic.2018.8824762.

19. Werner ME, Surti S, Karp JS, Implementation and evaluation of a 3D PET single scatter simulation with TOF modeling, in IEEE Nuclear Science Symposium Conference Record, 2006, vol. 3, pp. 1768–1773, https://doi.org/10.1109/NSSMIC.2006.354238.

20. Accorsi R, Adam L-E, Werner ME, et al. Optimization of a fully 3D single scatter simulation algorithm for 3D PET. Phys Med Biol 2004;49(12):2577–98.

21. Watson CC, Hu J, Zhou C, Extension of the SSS PET scatter correction algorithm to include double scatter, in 2018 IEEE Nuclear Science Symposium and Medical Imaging Conference Proceedings (NSS/MIC), 2018, https://doi.org/10.1109/nssmic.2018.8824475.

22. Watson CC. Extension of single scatter simulation to scatter correction of time-of-flight PET. IEEE Trans Nucl Sci 2007;54(5):1679–86.

23. Zhang X, Xie Z, Berg E, et al. Total-Body Dynamic Reconstruction and Parametric Imaging on the uEXPLORER. J Nucl Med July 2019. https://doi.org/10.2967/jnumed.119.230565. jnumed.119.230565.

24. Prasad R, Zaidi H. Scatter characterization and correction for simultaneous multiple small-animal PET imaging. Mol Imaging Biol 2014;16(2):199–209.

25. Knoll GF. Radiation detection and measurement. John Wiley; 2010.

26. Schmall JP, Karp JS, Werner M, et al. Parallax error in long-axial field-of-view PET scanners—a simulation study. Phys Med Biol 2016;61(14): 5443–55.

27. Borasi G, Fioroni F, Del Guerra A, et al. PET systems: the value of added length. Eur J Nucl Med Mol Imaging 2010;37(9):1629–32.

28. Harrison R, Gillispie S, Schmitz R, et al. Modeling block detectors in SimSET. J Nucl Med 2008; 49(Suppl 1):410P.

29. Mohammadi I, Castro IFC, Correia PMM, et al. Minimization of parallax error in positron emission tomography using depth of interaction capable detectors: methods and apparatus. Biomed Phys Eng Express 2019;5(6):062001.

30. Casey ME, Hoffman EJ. Quantitation in positron emission computed tomography: 7. A technique to reduce noise in accidental coincidence measurements and coincidence efficiency calibration. J Comput Assist Tomogr 1986;10(5): 845–50.

31. Nehmeh SA, Erdi YE. Respiratory motion in positron emission tomography/computed tomography: a review. Semin Nucl Med 2008;38(3):167–76.

32. Bai W, Brady M. Motion correction and attenuation correction for respiratory gated PET images. IEEE Trans Med Imaging 2011;30(2):351–65.

33. Polycarpou I, Tsoumpas C, King AP, et al. Impact of respiratory motion correction and spatial resolution on lesion detection in PET: a simulation study based on real MR dynamic data. Phys Med Biol 2014;59(3): 697–713.

34. Pépin A, Daouk J, Bailly P, et al. Management of respiratory motion in PET/computed tomography. Nucl Med Commun 2014;35(2):113–22.

35. Noonan PJ, Howard J, Hallett WA, et al. Repurposing the Microsoft Kinect for Windows v2 for external head motion tracking for brain PET. Phys Med Biol 2015;60(22):8753–66.

36. Heß M, Büther F, Gigengack F, et al. A dual-Kinect approach to determine torso surface motion for respiratory motion correction in PET. Med Phys 2015; 42(5):2276–86.

37. Polycarpou I, Tsoumpas C, Marsden PK. Analysis and comparison of two methods for motion correction in PET imaging. Med Phys 2012; 39(10):6474.

38. Low DA, White BM, Lee PP, et al. A novel CT acquisition and analysis technique for breathing motion modeling. Phys Med Biol 2013;58(11):L31–6. https://doi.org/10.1088/0031-9155/58/11/L31.

39. Hutchcroft W, Wang G, Chen KT, et al. Anatomically-aided PET reconstruction using the kernel method. Phys Med Biol 2016;61(18):6668–83.

40. Wang G, Qi J. PET image reconstruction using kernel method. IEEE Trans Med Imaging 2015; 34(1):61–71.

41. Deidda D, Karakatsanis NA, Robson PM, et al. Hybrid PET-MR list-mode kernelized expectation maximization reconstruction. Inverse Probl 2019; 35(4):044001. https://doi.org/10.1088/1361-6420/ab013f.

42. Wadhwa P, Thielemans K, Efthimiou N, et al. PET image reconstruction using physical and mathematical modelling for time of flight PET-MR scanners in the STIR library. Methods 2020. https://doi.org/10.1016/j.ymeth.2020.01.005.

43. Matej S, Lewitt RM. Practical considerations for 3-D image reconstruction using spherically symmetric volume elements. IEEE Trans Med Imaging 1996; 15(1):68–78.

44. Pantel AR, Viswanath V, Daube-Witherspoon ME, et al. PennPET explorer: Human imaging on a whole-body imager. J Nucl Med 2020;61(1): 144–51. https://doi.org/10.2967/jnumed.119.231845.

45. Viswanath V, Witherspoon MED, Karp JS, et al. Numerical observer study of lesion detectability for a long axial field-of-view whole-body {PET} imager using the {PennPET} Explorer. Phys Med Biol 2020; 65(3):35002.

46. Segars WP, Sturgeon G, Mendonca S, et al. 4D XCAT phantom for multimodality imaging research. Med Phys 2010;37(9):4902–15.

47. Thielemans K, Tsoumpas C, Mustafovic S, et al. STIR: Software for tomographic image reconstruction release 2. Phys Med Biol 2012;57(4):867–83. https://doi.org/10.1088/0031-9155/57/4/867.

48. Zhang X, Badawi R, Cherry S, et al. Development and Evaluation of Penalized image reconstruction for the total-body EXPLORER. J Nucl Med 2018; 59(supplement 1):1773.

49. Zhang X, Cherry SR, Xie Z, et al. Subsecond total-body imaging using ultrasensitive positron emission tomography. Proc Natl Acad Sci U S A 2020;117(5): 2265–7.

50. Vaquero JJ, Kinahan P. Positron emission tomography: current challenges and opportunities for technological advances in clinical and preclinical imaging systems. Annu Rev Biomed Eng 2015; 17(1):385–414.

51. Karakatsanis NA, Lodge MA, Tahari AK, et al. Dynamic whole-body PET parametric imaging: I. Concept, acquisition protocol optimization and clinical application. Phys Med Biol 2013;58(20): 7391–418.

52. Rahmim A, Lodge MA, Karakatsanis NA, et al. Dynamic whole-body PET imaging: principles, potentials and applications. Eur J Nucl Med Mol Imaging 2019;46(2):501–18.

53. Zhou J, Qi J. Fast and efficient fully 3D PET image reconstruction using sparse system matrix factorization with GPU acceleration. Phys Med Biol 2011; 56(20):6739–57. https://doi.org/10.1088/0031-9155/56/20/015.

54. Hogg D, Thielemans K, Spinks T, et al, Maximum-likelihood estimation of normalisation factors for PET, in 2001 IEEE Nuclear Science Symposium Conference Record (Cat. No.01CH37310), vol. 4, pp. 2065–2069, doi: 10.1109/NSSMIC.2001.1009231.

55. Niknejad T, Tavernier S, Varela J, Thielemans K. Validation of 3D model-based Maximum-Likelihood estimation of normalisation factors for partial ring Positron Emission Tomography. In: 2016 IEEE Nuclear Science Symposium, Medical Imaging Conference and Room-Temperature Semiconductor Detector Workshop, NSS/MIC/RTSD 2016vol. 2017. Institute of Electrical and Electronics Engineers Inc; 2017. https://doi.org/10.1109/NSSMIC.2016. 8069577.

56. Gravel P, Li Y, Matej S. Effects of TOF resolution models on edge artifacts in PET reconstruction from limited-angle data. IEEE Trans Radiat Plasma Med Sci 2020;1. https://doi.org/10.1109/trpms. 2020.2989209.

57. Daube-Witherspoon ME, Viswanath V, Surti S, Karp JS. Reconstruction performance for long axial field-of-view PET scanners with large axial gaps. Proc.SPIE. 2019;11072. https://doi.org/10.1117/12. 2533946.

58. Karakatsanis NA, Member S, Zein SA, et al. Positron Emission Tomography with Sparse Block Rings and Continuous Bed Motion ODERN clinical Positron Emission Tomography. 2019 IEEE Nucl Sci Symp Med Imaging Conf. 2019:1-6. https://doi.org/10. 1109/NSS/MIC42101.2019.9059913.

59. Akl MA, Bouhali O, Toufique Y, et al. Monte Carlo sensitivity study of a long axial FOV PET scanner with patient adaptive rings. In: 2019 IEEE Nuclear Science Symposium and Medical Imaging Conference (NSS/MIC). IEEE; 2019. https://doi.org/10. 1109/nss/mic42101.2019.9059834.

60. Efthimiou N, Whitehead AC, Stockhoff M, et al. Preliminary investigation of the impact of Axial Ring Splitting on Image Quality for the Cost Reduction of Total-Body PET. In: 2019 IEEE Nuclear Science Symposium and Medical Imaging Conference (NSS/MIC). IEEE; 2019. https://doi.org/10.1109/nss/mic42101.2019.9059650.

61. Yamaya T, Yoshida E, Inadama N, et al. A Multiplex "OpenPET" Geometry to Extend Axial FOV Without Increasing the Number of Detectors. IEEE Trans Nucl Sci 2009;56(5):2644–50. https://doi.org/10. 1109/tns.2009.2027437.

Reinventing Molecular Imaging with Total-Body PET, Part II: Clinical Applications

Babak Saboury, MD, MPH[a,b,c], Michael A. Morris, MD, MS[a,b],
Moozhan Nikpanah, MD[a], Thomas J. Werner, MS[c],
Elizabeth C. Jones, MD, MPH, MBA[a], Abass Alavi, MD[c,*]

KEYWORDS

- Total-body PET • Oncoradiology • Oncology • Inflammation imaging • Vascular imaging

KEY POINTS

- Total-body PET scans will make immuno-PET imaging and multitracer profiling feasible through delayed imaging and reduced radiation dose.
- As a result, multidimensional evaluation of disease heterogeneity in vivo will be practical in the clinic.
- Total-body PET dynamic whole body imaging allows simultaneous functional and molecular evaluation of multiple organ systems, a concept termed systems biology imaging.
- Total-body PET systems biology imaging allows the further development and clinical implementation of more robust global disease assessment capabilities.

INTRODUCTION

Total-body PET (TB-PET) imaging is an evolving technology addressing the limitations of conventional PET imaging. With a fundamentally novel approach for its geometric coverage to encompass the entire body, TB-PET imaging has the potential to dramatically increase the effective sensitivity of PET scans. The increased sensitivity could be used for different strategies, such as enhancing the signal-to-noise ratio, improving temporal resolution, or requiring less radioactivity at the time of imaging (**Table 1**).

In Part I of this 2-part article (see Babak Saboury and colleagues' article, "Reinventing Molecular Imaging with Total-Body PET, Part I: Technical Revolution in Evolution," elsewhere in this issue), we provided an overview of the technologic gains of the TB-PET scanner. In this second part, we discuss the practical advantages that this technology can bring about to specific clinical applications of PET imaging (**Fig. 1**).[1,2]

PRACTICAL CLINICAL APPLICATIONS

Conventional PET imaging techniques have been shown to suffer from significant limitations in clinical use to assess disorders that are diffuse in nature and involve many structures throughout the body. The major shortcomings are due to the limited sensitivity and limited field of view of approximately 20 to 30 cm, which requires imaging the entire body in a fractionated manner over an hour or longer to determine the extent of the disease at its various stages.[3] However, based on the experience that has been gained over the years, most disease abnormalities are best assessed by imaging the entire body to detect

Sources of funding: None.
[a] Department of Radiology and Imaging Sciences, Clinical Center, National Institutes of Health, 9000 Rockville Pike, Bethesda, MD 20892, USA; [b] Department of Computer Science and Electrical Engineering, University of Maryland, Baltimore County, Baltimore, MD, USA; [c] Department of Radiology, Hospital of the University of Pennsylvania, 3400 Spruce St, Philadelphia, PA 19104, USA
* Corresponding author. 3400 Spruce Street, Philadelphia, PA 19104.
E-mail address: abass.alavi@pennmedicine.upenn.edu

PET Clin 15 (2020) 463–475
https://doi.org/10.1016/j.cpet.2020.06.013
1556-8598/20/© 2020 Elsevier Inc. All rights reserved.

Table 1
Improved sensitivity of the TB-PET scanner can result in better signal-to-noise ratio (SNR), enhanced temporal resolution (T), or reduction of the required dose of the radiotracer (A)

Eq. 1

$$SNR_{phys} \approx k\sqrt{S \times A \times T}$$

SNR_{phys}: *Signal-to-Noise Ratio (physical system)*

S: *Effective Sensitivity*

A: *Radioactivity at the time of imaging*

T: *Imaging time*

Eq. 2

$\uparrow S \xrightarrow{SNR_{phys}: Cte}$
$\downarrow A$:
    a. *Lower injected dose* $\longrightarrow$ *ImmunoPET could be a clinical reality (sub mSv dose for multiple PET)*
    b. *Delayed imaging to increase biological SNR* [$\uparrow SNR_{bio}$]
$\downarrow T$: **c.** *Better temporal resolution* $\longrightarrow$ *Clinically feasible dynamic imaging*
    (kinetic parameters; extension of DTP paradigm)

unexpected lesions that may or may not be related to the primary sites. This is particularly applicable to the adult population, who are prone to developing many age-related maladies. Among these, we would like to emphasize the role of TB-PET imaging in examining patients with cancer, inflammatory and immunologic disorders, cardiovascular disease, and osteoporosis, which are known to involve many structures and organs in the body.

Global Disease Assessment and Systems Biology

The concept of a global disease assessment (GDA),[4] with the aim of quantifying the total burden of disease by combination of structural and molecular information, has gained popularity in recent years.[5–7] GDA is a method whereby a single or composite quantitative value, the Global Disease Score,[8] represents the burden of an ongoing disease process over the course of disease beginning at a baseline point and compared throughout subsequent therapeutic interventions (**Figs. 2** and **3**).[9,10] Hybrid molecular and structural imaging with PET and computed tomography (CT) scans or MR imaging as a single imaging instrument seems to be the approach of choice for such novel applications. GDA methodology has been adopted for assessing regional and global disease activity in many disorders, particularly those that are systemic in nature. Novel approaches have been described in the literature that demonstrate

this technique's unique ability to quantify the degree of abnormality in various organs and throughout the body. Data from the approach have similarly demonstrated great importance in patients with cancer, atherosclerosis, systemic inflammation, and musculoskeletal disorders.[11–18]

TB-PET imaging will be of unique importance in improving temporal resolution to better reflect overall disease burden and will allow for better management of many serious, disabling, and potentially fatal diseases and disorders. TB-PET imaging has the potential to expand the concept of dual time point–derived GDA by extracting the kinetic parameters. Both dynamic whole body imaging and the ability to perform more delayed imaging provide a mechanism to study whole body pathobiology kinetics.[8] GDA-based biological systems state quantification and systems interrelation characterization through time is the basis for a systems biology approach to medical imaging.

In clinical practice, TB-PET could be used for faster performance, a decreased patient dose, and enhanced capacity to make delayed imaging and dynamic whole body imaging possible. These technical capabilities lead to a unique usefulness: making systems biology imaging a reality. The human body is a complex, dynamic system with inherent interconnectedness; the boundaries between organs and systems have faded by new advancements in our understanding of the pathologic basis of disorders. The significant role of the immune system in disease makes this

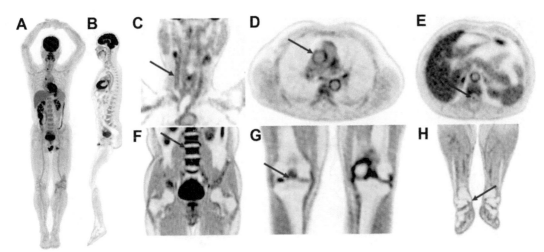

Fig. 1. Total-body PET scan of a patient who was injected with 290 MBq of ^{18}F-FDG. A 20-minute list-mode scan was performed at 82 minutes after injection on the EXPLORER scanner. (*A*) Total-body maximum intensity projection (MIP). (*B*) Total-body sagittal view that was generated from the 20-minute scan. Selected views including (*C*) head and neck view, showing walls of the right carotid artery (*arrow*). (*D*) Chest view, demonstrating walls of ascending aorta (*arrow*), (*E*) midthoracic view, showing spinal canal (*arrow*), (*F*) abdominal and pelvic view, indicating clear delineation of the superior endplate of L3 (*arrow*), (*G*) knees, showing bone spur on the right side (*arrow*), and (*H*) lower extremities, indicating defined medial tibial malleolus of the right side (*arrow*). (Originally published in Badawi RD et al. First Human Imaging Studies with the EXPLORER Total-Body PET Scanner. J Nucl Med 2019;60:299-303. © SNMMI.)

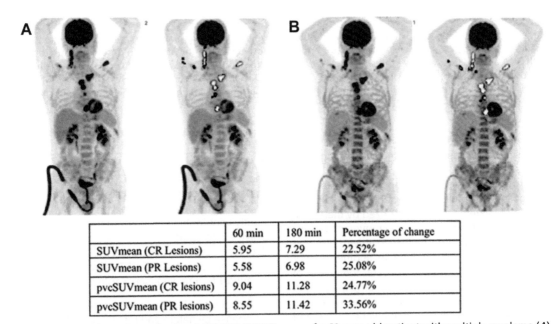

	60 min	180 min	Percentage of change
SUVmean (CR Lesions)	5.95	7.29	22.52%
SUVmean (PR Lesions)	5.58	6.98	25.08%
pvcSUVmean (CR lesions)	9.04	11.28	24.77%
pvcSUVmean (PR lesions)	8.55	11.42	33.56%

Fig. 2. Maximum intensity projection (MIP) FDG PET/CT scans of a 60-year-old patient with multiple myeloma (*A*) pretreatment 1 hour and (*B*) pretreatment 3 hours after administration of FDG. Table shows the percentage change of mean standardized uptake value (SUV$_{mean}$) and partial volume correction (pvc) of the SUV$_{mean}$ of the complete response (CR) and partial response (PR) lesions from 1-hour to 3-hour scans. (Originally published in Raynor, William Y., Abdullah Al-Zaghal, Mahdi Zirakchian Zadeh, Siavash Mehdizadeh Seraj, and Abass Alavi. 2019. "Metastatic Seeding Attacks Bone Marrow, Not Bone: Rectifying Ongoing Misconceptions." PET Clinics 14 (1): 135–44.)

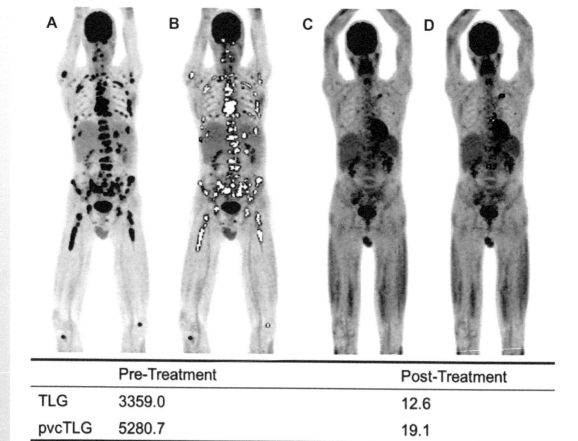

	Pre-Treatment	Post-Treatment
TLG	3359.0	12.6
pvcTLG	5280.7	19.1

Fig. 3. FDG PET examinations in a patient with multiple myeloma showing maximum intensity projection (MIP) images at baseline (*A*) with GDA applied (*B*), and on follow-up 2 months after high-dose chemotherapy (*C*) with GDA applied (*D*). Adaptive thresholding algorithm was used (ROVER software; ABX GmbH). (Originally published in Raynor, W.Y., Zadeh, M.Z., Kothekar, E., Yellanki, D.P. and Alavi, A., 2019. Evolving Role of PET-Based Novel Quantitative Techniques in the Management of Hematological Malignancies. PET clinics, 14(3), pp.331-340.)

interconnectedness much more explainable. Cardiovascular manifestations of the autoimmune disorders are only the tip of the iceberg.[19,20]

In complex systems theory, a system is composed of multiple interconnected subsystems. Subsystems are characterized by their state at each given time. The relation between subsystems only depends on their respective state and subsystems are not exposed to another's inner complexity. GDA thereby reflects the state of each system. This decrease in complexity is an essential prerequisite of building the system of subsystems, providing a framework to expand our understanding of the whole. The study of the interrelation of subsystem states at 1 time (synchronous) and through time (metachronous) was limited by the spatial and temporal constraints of conventional PET imaging. TB-PET imaging is a tool for systems biology par excellence.[21,22]

Oncology

Dose reduction

The increased sensitivity of TB-PET imaging can be used to decrease the required amount of activity at the time of imaging. This property will significantly contribute to decreasing the radiation dose delivered to patients. This capability opens the door for 3 particular use cases: multitracer PET imaging, shorter follow-up PET imaging, as well as immuno-PET imaging (see **Table 1**, Equation 2a).

1. By now, it is clear that cancer is a heterogeneous disease by nature and that tumor heterogeneity is the hallmark of treatment failure.[23] Using multiple tracers for imaging the tumor biology has a potential advantage.[24] Previously, the exposure dose was one of the drawbacks preventing this type of PET imaging. Some researchers alluded to this potential possible in routine standard of

care, such as the benefits of synergistic PET imaging for prognostication, as demonstrated by fludeoxyglucose (FDG) and HER2 PET in the ZEPHIR trial (**Fig. 4**).[25,26]

2. Treatment response follow-up by molecular imaging has shown value for personalized patient management, yet the exposure dose has also played a negative role in the expansion of this paradigm.

3. It is almost impossible to justify the radiation exposure of immuno-PET imaging in daily clinical practice outside of research studies. Attempting to characterize tumor heterogeneity with multiple immuno-PET tracers in series with conventional PET imaging could expose the patients to more than 100 mSv on conventional PET imaging. This factor could dramatically change in the TB-PET imaging era.

Delayed imaging

In addition to radiation dose reduction, the need for a lesser amount of radiotracer in TB-PET imaging provides opportunities for delayed imaging where the sensitivity of the scanner for detecting the metabolic activity is of utmost importance (see **Table 1**, Equation 2b). As described in Part I of this 2-part article (see Babak Saboury and colleagues' article, "Reinventing Molecular Imaging with Total-Body PET, Part I: Technical Revolution in Evolution," elsewhere in this issue), delayed imaging can improve the biological signal-to-noise ratio. Based on numerous research studies that have been conducted during the past 2 decades, it has become apparent that the degree of uptake of FDG in malignant tissues increases over time and reaches a plateau at around 4 to 5 hours after

administration of the compound.[27–29] Basu and colleagues[29] showed a continuous increase in FDG uptake of the lung cancer lesions up to 8 hours after injection. This phenomenon not only allows detecting the presence of cancer activity at the primary sites, but also improves the sensitivity of the technique for accurately staging the disease by visualizing metastases to the lymph nodes and different organs in the body. In addition, our group demonstrated FDG uptake decreases significantly from 1 to 3 hours after injection in the majority of normal tissues, except heart and bone marrow.[30] This property further enhances the contrast between tumor site activity and the surrounding background.[30] However, the bone marrow retention of FDG could be detrimental in detection of bone marrow metastatic lesions in delayed imaging, and this drawback should be considered in study designs. Overall, delayed imaging enhances the impact of FDG-PET imaging in the management of patients with various malignancies at various stages of the disease. Using the principles that our group previously described, some of the researchers speculated that TB-PET imaging could improve detection of micrometastases, which are smaller than 5 mm.[31]

Dynamic imaging

The combination of full field of view and enhanced temporal resolution in TB-PET imaging would allow improved dynamic quantification of radiotracer uptake over time (see **Table 1**, Equation 2c). The extraction of kinetic analysis parameters has already been clearly proven in the realm of FDG PET imaging. Our group extensively demonstrated the value of multiple time-point imaging in

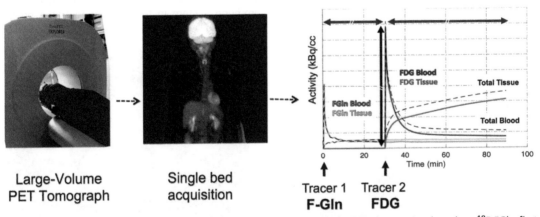

Fig. 4. Time–activity curves in a patient imaged in the prototype PennPET Explorer using low-dose ^{18}F-FGln first (*left*), followed by higher dose ^{18}F-FDG (*right*) for dual tracer PET imaging in series to model both glutamine and glucose metabolism in a single bed position, in a single encounter. (Originally published in Mankoff, David A., Austin R. Pantel, Varsha Viswanath, and Joel S. Karp. 2019. "Advances in PET Diagnostics for Guiding Targeted Cancer Therapy and Studying In Vivo Cancer Biology." Current Pathobiology Reports 7 (3): 97–108.)

tumor biology characterization.[28,32,33] Tumors with an increasing standardized uptake value over time are suggested to be more aggressive than those with a decreasing standardized uptake value over time.[34] There is limited literature available on the investigation of dynamic changes in other radiotracers within a single patient encounter, which is an area of important future investigation.

Systems Biology Approach to Cancer Imaging

As patients begin to live longer with chronic malignancies, dynamic imaging with TB-PET scans will also help to manage multisystemic effects of oncologic processes as well as side effects of treatments on body organs and systems (cancer as a chronic disease paradigm). A similar paradigm can be exemplified in the changing approach to patients with human immunodeficiency virus infection as more effective treatments became available.

Atherosclerosis

Patients with malignancies have a high incidence of atherosclerosis.[35–37] Currently, this serious complication is a major domain of research and interest in the population with cancer, particularly in patients with prostate cancer, hematologic malignancies, and some others whose disease can be controlled for an extended period of time. Clearly, the high incidence of atherosclerosis in these patients may lead to significant morbidity and mortality that are unrelated to their underlying disorders.[38,39] Both FDG[40] and ^{18}F-sodium fluoride (NaF),[41–43] which are commonly used for PET imaging of patients with various malignancies, are optimally suited for detecting atherosclerotic plaques in the arterial system throughout the body. Again, delayed imaging with total-body machines allows significant clearance of these tracers

from the circulation and therefore optimal visualization of atherosclerotic plaques. As such, total-body imaging at delayed time points may improve the ability to detect and treat vascular complications of various cancers with higher sensitivity and specificity.[44]

Venous thrombosis

It is well-established that the second most common cause of death among patients with cancer is pulmonary embolism. Most malignancies (with a higher incidence in certain cancers) are associated with a high incidence of clot formation in the venous system throughout the body. Research and clinical studies have shown high uptake of FDG in active clots throughout the body (**Fig. 5**).[45–47] This is due to the presence of activated white cells and platelets in actively forming clots. Therefore, FDG-PET imaging for assessing patients with cancer will allow detecting the presence of clots throughout the body, including in the lower extremities (**Fig. 6**). As such, by adopting the limited body imaging protocols, many instances of venous thrombosis in the lower extremities are frequently missed. Therefore, total-body imaging by dedicated TB-PET systems will play a major role in the early detection and treatment of venous thromboembolism in patients with malignant disorders.

Hyperinflammatory state

The process of oncogenesis is not merely invasion of tumor cells throughout the body. There is extensive interaction between the immune system and tumor cells, which results in significant control of the disease. This paradigm of healing from within resulted in novel treatment options, from immune-check-point inhibitors to chimeric antigen receptor T-cell therapy.[48,49] Engagement of the immune system in this prolonged battle on the one hand and effects of treatment options, on

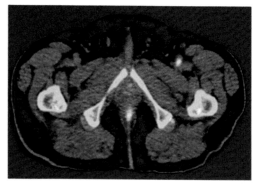

Fig. 5. Patient with a history of new non-occlusive thrombus involving the left renal vein with concern for deep vein thrombosis involving the left common femoral vein. (*left*) Axial contrast-enhanced CT scan, and (*right*) axial fused ^{18}F-FDG PET/CT scan showing increased FDG uptake within the filling defect within the left common femoral vein (*arrow*) suspected to correspond with deep vein thrombosis in this location.

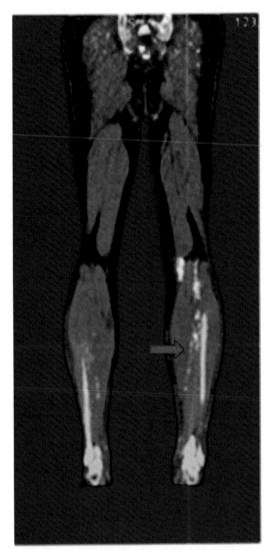

Fig. 6. A 65-year-old man with melanoma on the left upper back, on BRAF/MEK inhibitor since April 2012, which was held on December 21, 2012, secondary to toxicity, with biopsy-proven gastric metastasis and left axillary nodal metastasis. One day before the PET scan, the patient had 2+ edema from the mid-upper arm to the hand and 1+ edema in the left calf and foot. A coronal fused ^{18}F-FDG PET/CT image shows increased metabolic activity within the left lower leg veins (*arrow*) corresponding with an acute deep vein thrombosis.

the other hand, create dysregulation of immune system function, which may result in a subclinical inflammatory state in many organ systems.[48–50] This condition could have long-term negative effects and monitoring this condition could provide invaluable insight in the preventive aspects of chronic cancer care. Although FDG-PET plays a major role in this process, it has certain limitations where the adjacent biological process is also

hypermetabolically active. To overcome this limitation, one approach is to use positron-emitting nanoparticles to image macrophages.[51]

Bone metabolism

Cancer-induced bone loss, through either cytokine dysregulation caused by oncogenesis or calcium metabolism alteration caused by treatment, is a well-established phenomenon. Bone fragility and resulting fractures play an important role in mortality and morbidity of oncology patients. NaF-PET imaging provides invaluable information regarding bone turnover[52] and various quantitative methods have been investigated.[53,54] Evaluation of bone turnover in each patient's follow-up imaging examinations could prevent many devastating disease-related fractures.

Metastasis beyond eyes-to-thighs field of view

Although the claim of distal extremity bone marrow metastasis has been mentioned as the grounds for extending the PET field of view beyond conventional base-of-skull to mid-thigh, there is sparse red marrow below the knee in the adult population and the chance of having bone marrow metastasis in such a milieu is extremely rare. Until strong experimental evidence shows contrary, this possibility cannot be a justifying reason for extension of the field of view. However, in pediatric imaging, the presence of red marrow in distal extremities significantly increases such a possibility and mandates head-to-toe imaging.

Inflammation

Autoimmune disorders are multisystemic by definition,[55] even though the primary manifestation could be in one organ-system. For example, rheumatoid arthritis involves many other systems beyond synovium and joints. Even the joint involvement is not limited to 1 location or even the appendicular skeleton. The patient with rheumatoid arthritis may present with joint problems, but may also develop interstitial lung disease, or C1 to C2 subluxation. Any attempt to quantify rheumatoid arthritis burden of disease by local imaging, such as hand radiographs, is prone to fundamental problems. The lack of a comprehensive imaging biomarker to capture the totality of this disease is a major pitfall in treatment monitoring (hand radiographs are not sufficient). As such, we believe assessing inflammation in various organs and structures as well as osseous abnormalities that are associated with musculoskeletal diseases and disorders will benefit significantly from total-body imaging with PET. Although FDG will be of great value for assessing inflammation and muscle metabolism (**Fig. 7**),

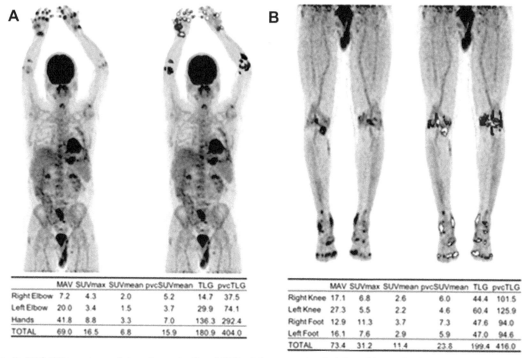

	MAV	SUVmax	SUVmean	pvcSUVmean	TLG	pvcTLG
Right Elbow	7.2	4.3	2.0	5.2	14.7	37.5
Left Elbow	20.0	3.4	1.5	3.7	29.9	74.1
Hands	41.8	8.8	3.3	7.0	136.3	292.4
TOTAL	69.0	16.5	6.8	15.9	180.9	404.0

	MAV	SUVmax	SUVmean	pvcSUVmean	TLG	pvcTLG
Right Knee	17.1	6.8	2.6	6.0	44.4	101.5
Left Knee	27.3	5.5	2.2	4.6	60.4	125.9
Right Foot	12.9	11.3	3.7	7.3	47.6	94.0
Left Foot	16.1	7.6	2.9	5.9	47.0	94.6
TOTAL	73.4	31.2	11.4	23.8	199.4	416.0

Fig. 7. FDG-PET maximum intensity projection (MIP) of the upper body (*A*) and lower body (*B*) of a patient with rheumatoid arthritis. Synovial inflammation was assessed by segmenting FDG-avid joints using an adaptive thresholding algorithm (ROVER software, ABX GmbH, Radeberg, Germany). Metabolically active volume (MAV), max standardized uptake value (SUV$_{max}$), mean SUV (SUV$_{mean}$), partial volume-corrected SUV$_{mean}$ (pvcSUV$_{mean}$), total lesion glycolysis (TLG), and partial volume-corrected TLG (pvcTLG) were calculated and summed for each segmented region. The overall pvcTLG for this patient was 820.0.

NaF will allow the detection of osseous abnormalities and calcium aberrancies in patients with systemic inflammation (**Fig. 8**). Improved temporal resolution with a 1-minute or less acquisition time is also an advantage that will lead to decreased motion artifact and partial volume effects. This property could be particularly helpful for evaluation of inflammatory diseases of the bowel.[1,56,57] Inflammatory vasculitides often affect multiple body regions.[44]

In addition to autoimmune disorders, viral infections have proven over and over again to be a multisystem disease. The emerging evidence by studying severe acute respiratory syndrome coronavirus-2 pathogenesis (coronavirus disease-2019 disease) is a salient example to remind us that viruses have systemic effects on the body beyond the primary site of infection that may initially go unrecognized.[58,59] Similarly, total-body human immunodeficiency virus burden in vivo has been suggested using TB-PET imaging.[60]

Cardiovascular

Atherosclerosis, as the most common cause of morbidity and mortality in the elderly population, is a systemic disease and frequently involves many arteries throughout the body.[61,62] Although cardiac and cerebral complications of atherosclerosis are the main causes of morbidity and mortality in the affected population, no other organ is immune to the serious consequences of this disease. Therefore, there is a dire need for an imaging modality that allows screening the entire body for detecting and characterizing atherosclerotic plaques in their early stages and before they cause significant and irreversible damage to various organs in the body. During the past 5 decades structural imaging techniques such as CT, MR imaging, and ultrasound imaging have been extensively used for detection of this disease but they are known to suffer from many shortcomings.[63–65] It is well-established that these modalities are insensitive for the early detection of the plaques and assessing their response to medical and other interventions. During the past 2 decades, attempts have been made to detect and quantify this common disease at the molecular and cellular levels and before it causes structural changes in the arterial system.[66] In particular, PET/CT scans and PET/MR scans have been used to visualize and quantify inflammation and calcification in plaques

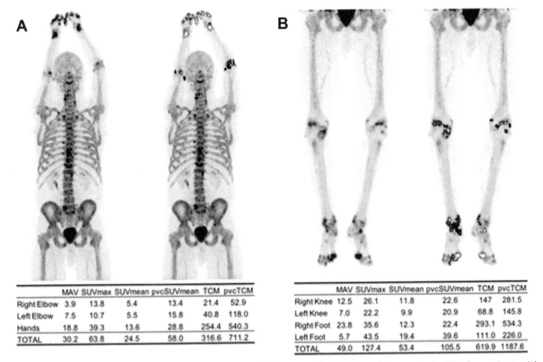

	MAV	SUVmax	SUVmean	pvcSUVmean	TCM	pvcTCM
Right Elbow	3.9	13.8	5.4	13.4	21.4	52.9
Left Elbow	7.5	10.7	5.5	15.8	40.8	118.0
Hands	18.8	39.3	13.6	28.8	254.4	540.3
TOTAL	30.2	63.8	24.5	58.0	316.6	711.2

	MAV	SUVmax	SUVmean	pvcSUVmean	TCM	pvcTCM
Right Knee	12.5	26.1	11.8	22.6	147	281.5
Left Knee	7.0	22.2	9.9	20.9	68.8	145.8
Right Foot	23.8	35.6	12.3	22.4	293.1	534.3
Left Foot	5.7	43.5	19.4	39.6	111.0	226.0
TOTAL	49.0	127.4	53.4	105.5	619.9	1187.6

Fig. 8. NaF-PET maximum intensity projection (MIP) of the upper body (*A*) and lower body (*B*) of a patient with rheumatoid arthritis. Focal areas of high bone formation in the joints were segmented using an adaptive thresholding algorithm (ROVER software, ABX GmbH, Radeberg, Germany). Metabolically active volume (MAV), maximum standardized uptake value (SUV$_{max}$), mean SUV (SUV$_{mean}$), partial volume-corrected SUV$_{mean}$ (pvcSUV$_{mean}$), total calcium metabolism (TCM), and partial volume-corrected TCM (pvcTCM) were calculated and summed for each segmented region. The overall pvcTCM for this patient was 1898.8.

throughout the body.[67,68] FDG-PET imaging has been successfully used to detect inflammation in various organs owing to a variety of causes. Activated inflammatory cells, such as those within atherosclerotic plaques, are highly glycolytic and as such are readily visualized by FDG-PET. Similarly, molecular calcification can be assessed by radioactive fluoride (NaF) in various arteries far in advance of macroscopic calcification that is visualized by CT imaging.[69] By now, the NaF-PET technique has been shown to be very sensitive for detecting early evidence for atherosclerosis in the arterial system throughout the body.[43] As noted elsewhere in this article, delayed imaging (hours after the administration of either FDG or NaF) is essential to achieve successful results.[70–72]

TB-PET imaging instruments are well-suited for assessing patients with atherosclerosis at various stages of the disease. This imaging methodology allows early detection of many diseases and disorders, as well as also careful monitoring of disease course after various interventions. Novel quantitative techniques that have been developed in recent years allow measurement of GDA and

provide a single number for disease affecting each organ as well as the entire body. This measurement has been termed the athero burden, when the approach is adopted in patients with suspected or proven atherosclerosis. We believe systematic quantification will be of great value for the management of affected patients.

Osteoporosis

Osteoporosis is a major source of morbidity and mortality in the elderly population, particularly in postmenopausal women. Osteoporosis can also manifest in patients with cancer as osteoblasts are exposed to chemotherapeutic agents. This metabolic disorder commonly manifests pathologically in the spine and the lower extremities and is associated with significant fractures and complications related to immobility such as pulmonary embolism and high mortality. NaF-PET imaging is increasingly used for early detection of osteoporosis far in advance of its detectability by structural imaging techniques such as dual energy x-ray absorptiometry scans (**Fig. 9**). It is apparent that the diffuse nature of this disorder requires total-body metabolic assessment with a modality that can

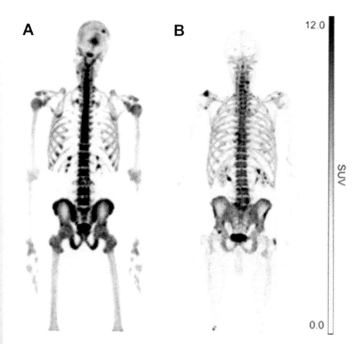

Fig. 9. NaF-PET maximum intensity projections (MIP) portraying active calcification in a 36-year-old man (*A*) and a 76-year-old man (*B*). Systemic osteoblastic metabolism was assessed by measuring NaF uptake at the femoral neck and in the whole skeleton. The mean standardized uptake value (SUV_{mean}) in the femoral neck and whole skeleton of the younger subject was 6.7 and 5.2, respectively, whereas the SUV_{mean} in the femoral neck and whole skeleton of the older subject was 1.8 and 2.4, respectively.

readily screen for this serious disease. It is possible that TB-PET scanning with NaF will become the modality of choice for both early detection of osteoporosis by innovative global assessment techniques and for the early assessment of response in this population.

Metabolic bone disease could be characterized by NaF TB-PET imaging with sub-mSv patient exposures. Whole body bone metabolism and mineral content could be quantified synergistically by combining TB-PET imaging with photon-counting CT scans.

Other Applications

In pediatric imaging, TB-PET can make the entire body image acquisition extremely fast[73] compared with the conventional PET-CT instruments with a limited field of view. Longer scans require appropriate measures to decrease the movement of the patient, such as sedation. The need for sedation has deprived pediatric patients of the benefits of many useful imaging techniques. TB-PET imaging can change this challenging situation. In addition to a shorter study time, this technology could significantly decrease the radiation dose. In modern oncology practice, 84% of pediatric patients live for more than 5 years after their diagnosis compared with 58% in the 1970s,[74] and we should be cognizant of the realities of radiation exposure over the long term in these patients.

SUMMARY

TB-PET provides clinicians the ability to take a comprehensive approach to medical imaging and for imaging scientists may use a systems biology approach to analyze the TB PET images and data. The entire tracer physiology within the patient's body over a given scan time interval can be portrayed, telling a more complete story of the patient's disease process. This information was always present in PET imaging; however, we were limited in our ability to listen. After the injection of a radiotracer to the patient, the patient has paid a fixed cost of radiation exposure. It is our ethical and professional obligation as physicians to obtain as much information as possible for asking the patient to expose himself or herself to that cost. Decreased scan times, lower tracer dose, economies of scale, and added clinical usefulness will also contribute to the economics of TB-PET imaging, which is projected to be a 5- to 6-fold capital investment over conventional PET/CT scans or in the neighborhood of $10 million.[1]

Conventional PET imaging has less signal and therefore less bandwidth compared with TB-PET imaging, as if taking the medical history of a patient, but only listening to 1 word in each sentence. TB-PET imaging allows molecular imaging physicians to sharpen their ears as they listen to the patient, as Osler famously said, "listen to your patient, he is telling you the diagnosis."[75]

Molecular imaging physicians can be more attentive to the patient and his or her disease process through the lens of TB-PET imaging.

Enhanced reimbursement from the TB PET needs to be justified by evidence based studies of the benefits of the TB PET over conventional PET. Various new types of PET examinations made possible by TB-PET imaging need reimbursed commensurate with their clinical value. These new examinations may even be able to occur during the same clinical encounter (performed on the same day, but requiring additional scanner resources and time) or ordered retrospectively after the original data has been acquired (similar to adding an additional laboratory test to a previously acquired phlebotomy sample). Examples include but are not limited to delayed PET imaging, dynamic whole body PET imaging (GDA), organ or tissue-specific physiologic activity quantification (eg, glomerular filtration rate, quantitative pulmonary perfusion, among others).

CONFLICTS OF INTEREST

None.

REFERENCES

1. Cherry SR, Jones T, Karp JS, et al. Total-body PET: maximizing sensitivity to create new opportunities for clinical research and patient care. J Nucl Med 2018;59(1):3–12.
2. Badawi RD, Shi H, Hu P, et al. First human imaging studies with the EXPLORER total-body PET scanner. J Nucl Med 2019;60(3):299–303.
3. Alavi A, Werner TJ, Høilund-Carlsen PF. What can Be and what cannot Be accomplished with PET: rectifying ongoing Misconceptions. Clin Nucl Med 2017;42(8):603.
4. Alavi A, Newberg AB, Souder E, et al. Quantitative analysis of PET and MRI data in normal aging and Alzheimer's disease: atrophy weighted total brain metabolism and absolute whole brain metabolism as reliable discriminators. J Nucl Med 1993;34(10):1681–7.
5. Saboury B, Salavati A, Brothers A, et al. FDG PET/CT in Crohn's disease: correlation of quantitative FDG PET/CT parameters with clinical and endoscopic surrogate markers of disease activity. Eur J Nucl Med Mol Imaging 2014;41(4):605–14.
6. Basu S, Saboury B, Werner T, et al. Clinical utility of FDG–PET and PET/CT in non-malignant thoracic disorders. Mol Imaging Biol 2011;13(6):1051–60.
7. Abdulla S, Salavati A, Saboury B, et al. Quantitative assessment of global lung inflammation following radiation therapy using FDG PET/CT: a pilot study. Eur J Nucl Med Mol Imaging 2014;41(2):350–6.
8. Høilund-Carlsen PF, Edenbrandt L, Alavi A. Global disease score (GDS) is the name of the game! Eur J Nucl Med Mol Imaging 2019;46(9):1768–72.
9. Raynor WY, Al-Zaghal A, Zadeh MZ, et al. Metastatic seeding Attacks bone marrow, not bone: rectifying ongoing misconceptions. PET Clin 2019;14(1):135–44.
10. Raynor WY, Zadeh MZ, Kothekar E, et al. Evolving role of PET-based novel quantitative techniques in the management of hematological malignancies. PET Clin 2019;14(3):331–40.
11. Raynor WY, Jonnakuti VS, Zirakchian Zadeh M, et al. Comparison of methods of quantifying global synovial metabolic activity with FDG-PET/CT in rheumatoid arthritis. Int J Rheum Dis 2019;22(12):2191–8.
12. Khosravi M, Peter J, Wintering NA, et al. 18F-FDG is a superior indicator of cognitive performance compared to 18F-florbetapir in Alzheimer's disease and mild cognitive impairment evaluation: a global quantitative analysis. J Alzheimers Dis 2019;70(4):1197–207.
13. Saboury B, Parsons MA, Moghbel M, et al. Quantification of aging effects upon global knee inflammation by 18F-FDG-PET. Nucl Med Commun 2016;37(3):254–8.
14. Peter J, Houshmand S, Werner TJ, et al. Applications of global quantitative 18F-FDG-PET analysis in temporal lobe epilepsy. Nucl Med Commun 2015;1. https://doi.org/10.1097/mnm.0000000000000440.
15. Fardin S, Gholami S, Samimi S, et al. Global quantitative techniques for positron emission tomographic assessment of disease activity in cutaneous T-cell lymphoma and response to treatment. JAMA Dermatol 2016;152(1):103–5.
16. Marin-Oyaga VA, Salavati A, Houshmand S, et al. Feasibility and performance of an adaptive contrast-oriented FDG PET/CT quantification technique for global disease assessment of malignant pleural mesothelioma and a brief review of the literature. Hell J Nucl Med 2015;18(1):11–8.
17. Basu S, Zaidi H, Salavati A, et al. FDG PET/CT methodology for evaluation of treatment response in lymphoma: from "graded visual analysis" and "semiquantitative SUVmax" to global disease burden assessment. Eur J Nucl Med Mol Imaging 2014;41(11):2158–60.
18. Seraj SM, Ayubcha C, Zadeh MZ, et al. The evolving role of PET-based novel quantitative techniques in the interventional radiology procedures of the liver. PET Clin 2019;14(4):419–25.
19. Sherer Y, Shoenfeld Y. Mechanisms of disease: atherosclerosis in autoimmune diseases. Nat Clin Pract Rheumatol 2006;2(2):99–106.
20. Diani M, Altomare G, Reali E. T helper cell subsets in clinical manifestations of psoriasis. J Immunol Res 2016;2016:7692024.

21. Pinu FR, Beale DJ, Paten AM, et al. Systems biology and multi-omics integration: viewpoints from the metabolomics research community. Metabolites 2019; 9(4). https://doi.org/10.3390/metabo9040076.

22. Mardinoglu A, Boren J, Smith U, et al. Systems biology in hepatology: approaches and applications. Nat Rev Gastroenterol Hepatol 2018;15(6): 365–77.

23. Hanahan D, Weinberg RA. Hallmarks of cancer: the next generation. Cell 2011;144(5):646–74.

24. Basu S, Kwee TC, Gatenby R, et al. Evolving role of molecular imaging with PET in detecting and characterizing heterogeneity of cancer tissue at the primary and metastatic sites, a plausible explanation for failed attempts to cure malignant disorders. Eur J Nucl Med Mol Imaging 2011; 38(6):987–91.

25. Mankoff DA, Pantel AR, Viswanath V, et al. Advances in PET Diagnostics for guiding targeted cancer therapy and studying in vivo cancer biology. Curr Pathobiol Rep 2019;7(3):97–108.

26. Surti S, Pantel AR, Karp JS. Total Body PET: Why, How, What for? IEEE Transactions on Radiation and Plasma Medical Sciences 2020;4(3):283–92. Available at: https://ieeexplore.ieee.org/abstract/document/9056798/?casa_token=NTPSPgSONToA AAAA:zifFWCuiZyM0xSEYlo9QNC_EdO0iThLYJwM V_Scs5qtYpvcfPAFAGQy1tkPLTamVsaRjkqosAQ.

27. Pauwels EK, Ribeiro MJ, Stoot JH, et al. FDG accumulation and tumor biology. Nucl Med Biol 1998; 25(4):317–22.

28. Zhuang H, Pourdehnad M, Lambright ES, et al. Dual time point 18F-FDG PET imaging for differentiating malignant from inflammatory processes. J Nucl Med 2001;42(9):1412–7.

29. Basu S, Kung J, Houseni M, et al. Temporal profile of fluorodeoxyglucose uptake in malignant lesions and normal organs over extended time periods in patients with lung carcinoma: implications for its utilization in assessing malignant lesions. Q J Nucl Med Mol Imaging 2009;53(1):9.

30. Cheng G, Alavi A, Lim E, et al. Dynamic changes of FDG uptake and clearance in normal tissues. Mol Imaging Biol 2013;15(3):345–52.

31. Cherry SR, Badawi RD, Karp JS, et al. Total-body imaging: transforming the role of positron emission tomography. Sci Transl Med 2017;9(381). https://doi.org/10.1126/scitranslmed.aaf6169.

32. Hustinx R, Smith RJ, Benard F, et al. Dual time point fluorine-18 fluorodeoxyglucose positron emission tomography: a potential method to differentiate malignancy from inflammation and normal tissue in the head and neck. Eur J Nucl Med 1999;26(10): 1345–8.

33. Cheng G, Torigian DA, Zhuang H, et al. When should we recommend use of dual time-point and delayed time-point imaging techniques in FDG PET? Eur J Nucl Med Mol Imaging 2013;40(5):779–87.

34. Viswanath V, Daube-Witherspoon ME, Schmall JP, et al. Development of pet for total-body imaging. Acta Phys Pol B 2017;48(10):1555–66.

35. Ross JS, Stagliano NE, Donovan MJ, et al. Atherosclerosis and cancer: common molecular pathways of disease development and progression. Ann N Y Acad Sci 2001;947:271–92 [discussion: 292–3].

36. Ross JS, Stagliano NE, Donovan MJ, et al. Atherosclerosis: a cancer of the blood vessels? Pathol Patterns Rev 2001;116(suppl_1):S97–107.

37. Tapia-Vieyra JV, Delgado-Coello B, Mas-Oliva J. Atherosclerosis and cancer; A resemblance with far-reaching implications. Arch Med Res 2017; 48(1):12–26.

38. Ogawa A, Kanda T, Sugihara S, et al. Risk factors for myocardial infarction in cancer patients. J Med 1995;26(5–6):221–33.

39. Dardiotis E, Aloizou A-M, Markoula S, et al. Cancer-associated stroke: pathophysiology, detection and management. Int J Oncol 2019;54(3):779–96.

40. Yun M, Yeh D, Araujo LI, et al. F-18 FDG uptake in the large arteries. Clin Nucl Med 2001;26(4):314–9.

41. Beheshti M, Saboury B, Mehta NN, et al. Detection and global quantification of cardiovascular molecular calcification by fluoro18-fluoride positron emission tomography/computed tomography–a novel concept. Hell J Nucl Med 2011;14(2):114–20.

42. Moghbel M, Al-Zaghal A, Werner TJ, et al. The role of PET in evaluating atherosclerosis: a critical review. Semin Nucl Med 2018;48(6):488–97.

43. Høilund-Carlsen PF, Sturek M, Alavi A, et al. Atherosclerosis imaging with 18F-sodium fluoride PET: state-of-the-art review. Eur J Nucl Med Mol Imaging 2020;47(6):1538–51.

44. Schmall JP, Karp JS, Alavi A. The potential role of total body PET imaging in assessment of atherosclerosis. PET Clin 2019;14(2):245–50.

45. Sydow BD, Srinivas SM, Newberg A, et al. Deep venous thrombosis on F-18 FDG PET/CT imaging. Clin Nucl Med 2006;31(7):403–4.

46. Sharma P, Kumar R, Singh H, et al. Imaging thrombus in cancer patients with FDG PET–CT. Jpn J Radiol 2012;30(2):95–104.

47. Hess S, Madsen PH, Basu S, et al. Potential role of FDG PET/CT imaging for assessing venous thromboembolic disorders. Clin Nucl Med 2012;37(12):1170–2.

48. Bukhari A, Kesari V, Sirous R, et al. Increased cortical glycolysis following CD19 CART therapy: a radiographic surrogate for an altered blood-brain barrier. Blood 2019;134(Supplement_1):4454.

49. Holtzman NG, Bentzen SM, Kesari V, et al. Immune effector cell-associated neurotoxicity syndrome (ICANS) after CD19-directed chimeric antigen receptor T-cell therapy (CAR-T) for large B-cell

lymphoma: predictive biomarkers and clinical outcomes. Blood 2019;134(Supplement_1):3239.

50. Basu S, Kwee TC, Torigian D, et al. Suboptimal and inadequate quantification: an alarming crisis in medical applications of PET. Eur J Nucl Med Mol Imaging 2011;38(7):1381.

51. Lu HD, Wang LZ, Wilson BK, et al. Copper loading of preformed nanoparticles for PET-imaging applications. ACS Appl Mater Interfaces 2018;10(4):3191–9.

52. Blake GM, Siddique M, Frost ML, et al. Imaging of site specific bone turnover in osteoporosis using positron emission tomography. Curr Osteoporos Rep 2014;12(4):475–85.

53. Raijmakers P, Temmerman OPP, Saridin CP, et al. Quantification of F-18-Fluoride kinetics: evaluation of simplified methods. J Nucl Med 2014;55(7):1122–7.

54. Al-beyatti Y, Siddique M, Frost ML, et al. Precision of F-18-fluoride PET skeletal kinetic studies in the assessment of bone metabolism. Osteoporos Int 2012;23(10):2535–41.

55. Rankin LC, Artis D. Beyond host defense: emerging functions of the immune system in regulating complex tissue physiology. Cell 2018;173(3):554–67.

56. Wibmer AG, Hricak H, Ulaner GA, et al. Trends in oncologic hybrid imaging. Eur J Hybrid Imaging 2018;2(1):1.

57. Chen DL. Promising advances for imaging lung macrophage recruitment. Am J Respir Crit Care Med 2020;201(1):11–3.

58. Mao L, Jin H, Wang M, et al. Neurologic manifestations of hospitalized patients with coronavirus disease 2019 in Wuhan, China. JAMA Neurol 2020. https://doi.org/10.1001/jamaneurol.2020.1127.

59. Carod-Artal FJ. Neurological complications of coronavirus and COVID-19. Rev Neurol 2020;70(9):311–22.

60. Henrich TJ, Hsue PY, VanBrocklin H. Seeing is believing: nuclear imaging of HIV persistence. Front Immunol 2019;10:2077. Available at: https://apps.webofknowledge.com//full_record.do?product=WOS&search_mode=CitingArticles&qid=27&SID=7EqLigFTSJIT32iWyNA&page=3&doc=22.

61. Lloyd-Jones D, Adams R, Carnethon M, et al. Heart disease and stroke statistics–2009 update: a report from the American Heart Association Statistics Committee and stroke statistics subcommittee. Circulation 2009;119(3):480–6.

62. Lozano R, Naghavi M, Foreman K, et al. Global and regional mortality from 235 causes of death for 20 age groups in 1990 and 2010: a systematic analysis for the Global Burden of Disease Study 2010. Lancet 2012;380(9859):2095–128.

63. Wilms G, Baert AL. The history of angiography. J Belge Radiol 1995;78(5):299–302.

64. Agatston AS, Janowitz WR, Hildner FJ, et al. Quantification of coronary artery calcium using ultrafast computed tomography. J Am Coll Cardiol 1990;15(4):827–32.

65. Willemink MJ, van der Werf NR, Nieman K, et al. Coronary artery calcium: a technical argument for a new scoring method. J Cardiovasc Comput Tomogr 2019;13(6):347–52.

66. Alavi A, Werner TJ, Høilund-Carlsen PF. PET-based imaging to detect and characterize cardiovascular disorders: unavoidable path for the foreseeable future. J Nucl Cardiol 2018;25(1):203–7.

67. Alavi A, Werner TJ, Høilund-Carlsen PF. What can be and what cannot be accomplished with PET to detect and characterize atherosclerotic plaques. J Nucl Cardiol 2018;25(6):2012–5.

68. McKenney-Drake ML, Moghbel MC, Paydary K, et al. 18F-NaF and 18F-FDG as molecular probes in the evaluation of atherosclerosis. Eur J Nucl Med Mol Imaging 2018;45(12):2190–200.

69. Raynor WY, Borja AJ, Rojulpote C, et al. 18F-sodium fluoride: an emerging tracer to assess active vascular microcalcification. J Nucl Cardiol 2020. https://doi.org/10.1007/s12350-020-02138-9.

70. Blomberg BA, Thomassen A, Takx RAP, et al. Delayed 18F-fluorodeoxyglucose PET/CT imaging improves quantitation of atherosclerotic plaque inflammation: results from the CAMONA study. J Nucl Cardiol 2014;21(3):588–97.

71. Blomberg BA, Thomassen A, Takx RAP, et al. Delayed sodium 18F-fluoride PET/CT imaging does not improve quantification of vascular calcification metabolism: results from the CAMONA study. J Nucl Cardiol 2014;21(2):293–304.

72. Kwiecinski J, Berman DS, Lee S-E, et al. Three-hour delayed imaging improves assessment of coronary 18F-sodium fluoride PET. J Nucl Med 2019;60(4):530–5.

73. Zhuang H, Alavi A. Evolving role of PET in pediatric disorders. PET Clin 2020;15(3):xv–xvii.

74. Viale PH. The American Cancer Society's facts & figures: 2020 edition. J Adv Pract Oncol 2020;11. https://doi.org/10.6004/jadpro.2020.11.2.1.

75. Waeber G. Just listen to your patient, he is telling you the diagnosis. In: Forum Médical Suisse. Vol 19. EMH Media; 2019:373-373.

An Update on the Role of Total-Body PET Imaging in the Evaluation of Atherosclerosis

Austin J. Borja, BA[a,b], Chaitanya Rojulpote, MD[a,c],
Emily C. Hancin, MS, BA[a,d], Poul Flemming Høilund-Carlsen, MD, DMSc[e,f],
Abass Alavi, MD[a,*]

KEYWORDS

- PET • 18F-FDG • 18F-NaF • Cardiovascular disease • Atherosclerosis • Plaque burden
- Total-body PET imaging

KEY POINTS

- Total-body PET imaging has demonstrated increased sensitivity and specificity in atherosclerosis.
- Recent evidence points toward 18F-sodium fluoride as the radiotracer of choice over 18F-fluoro-deoxyglucose for evaluation of atherosclerotic plaque burden.
- Global disease assessment may be used as an adjunct tool in atherosclerosis PET imaging.

INTRODUCTION

Atherosclerosis is one of the most prevalent diseases in the United States, and approximately 735,000 Americans experience atherosclerosis-related myocardial infarctions every year.[1] This pathology is characterized by the obstruction of arteries by low-density lipoproteins (LDLs), which then leads to a sustained inflammatory response in endothelial cells.[2] Monocytes subsequently phagocytose and oxidize LDLs, generating cholesterol-laden plaques that progressively occlude the vessel and cause chronic ischemia.[3] These plaques also may detach acutely from the arterial walls and embolize in the brain, heart, lungs, and extremities.[4] It is expected that, by 2035, the health care costs and productivity losses associated with cardiovascular diseases, including atherosclerosis, will reach over $1.1 trillion.[5] Thus, it is critical to identify more sensitive and specific methods for the assessment of atherosclerosis. Specifically, modalities that can characterize pathologic changes on the molecular level may both improve clinical outcomes and reduce the associated costs for patients before more serious cardiovascular diseases develop.

PET, combined with computed tomography (CT), has been used widely to examine the effects of atherosclerosis on the vasculature.[6–8] Fused PET/CT is both a structural and a functional imaging modality and, therefore, is able to detect the microscopic biochemical changes associated with the development of plaques and inflammation (Fig. 1).[7] 18F-fluorodeoxyglucose (FDG), a glucose analog, is a common tracer used in PET/

a Department of Radiology, Hospital of the University of Pennsylvania, 3400 Spruce Street, Philadelphia, PA 19104, USA; b Perelman School of Medicine at the University of Pennsylvania, 3400 Civic Center Blvd, Philadelphia, PA 19104, USA; c Department of Internal Medicine, The Wright Center for Graduate Medical Education, 501 S Washington Ave Suite 1000, Scranton, PA 18505, USA; d Lewis Katz School of Medicine at Temple University, 3500 N Broad St, Philadelphia, PA 19140, USA; e Department of Nuclear Medicine, Odense University Hospital, J. B. Winsløws Vej 4, 5000 Odense C, Denmark; f Department of Clinical Research, University of Southern Denmark, Winsløwparken 19, 3. salOdense C - DK-5000, Denmark
* Corresponding author. Department of Radiology, Hospital of the University of Pennsylvania, 3400 Spruce Street, Philadelphia, PA 19104, USA.
E-mail address: abass.alavi@pennmedicine.upenn.edu

PET Clin 15 (2020) 477–485
https://doi.org/10.1016/j.cpet.2020.06.006
1556-8598/20/© 2020 Elsevier Inc. All rights reserved.

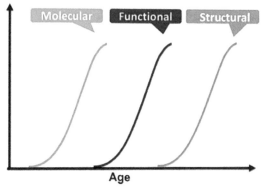

Fig. 1. This figure graphically illustrates the probable sequence of biological events as they relate to many disorders. Functional activities refer to physiologic alterations, such as blood flow and organ motility. This pattern is relevant particularly to the assessment of atherosclerosis in the coronary arteries as well as other arteries. As such, molecular imaging with PET may provide early evidence of the disease process. (Reproduced with permission from Moghbel et al.[7])

CT to identify inflammatory processes throughout the body. Lesions of increased FDG uptake reflect focal spikes in cellular metabolism in conditions, such as malignancy, infection, and autoimmune disease.[9] 18F-sodium fluoride (NaF) also has been utilized in numerous PET/CT studies as a marker for molecular calcification. NaF has been identified as a more sensitive and specific marker than FDG in the assessment of arterial calcification and plaque development.[10–12]

Total-body PET/CT imaging has taken the standard parameters of PET/CT to new heights. Specifically, total-body PET instruments aim to capture the

entire body without any gantry movements (Fig. 2).[13,14] By increasing the geometric coverage of the scans to encompass the entire body, total-body PET/CT has the potential to increase sensitivity within certain pathologies by as much as 40-fold or in practice for most imaging procedures by a factor of 8.[15] Moreover, through this technology, radiotracer uptake can be quantified simultaneously across the entire body.[16] As a result, total-body imaging will be best suited for pathologies that affect and therefore, may be quantified, across the entire body, including hematologic malignancies, inflammatory and osseous musculoskeletal disease, and cardiovascular disease.[17] This may be helpful particularly in monitoring the development of atherosclerosis and related sequelae, which may be missed in single-organ PET.[18,19]

This review aims at presenting the most recent findings surrounding the importance of total-body PET imaging in the diagnosis and treatment of atherosclerosis. These data demonstrate the feasibility of total-body PET imaging in the clinical setting, and they show that it is a highly preferred technique in the surveillance of atherosclerotic plaque development and subsequent disease progression. This information is of critical importance to physicians, who rely on the development of refined imaging techniques to improve patient outcomes, preventative measures, and treatment plans.

LIMITATIONS OF 18F-FLUORODEOXYGLUCOSE–PET IN THE ASSESSMENT OF ATHEROSCLEROSIS

Previous studies have utilized FDG to identify atherosclerosis indirectly by intimal inflammation.

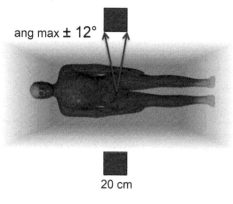

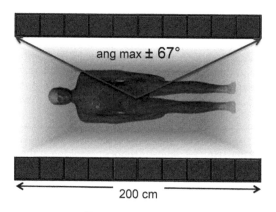

Standard whole-body PET   **Total-body PET**

Fig. 2. In total-body PET, the patient is surrounded by detectors across the length of the entire body. As result, the entire body can be imaged simultaneously with no movement of the imaging bed. In addition, the wider axial acceptance angle (ang max) in total-body increases photon sensitivity over standard PET. As such, the major potential for total-body PET whole-body pathologies. (Reproduced with permission from Schmall et al.[13])

Ben-Haim and colleagues[20] used total-body FDG-PET/CT in 122 cancer patients over age 50 to assess FDG uptake and CT calcifications in the vasculature. They determined that CT calcifications were found more commonly in patients presenting with hyperlipidemia or hypertension and in smokers, and they found that there was increased FDG-PET/CT uptake in patients with hypertension and marginally increased in those presenting with cardiovascular disease. In addition, de Boer and colleagues[21] performed total-body FDG-PET/CT to assess subclinical arterial inflammation in patients with type 2 diabetes mellitus. They determined that FDG uptake was significantly associated with determinants of arterial stiffness, as assessed by central systolic blood pressure, carotid-femoral pulse wave velocity, and augmentation index. Kim and colleagues[22] studied patients presenting with cerebral atherosclerosis and examined the association between atherosclerotic plaque presence and bone marrow activity. Using FDG-PET/CT across the whole body, they determined that the cavernous internal carotid artery showed increased FDG uptake in patients with cerebral atherosclerosis. The same patients also demonstrated significantly decreased FDG uptake in the lumbar vertebrae, which further points to the systemic influence of atherosclerosis. These studies prove that total-body FDG-PET imaging is feasible for detecting inflammatory plaques within atherosclerosis.

Other groups, however, have highlighted the limitations of FDG-PET. For instance, Sánchez-Roa and colleagues[23] examined total-body FDG-PET/CT scans within 22 patients referred for oncological evaluation and with a history of coronary artery disease. They determined that patients with coronary artery disease are at an increased risk for increased FDG uptake of the thoracic aorta, abdominal aorta, and the carotid arteries. The investigators further found, however, that focal FDG uptake rarely was associated with calcification, emphasizing a key restriction on FDG-PET for this pathology. Moreover, Wassélius and colleagues[24] studied 28 patients who underwent 2 whole-body FDG-PET/CT scans within 7 months apart. Comparing the appearance of vascular plaques between the 2 scans, they calculated a correlation of nearly 100% for calcified inactive plaques but only 50% FDG-accumulating plaques. These data demonstrate that FDG uptake is feasible for inflammatory atherosclerotic lesions but not for quiescent plaques.

TOTAL-BODY 18F-SODIUM FLUORIDE–PET IN THE ASSESSMENT OF ATHEROSCLEROSIS

Recent evidence suggests that other radiotracers, namely NaF, may be superior to FDG in the

evaluation of atherosclerosis. For example, arterial blood pool activity has been demonstrated to negatively influence the efficacy of assessing plaque accumulation by FDG-PET. Saboury and colleagues[25] examined 9 lung cancer patients, they obtained FDG-PET images at 1 hour, 2 hours, and 3 hours post-FDG injection. They concluded that FDG-PET images obtained 1 and 2 hours after FDG administration were particularly difficult to interpret in assessing atherosclerotic plaque burden. In addition, Blomberg and colleagues[26] used total-body PET scans in a prospective assessment of 40 patients at 90 minutes and 180 minutes after FDG administration, and they found that the 180-minute time point was more effective in identifying inflammation associated with atherosclerotic plaques. These findings may be due to the decrease in blood-pool activity over time, suggesting the benefits of delayed time-point FDG-PET imaging. On the other hand, another study by Blomberg and colleagues[27] in the same cohort of patients demonstrated that NaF-PET does not suffer from this same limitation.

Other research has directly demonstrated that NaF, but not FDG, is associated with atherosclerotic risk factors. Arani and colleagues[28] determined that NaF uptake within the abdominal aorta was significantly correlated with age and Framingham risk score, but they found that FDG did not exhibit the same association with cardiovascular risk factors. In addition, Blomberg and colleagues[29] determined that vascular calcium metabolism in the thoracic aorta, as measured by NaF-PET/CT, was significantly associated with cardiovascular risk. In contrast, arterial inflammation in these same regions, as measured by FDG uptake, was not significantly correlated with cardiovascular risk. Finally, Castro and colleagues[30] found that NaF uptake in the left common carotid artery was significantly associated with cardiovascular risk factors, such as increased age, hypercholesterolemia, and hypertension, whereas the uptake values were correlated inversely with level of physical activity. Emamzadehfard and colleagues,[31] however, were unable to find a correlation between carotid FDG uptake and cardiovascular risk factors. These data indicate that NaF is a more powerful indicator of atherosclerotic calcifications and, therefore, FDG may be best used in a supplementary role for active inflammation.

NaF has been used as a tracer to measure whole-body plaque burden with substantial success. Rojulpote and colleagues[32] studied 75 healthy controls and 44 subjects with cardiovascular risk factors, demonstrating that NaF uptake across the common iliac, external iliac, femoral,

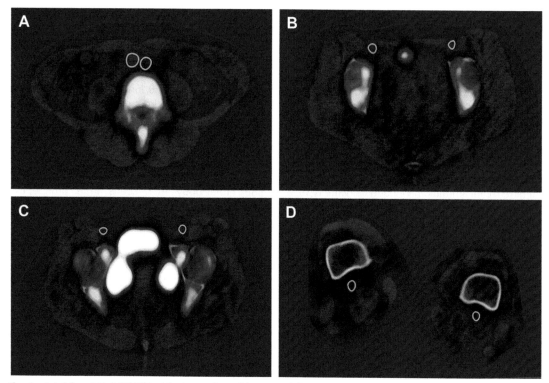

Fig. 3. Axial fused NaF-PET/CT with the region of interest delineating lower extremity arteries in a healthy control. Using a previously established methodology, the manually delineated region of interest determined the NaF uptake in the (*A*) common iliac artery, (*B*) external iliac artery, (*C*) femoral artery, and (*D*) popliteal artery.

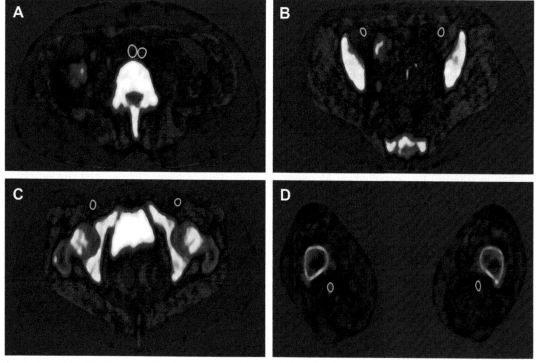

Fig. 4. Axial fused NaF-PET/CT with the region of interest delineating lower extremity arteries in a high-risk subject. Using a previously established methodology, the manually delineated region of interest determined the NaF uptake in the (*A*) common iliac artery, (*B*) external iliac artery, (*C*) femoral artery, and (*D*) popliteal artery.

and popliteal arteries was associated with atherosclerotic risk (**Figs. 3** and **4**). Further investigation from this group has expanded the analysis to include the common carotid and coronary arteries; aortic arch; and ascending, descending, and abdominal aorta (**Figs. 5** and **6**). Individual vessels' segmental mean standardized uptake value (SUVmean) analyzed in a healthy control and a high-risk subject is presented in **Table 1**, with total-body NaF arterial uptake derived as the sum of the SUVmean of all arteries examined.

In addition, Derlin and colleagues[33] performed a retrospective analysis using NaF-PET/CT scans in a cohort of 75 patients and determined that whole-body atherosclerosis burden can provide accurate information about the degree of mineral deposition and the associated structural and functional changes in arterial walls. Furthermore, de Oliveira-Santos and colleagues[34] studied a cohort of patients at high risk for cardiovascular disease as determined by risk score in order to assess how well NaF-PET/CT measurements across the entire body correlated with the identification of risk. They found that, although there was no association between coronary NaF uptake and calcium score, there did exist a significant relationship

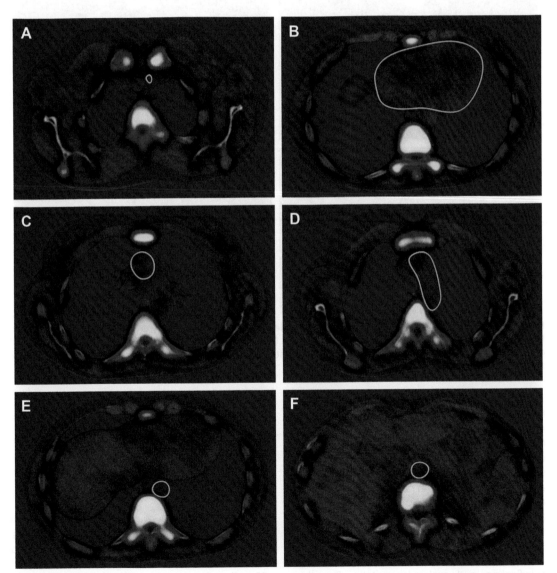

Fig. 5. Axial fused NaF-PET/CT with regions of interest delineating upper extremity arteries in a healthy control. Manually delineated region of interest determined the NaF uptake in the (*A*) common carotid artery, (*B*) global coronary arteries (which excluded aortic valve, skeletal structures, and aortic wall), (*C*) ascending aorta, (*D*) aortic arch, (*E*) descending aorta, and (*F*) abdominal aorta.

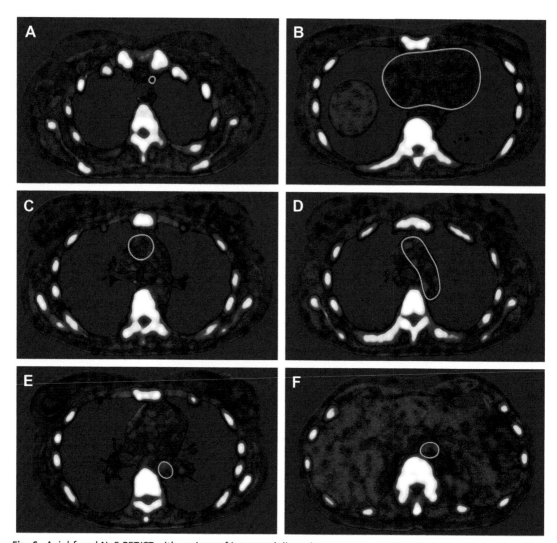

Fig. 6. Axial fused NaF-PET/CT with regions of interest delineating upper extremity arteries in a high-risk subject. Manually delineated region of interest determined the NaF uptake in the (*A*) common carotid artery, (*B*) global coronary arteries (which excluded aortic valve, skeletal structures, and aortic wall), (*C*) ascending aorta, (*D*) aortic arch, (*E*) descending aorta, and (*F*) abdominal aorta.

between NaF uptake and both thoracic fat volume and cardiovascular risk factors. Finally, Kurata and colleagues[35] utilized NaF-PET/CT scans in 29 cancer patients. Of these 29 patients, 8 of them had scans with significantly increased NaF uptake across the whole body, in particular the abdominal aorta, descending thoracic aorta, and the aortic arch; 91% of the lesions that took up NaF also were recognized as areas of calcification, which suggests that NaF is a particularly effective tracer to use in total-body PET/CT in the colocalization of calcification and molecular uptake. Together, these studies demonstrate the feasibility of NaF-PET/CT scanners for atherosclerosis imaging. Moving forward, the authors expect total-body

PET imaging to become the gold standard in the systemic imaging of atherosclerotic developments, particularly with the use of NaF as a tracer.

OTHER TRACERS FOR TOTAL-BODY PET IMAGING

Tracers besides FDG and NaF also have been used in atherosclerosis PET imaging across the body. For example, Derlin and colleagues[36] used 11C-acetate PET/CT across the whole body of 36 patients to determine if it could be used as a method to detect the presence of plaques. They found that 29.1% of the lesions marked by 11C-acetate uptake were colocalized with arterial

Table 1
Global arterial 18F-sodium fluoride mean standardized uptake value representing microcalcification in multiple arteries of a healthy control and a high-risk subject

Vessel	Healthy Subject (18F-Sodium Fluoride Mean Standardized Uptake Value)	High-Risk Subject (18F-Sodium Fluoride Mean Standardized Uptake Value)
Carotid artery	0.41	0.73
Coronary arteries	0.59	0.76
Ascending aorta	0.53	1.05
Aortic arch	0.49	1.24
Descending aorta	0.52	1.23
Abdominal aorta	1.08	0.97
Common iliac artery	1.40	1.89
External iliac artery	1.29	1.66
Femoral artery	1.43	1.62
Popliteal artery	0.98	1.53
Total body arterial uptake	8.74	12.70

calcification, suggesting some potential for this modality to be used in conjunction with other techniques for the identification of plaques. In addition, Kato and colleagues[37] analyzed 11C-choline scans of the entire body within 93 male patients between 60 years old and 80 years old with prostate cancer. They detected 11C-choline uptake in 95% of patients, and 94% of vessel segments demonstrated calcification. Only 6% of the calcifications, however, were colocalized with 11C-choline uptake. These findings suggest that 11C-choline is less accurate in localizing calcification secondary to atherosclerosis. Taken together, these studies data present a possibility for the use of alternatives in tandem with FDG or NaF in total-body PET imaging.

GLOBAL DISEASE ASSESSMENT

In conjunction with total-body PET/CT, the authors believe that global disease assessment is critical toward an accurate and reproducible measure for plaque burden. PET/CT imaging has been utilized in several vascular pathologies, including atherosclerosis, to calculate global disease burden.[38,39] Moreover, global assessment can be utilized longitudinally to monitor disease progression and therapeutic efficacy.[40] In contrast, single measurements of maximum standardized uptake value (SUVmax) frequently are inaccurate and can be manipulated easily by scanner condition heterogeneity and random scatter.[41] Therefore, the authors believe that global disease assessment is a powerful complement to total-body PET imaging.

SUMMARY

Atherosclerosis is a major source of morbidity and mortality worldwide. Recent studies have pointed toward molecular imaging by total-body PET/CT as the gold standard for the determination of total atherosclerotic plaque burden. In addition, the measurement of microcalcifications by NaF uptake is more sensitive and specific to atherosclerosis than the quantification of vessel wall inflammation using FDG. Finally, global disease assessment may be employed to deliver robust, reproducible values regarding disease severity. Moving forward, the authors envision prospective, multicenter studies to further demonstrate the utility of these methodologies in the evaluation of atherosclerosis.

DISCLOSURE

The authors declare no conflicts of interest.

REFERENCES

1. Pahwa R, Jialal I. Atherosclerosis. StatPearls. Treasure Island (FL): StatPearls Publishing; 2019.
2. Rafieian-Kopaei M, Setorki M, Doudi M, et al. Atherosclerosis: process, indicators, risk factors and new hopes. Int J Prev Med 2014;5:927–46.
3. Bergheanu SC, Bodde MC, Jukema JW. Pathophysiology and treatment of atherosclerosis. Neth Heart J 2017;25:231–42.
4. Wang Y, Qiu J, Luo S, et al. High shear stress induces atherosclerotic vulnerable plaque formation

through angiogenesis. Regen Biomater 2016;3: 257–67.

5. Dunbar SB, Khavjou OA, Bakas T, et al. Projected costs of informal caregiving for cardiovascular disease: 2015 to 2035: a policy statement from the American Heart Association. Circulation 2018;137:e558–77.

6. Sheikine Y, Akram K. FDG–PET imaging of atherosclerosis: do we know what we see? Atherosclerosis 2010;211:371–80.

7. Moghbel M, Al-Zaghal A, Werner TJ, et al. The role of PET in evaluating atherosclerosis: a critical review. Semin Nucl Med 2018;48:488–97.

8. Høilund-Carlsen PF, Moghbel MC, Gerke O, et al. Evolving role of PET in detecting and characterizing atherosclerosis. PET Clin 2019;14:197–209.

9. Matic N, Ressner M, Wiechec E, et al. In vitro measurement of glucose uptake after radiation and cetuximab treatment in head and neck cancer cell lines using 18F-FDG, gamma spectrometry and PET/CT. Oncol Lett 2019;18:5155–62.

10. Li X, Heber D, Wadsak W, et al. Combined 18F-FDG PET/CT and 18F-NaF PET/CT imaging in assessing vascular inflammation and osteogenesis in calcified atherosclerotic lesions. J Nucl Med 2016;57:68.

11. Seraj SM, Raynor W, Rojulpote C, et al. Assessing the feasibility of NaF or FDG as PET probes to evaluate atherosclerosis in rheumatoid arthritis patients. J Nucl Med 2019;60:1439.

12. McKenney-Drake ML, Moghbel MC, Paydary K, et al. 18F-NaF and 18F-FDG as molecular probes in the evaluation of atherosclerosis. Eur J Nucl Med Mol Imaging 2018;45:2190–200.

13. Schmall JP, Karp JS, Alavi A. The potential role of total body PET imaging in assessment of atherosclerosis. PET Clin 2019;14:245–50.

14. Schmall JP, Karp JS, Werner M, et al. Parallax error in long-axial field-of-view PET scanners-a simulation study. Phys Med Biol 2016;61:5443–55.

15. Cherry SR, Jones T, Karp JS, et al. Total-Body PET: maximizing sensitivity to create new opportunities for clinical research and patient care. J Nucl Med 2018;59:3–12.

16. Cherry SR, Badawi RD, Karp JS, et al. Total-body imaging: transforming the role of positron emission tomography. Sci Transl Med 2017;9. https://doi.org/10.1126/scitranslmed.aaf6169.

17. Berg E, Cherry SR. Innovations in instrumentation for positron emission tomography. Semin Nucl Med 2018;48:311–31.

18. Galkina E, Ley K. Immune and inflammatory mechanisms of atherosclerosis (*). Annu Rev Immunol 2009;27:165–97.

19. Aronow WS. Peripheral arterial disease of the lower extremities. Arch Med Sci 2012;8:375–88.

20. Ben-Haim S, Kupzov E, Tamir A, et al. Evaluation of 18F-FDG uptake and arterial wall calcifications using 18F-FDG PET/CT. J Nucl Med 2004;45:1816–21.

21. de Boer SA, Hovinga-de Boer MC, Heerspink HJ, et al. Arterial stiffness is positively associated with 18F-fluorodeoxyglucose positron emission tomography–assessed subclinical vascular inflammation in people with early type 2 diabetes. Diabetes Care 2016;39:1440–7.

22. Kim J-M, Lee ES, Park K-Y, et al. Decreased bone marrow activity measured by using 18 F-fluorodeoxyglucose positron emission tomography among patients with cerebral atherosclerosis. J Neurosonol Neuroimag 2019;11:78–83.

23. Sánchez-Roa PM, Rees JI, Bartley L, et al. Systemic atherosclerotic plaque vulnerability in patients with coronary artery disease with a single whole body FDG PET-CT scan. Asia Ocean J Nucl Med Biol 2020;8:18–26.

24. Wassélius J, Larsson S, Jacobsson H. Time-to-time correlation of high-risk atherosclerotic lesions identified with [(18)F]-FDG-PET/CT. Ann Nucl Med 2009; 23:59–64.

25. Saboury B, Blomberg B, Gharavi M, et al. Dynamic changes of blood pool activity in the arteries and the veins over time on FDG-PET/CT images: implications of this observation in assessing atherosclerotic lesions. J Nucl Med 2012;53:1855.

26. Blomberg BA, Thomassen A, Takx RA, et al. Delayed (1)(8)F-fluorodeoxyglucose PET/CT imaging improves quantitation of atherosclerotic plaque inflammation: results from the CAMONA study. J Nucl Cardiol 2014;21:588–97.

27. Blomberg BA, Thomassen A, Takx RA, et al. Delayed sodium 18F-fluoride PET/CT imaging does not improve quantification of vascular calcification metabolism: results from the CAMONA study. J Nucl Cardiol 2014;21:293–304.

28. Arani LS, Gharavi MH, Zadeh MZ, et al. Association between age, uptake of 18F-fluorodeoxyglucose and of 18F-sodium fluoride, as cardiovascular risk factors in the abdominal aorta. Hell J Nucl Med 2019;22:14–9.

29. Blomberg BA, de Jong PA, Thomassen A, et al. Thoracic aorta calcification but not inflammation is associated with increased cardiovascular disease risk: results of the CAMONA study. Eur J Nucl Med Mol Imaging 2017;44:249–58.

30. Castro S, Muser D, Acosta-Montenegro O, et al. Common carotid artery molecular calcification assessed by 18F-NaF PET/CT is associated with increased cardiovascular disease risk: results from the CAMONA study. J Nucl Med 2017;58:34.

31. Emamzadehfard S, Castro S, Werner T, et al. Does FDG PET/CT precisely detect carotid artery inflammation? J Nucl Med 2018;59:1550.

32. Rojulpote C, Seraj SM, Al-Zaghal A, et al. NaF PET/CT in assessing the atherosclerotic burden in major arteries supplying the lower limbs. J Nucl Med 2019; 60:1452.

33. Derlin T, Richter U, Bannas P, et al. Feasibility of 18F-sodium fluoride PET/CT for imaging of atherosclerotic plaque. J Nucl Med 2010;51:862–5.

34. de Oliveira-Santos M, Castelo-Branco M, Silva R, et al. Atherosclerotic plaque metabolism in high cardiovascular risk subjects - a subclinical atherosclerosis imaging study with 18F-NaF PET-CT. Atherosclerosis 2017;260:41–6.

35. Kurata S, Tateishi U, Shizukuishi K, et al. Assessment of atherosclerosis in oncologic patients using 18F-fluoride PET/CT. Ann Nucl Med 2013;27:481–6.

36. Derlin T, Habermann CR, Lengyel Z, et al. Feasibility of 11C-acetate PET/CT for imaging of fatty acid synthesis in the atherosclerotic vessel wall. J Nucl Med 2011;52:1848–54.

37. Kato K, Schober O, Ikeda M, et al. Evaluation and comparison of 11C-choline uptake and calcification in aortic and common carotid arterial walls with combined PET/CT. Eur J Nucl Med Mol Imaging 2009;36: 1622–8.

38. Rojulpote C, Borja AJ, Zhang V, et al. Role of 18F-NaF-PET in assessing aortic valve calcification with age. Am J Nucl Med Mol Imaging 2020;10: 47–56.

39. Borja AJ, Hancin EC, Zhang V, et al. Potential of PET/CT in assessing dementias with emphasis on cerebrovascular disorders. Eur J Nucl Med Mol Imaging 2020. https://doi.org/10.1007/s00259-020-04697-y.

40. Borja A, Werner T, Alavi A. Role of PET/CT in vascular dementia. J Nucl Med 2019;60:1153.

41. Høilund-Carlsen PF, Edenbrandt L, Alavi A. Global disease score (GDS) is the name of the game! Eur J Nucl Med Mol Imaging 2019;46:1768–72.

Diagnosis and Monitoring of Osteoporosis with Total-Body ^{18}F-Sodium Fluoride-PET/CT

Vincent Zhang, BA[a,1], Benjamin Koa, BS[a,b,1], Austin J. Borja, BA[a,c],
Sayuri Padmanhabhan, UGS[a], Abhijit Bhattaru, UGS[a],
William Y. Raynor, BS[a,b], Chaitanya Rojulpote, MD[a,d],
Siavash Mehdizadeh Seraj, MD[a], Thomas J. Werner, MS[a],
Chamith Rajapakse, PhD[a], Abass Alavi, MD[a,*],
Mona-Elisabeth Revheim, MD, PhD, MHA[a,e,f]

KEYWORDS

• PET/CT • Total-body PET/CT • NaF • Osteoporosis • Global Disease Assessment

KEY POINTS

• ^{18}F-Sodium Fluoride (NaF)-PET/CT currently is one imaging method of many for the assessment and management of metabolic bone diseases, such as osteoporosis.
• Quantitative analysis using NaF-PET/CT has excelled in preliminary studies, when measuring osteoporotic disease burden.
• NaF-PET/CT quantification can be enhanced through adopting the usage of total-body PET/CT and global disease assessment, to best illustrate total osteoporotic disease activity.

INTRODUCTION

Bone remodeling is an important physiologic process for replacing old bone with newer and healthier bone. This remodeling process requires the constant activity of osteoclasts, which degrade old bone, and osteoblasts, which form new bone and whose activity decreases with age.[1] Relative declining bone growth and increasing bone removal, therefore, contribute to lower bone density and hence can cause metabolic bone diseases. The World Health Organization categorizes metabolic bone diseases by bone mineral density (BMD) in the spine, hip, or forearm evaluated by dual-energy x-ray absorptiometry (DXA).[2] Osteopenia, prevalent in 18 million Americans, is characterized by a T-score that falls between −1.0 and −2.5. Likewise, osteoporosis is characterized by a T-score of −2.5 or lower.[3]

DXA is one of the most common methods for diagnosing metabolic bone diseases by measuring BMD in vivo. DXA, however, which originally was intended for the postmenopausal population, who are naturally at high risk for fracture, is being utilized among all demographics and is limited to producing only 2-dimensional, low-resolution scans.[4] Although BMD as measured by DXA generally is correlated with fracture risk,

[a] Department of Radiology, Hospital of the University of Pennsylvania, Philadelphia, PA, USA; [b] Drexel University College of Medicine, Philadelphia, PA, USA; [c] Perelman School of Medicine at the University of Pennsylvania, Philadelphia, PA, USA; [d] Department of Internal Medicine, The Wright Center for Graduate Medical Education, Scranton, PA, USA; [e] Division of Radiology and Nuclear Medicine, Oslo University Hospital, Oslo, Norway; [f] Institute of Clinical Medicine, Faculty of Medicine, University of Oslo, Oslo, Norway
[1] Shared first-author.
* Corresponding author. 3400 Spruce Street, Philadelphia, PA 19104.
E-mail address: abass.alavi@pennmedicine.upenn.edu

PET Clin 15 (2020) 487–496
https://doi.org/10.1016/j.cpet.2020.06.011

the inability to examine bone structure, quality, and cortical and trabecular bone separately results in large variation in fracture risk between individuals with similar DXA scores.[5] Additionally, there are frequent errors in acquisition and analysis, such as external artifacts, artifacts caused by degenerative changes, artifacts from ingested medications overlying bone, improper positioning, and misplacement of the region of interest (ROI), which can result in misdiagnosis and improper treatment.[6] Apart from DXA, bone turnover also can be measured through bone biopsy after double tetracycline labeling, but this is less common due to its invasiveness.[7] In terms of molecular imaging, technetium-99m (^{99m}Tc) bone scintigraphy using single-photon emission computed tomography (SPECT) and bone turnover markers often are used to detect skeletal abnormalities, but ^{18}F-sodium fluoride (NaF), a radiotracer that reflects calcification and skeletal metabolism, may be more effective for identifying certain metabolic bone diseases.[8–11] Despite this, ^{99m}Tc bone scintigraphy still is more practical and widely used primarily because it is significantly cheaper, but NaF can be more accurate for localization of lesions by a significant margin.[10]

Osteoblastic activity can be traced by NaF through positron emission tomography/computed tomography (PET/CT). With a half-life of 110 minutes, NaF is injected and 50% is retained by bone and 30% by red blood cells after a single pass-through.[11] Bone marrow uptake is negligible and NaF can freely diffuse across membranes so that the incorporation of NaF in the bone matrix can represent osteoblastic activity, the bone remodeling process, and blood flow. Quantitative measurements of bone blood flow and metabolism derived from NaF imaging correlate well with bone turnover.[9] High bone uptake of the radiotracer after injection allows for prompt total-body imaging. Therefore, the future use of such total-body PET machines will further the ease and accuracy of diagnosis for such diseases in a time-efficient and accurate manner.[12,13]

Due to its rapid plasma clearance, NaF offers a noninvasive technique for assessing rate of bone turnover in areas of high fracture risk like the hip and spine but also in cortical, trabecular, and subchondral bone.[14] After administration, NaF binds to elements in the osseous metabolic microarchitecture of the bone tissue and thus has high uptake in regions of increased bone formation activity. NaF uptake can be quantified by standardized uptake values (SUVs) that are normalized to both tracer dosage and body weight.[15] A method through which specific bones can be measured, and only those bones of interest, is through the use of ROIs to eliminate extraneous regions. An example can be when the entire pelvic girdle of a sample subject is whittled down to just the pelvis itself, enabling simple SUV quantification (**Fig. 1**). The maximum SUV (SUVmax) often is reported for tumors in oncology because the distribution of uptake throughout the ROI can vary, but in osteoporosis, where the uptake is more uniform, mean SUV (SUVmean) is reported because the tracer is distributed rather homogeneously.[16]

The Hawkins method provides a quantitative analysis of tracer clearance after the first 60 minutes of injection.[17] To calculate the time-activity curve (TAC) for the concentration of tracer in the bone ROI and arterial blood, arterial input must be found. The gold standard for arterial input is taking a direct arterial blood line, but it also can be determined with an image input function from an ROI placed against the abdominal aorta or with a population-derived curve. Following this, the Hawkins model TACs describe the bone plasma flow to bone tissue and plasma clearance to bone mineral compartment. The Patlak plot is another method that assumes the total amount of tracer in the bone ROI to calculate bone plasma clearance. This plot graphically measures normalized bone uptake to normalized time and the concentration of uptake in the ROI and is calculated using an equation.[18]

The problem with using the Hawkins method is that scanning for 60 minutes at a single site is

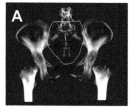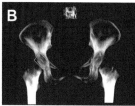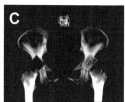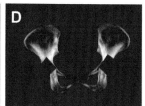

Fig. 1. Segmentation of the pelvic girdle. A maximum intensity projection of the CT scan with ROIs drawn to progressively remove the sacrum (*A*) and both femurs (*B and C*). From here, this CT scan (*D*) will be fused with the PET scan to allow for quantitative assessment of NaF uptake in the pelvis alone.

long and tedious and may lead to inaccurate scans. As an alternative to the Hawkins and Patlak methods, SUVs use a static scan that takes 5 minutes scans at each measurement site after NaF injection.[18] This inexpensive method allows for easy quantification of NaF uptake and does not require arterial sampling.

APPLICATION
Lumbar Spine

The lumbar spine is clinically reputed to have high intensity of osteoporosis. The lumbar spine is responsible for bearing the weight of the torso and head and is a common site for vertebral fractures. Bone growth weakens with age, causing fragile vertebral bones, possible scoliosis, and fractures due to increased weight stress and weak bone.[19] Postmenopausal women are more prone to osteoporosis, and NaF-PET has shown that the women who had osteoporotic T-values, versus osteopenic and normal levels, had lesser uptake in the lumbar spine.[20] Quantification of bone turnover typically is accomplished using SUVs or, alternatively, using the Hawkins method that calculates NaF clearance. Static PET scans acquire images 30 minutes and 60 minutes after injection and has been demonstrated to be the more accurate method for measuring NaF uptake in the bone.[21] Not only does NaF-PET show changes in certain bone diseases like osteoporosis but also it has been shown to have utility in other metabolic bone diseases like Paget disease.[22]

The most widely prescribed treatment of osteoporosis is bisphosphonates, and their effects in the lumbar spine can be monitored through NaF-PET/CT. Bisphosphonates, such as alendronate and risedronate, decrease bone resorption and bone ossification, but ossification decreases at a proportionally smaller rate, leading to increased overall bone growth.[23] A small study reported that SUV measurements from NaF-PET imaging of the lumbar spine, hip, and femoral region determined that the alendronate group was more effective in suppressing osteoblastic metabolism after discontinuation than risedronate, a finding that was further supported by measured BMD levels between the 2 groups and previous clinical studies.[24] The potential for observing and testing treatment in the lumbar spine using NaF-PET/CT can open new doors for diagnosing and treating metabolic bone diseases efficiently.

Hip

Decreased BMD in the hip can result in fractures that globally affect 18% of women and 6% of men and is associated with increased mortality.[25,26] Femoral neck fractures and intertrochanteric hip fractures are among the most common hip fractures due to the fragile cortex of the weight-bearing hip bone and progressive loss of bone tissue, which corresponds to the variable bone turnover rates throughout.[27] Cortical and trabecular bone has been shown to generate different uptake levels of NaF in the hip, due to the presence of microenvironments for bone formation, through biopsy and NaF-PET.[28–30] Frost and colleagues[31] have concluded that bone formation increases the most in the femoral shaft, than the total hip, pelvis, and spine as patients were treated with teriparatide, and that cortical bone was more sensitive to treatment than trabecular bone as measured with NaF-PET. DXA scanning found the exact opposite, with a greater increase in BMD after teriparatide therapy in trabecular bone compared with cortical, leading to the conclusion that perhaps increases in bone density may not necessarily translate to an increase in bone formation rate.

Certain treatments can be assessed by measuring bone turnover in the hip, pelvis, and femur. Uchida and colleagues[32] studied glucocorticoid-induced osteoporosis in the lumbar spine and femoral neck and gave alendronate to subjects over a 12-week period. In their study, the investigators found that SUV measurements using NaF-PET showed a decrease in osteoblastic metabolism, demonstrating that drug induced osteoporosis can be measured effectively with NaF-PET. Similarly, as discussed previously, antiresorptive agents, such as bisphosphonates, and anabolic agents, such as teriparatide, are common treatment therapies for osteoporosis that increase BMD and bone architecture and decrease fracture risk.[33] Thus, assessing treatment with NaF-PET can be utilized for measuring minute metabolic activity as a method of risk assessment for hip fractures.[34]

Tibia

The tibia is the most commonly fractured long bone in the body, typically fracturing after repetitive strain (stress fractures) or sudden major forces, such as those that occur in car accidents.[35–37] As a result, osteoporosis present in this bone tends to lead to the formation of fragility fractures, which can dramatically decrease the quality of life of patients, by forcing temporary disuse of the lower leg. Disuse occurs due to the forced immobilization of the limb, resulting from the placement of a lower leg cast.[38,39] This disuse then can compound the effects of osteoporosis by reducing BMD and further weakening the bone, thereby increasing patient susceptibility to future fractures.[40,41]

With the importance of the tibia noted, it thus is of great interest to study the effectiveness of NaF in quantifying regular or irregular bone formation in the tibia. In the existing literature, there remain 2 studies centered around NaF uptake in primarily the tibia. First, Wang and colleagues[42] have proved that in vivo molecular imaging centering around the tibia of osteoporotic rats can be effective. A significant decrease in NaF uptake was observed in the osteoporotic rat tibias, which confirmed the expectation that osteoporosis in the tibia would lead to decreased bone formation by osteoblasts. Likewise, Lundblad and colleagues[43] have come to a similar conclusion, through illustrating how NaF uptake is an accurate indicator of bone formation progression of the tibia in human subjects. Overall, both of these studies indicate a promising future for NaF-PET/CT in tracking tibia bone formation and thus possibly the effect of osteoporosis in the tibia.

Humerus

The humerus is the long bone of the upper arm. Given that the head of the humerus articulates with the glenoid cavity of the shoulder joint, the humerus is crucial for abduction of the arm and thus the basic motion of lifting the arm.[44,45] Despite its crucial function, the humerus remains one of the most commonly fractured bones in the body. These fractures typically either occur due to blunt trauma or pathologic risk factors, such as metastatic bone diseases or osteoporosis. Specifically, in the elderly, osteoporosis tends to be the underlying factor of the majority of the problems with the upper arm, because falls from an outstretched arm that lead to fracturing of the proximal humerus occur commonly.[46–49] The study of osteoporotic humeral bone is thus of great importance, given its clinical significance in the geriatric population.

With this said, few studies have used NaF-PET/CT to assess the humerus. Win and Aparici[50] calculated average normal SUVmax values of the humerus in normal skeletons, in order to effectively quantify and compare NaF uptake in the different bones of the body. In the humeral head, from 11 patients, the average normal SUVmax was found to be 1.82 with a range of 1.2 to 2.9, as determined by PET images reconstructed using ordered subset expectation maximization, with 2 iterative steps and 24 subsets obtained with a PET/CT scanner (GE Discovery STE 64-slice CT scanner; GE Healthcare, Waukesha, Wisconsin). From this standardized uptake of the healthy humerus, NaF uptake can be compared with osteoporotic bone and, therefore, assist in its diagnosis. Additionally, Wang and colleagues[42] have shown that NaF uptake is demonstrated in the humerus of rats and that it reaches a maximum level 60 minutes after injection. No significant difference was found, however, between NaF uptake in the humerus of osteoporotic rats compared with that of normal control rats. Regardless, no prospective studies have directly compared the expected difference in NaF uptake between the osteoporotic humerus and normal humerus in human subjects, therefore illustrating a future area of interest for NaF-PET/CT imaging of the skeletal system.

Calcaneus

The calcaneus, or heel bone, is a superficial osseous structure in the tarsus of the foot. Fracture of the calcaneus occurs most commonly from a fall from a height or a motor vehicle accident, and patients with low BMD are believed at higher risk for these injuries.[51] Only a few studies have attempted to use molecular imaging to examine the calcaneus. Link and colleagues[52] used magnetic resonance imaging (MRI) to investigate the calcaneus in 50 postmenopausal patients. Morphologic parameters, fractal dimensions, and BMD measured by high-resolution MRI (1.5T) were compared between 23 patients with low-energy osteoporotic hip fractures and 27 age-matched postmenopausal controls. For measurements performed in the axial plane, the fracture group was observed to have significantly lower bone volume–to–total volume ratio ($P = .0001$) and trabecular number ($P = .0019$) than controls. Moreover, fracture patients were noted to demonstrate significantly higher trabecular spacing in the calcaneus than controls ($P = .0018$), suggesting a major involvement of the calcaneus in osteoporosis.[52] Rebuzzi and colleagues[53] evaluated the potential of internal magnetic field gradient (IMFG) to quantify intertrabecular spacing to identify subjects as healthy, osteopenic, or osteoporotic, as classified by DXA scan; 55 women (8 healthy, 25 osteopenic, and 22 osteoporotic; mean age 62.9 ± 6.6 years) received MRI (3T) of the calcaneus. Calcaneal IMFG was found significantly different ($P<.01$, subtalar) between each cohort, suggesting the feasibility of IMFG to classify disease risk.[53] No studies have examined the association between osteoporosis and calcaneal NaF uptake by PET/CT. The aforementioned MRI studies demonstrate the involvement of the calcaneus in osteoporotic processes and, therefore, lay the foundation for future NaF-PET/CT studies into this osseous region.

TOTAL-BODY NaF-PET/CT

Currently, the gold standard for PET/CT imaging is whole-body scans using clinical PET systems covering an axial extension of 15 cm to 30 cm. These clinical PET/CT scanners rely on a single detector ring that moves up and down to create scans of the entire body in a single study. Given that this technology typically excludes 85% to 90% of the entire body outside of the field of view at any given time point and only uses a single detector ring (which misses much of the emitted ionizing radiation), the sensitivity remains relatively poor compared with other imaging modalities and region-specific PET/CT.[54,55] Furthermore, whole-body PET/CT imaging not only is time-consuming, due to the need to adequately position the single detector ring around every subsection of the body, but also requires a higher dose of radioactive tracer, because the single ring only occupies a small area and the signal decays rather.[56,57] Unsurprisingly, clinical use of whole-body PET/CT scanners also has been marred by concerns surrounding radiation exposure to patients.

The drawbacks of whole-body PET imaging in mind, Cherry and colleagues[12] and Badawi and colleagues[58] have developed a novel total-body PET/CT scanner, where proof-of-concept trials have shown increases in sensitivity, reductions in scanner time (to approximately 5 minutes vs almost an hour), and decreases in tracer dosage (by a factor of 10 to 20).[59] The last benefit is key, because decreasing tracer dosage by such a factor now can allow children and young adults to be scanned safely. This is crucial for the management and assessment of osteoporosis, given that, in the literature, not a single study has examined juvenile osteoporosis using whole-body NaF-PET/CT due to fears of excess radiation risk. Furthermore, this scanner significantly increases geometric coverage of the body, due to a longer axial field of view, which has been made possible due to advances in scintillation materials.

Even aside from these improvements, total-body PET/CT imaging of bone diseases holds several unique benefits over whole-body PET/CT imaging. First and foremost, whole-body PET/CT scanners remain a slight misnomer in that they typically scan only from the top of the cranium down to the mid-lower leg region; in other words, these scanners tend to exclude the foot and ankle region. As discussed previously, osteoporosis can induce fragility fractures in the calcaneus, creating a region of concern that cannot be assessed by whole-body PET/CT imaging.[60,61] In other words, whole-body NaF-PET/CT can assess only a

limited amount of osteoporotic bones, without tracking them all simultaneously and not allowing for dynamic total-body imaging. On the other hand, region-specific PET/CT can image each specific section of the body and eventually piece them together after quantitative analysis; however, this comes with its own drawbacks, such as the inability to study the body as an entire system in a single injection period. Furthermore, osteoarthritis and small joint arthritis are bone-related disorders that also have been successfully tracked and imaged using NaF-PET.[62–64] Because both these disorders also can affect the foot and ankle, they also are future areas of interest to study along with osteoporosis when using total-body NaF-PET/CT imaging. Secondly, a specific benefit of total-body NaF-PET/CT over whole-body NaF-PET/CT with regard to bone diseases is the vast increase in dynamic range: this allows for the radiotracer to be traced for an additional 5 to 6 half-lives on top of the original 3 half-lives of existing scanners. Specifically, for bone diseases, this could be useful by allowing the comparison of multitracer studies, where the radioactive signal of the first tracer would interfere minimally with that of the second.

In addition to metabolic bone diseases, PET-based methods have been proposed to assess a variety of benign musculoskeletal disorders. Bone formation as visualized with NaF has been proposed for assessing osteoarthritis,[65–70] rheumatoid arthritis,[14,64] ankylosing spondylitis,[71–73] bisphosphonate-associated osteonecrosis of the jaw,[74–76] and back pain.[77–79] Additionally, uptake of ^{18}F-fluorodeoxyglucose (FDG), a PET tracer that represents glycolytic activity, has demonstrated utility in assessing infection and inflammation in the musculoskeletal system. In particular, studies have used FDG-PET to visualize disease activity in inflammatory myopathies,[80–82] osteoarthritis,[83–86] rheumatoid arthritis,[87–89] prosthetic infections,[90–92] osteomyelitis and diabetic foot,[93–96] and polymyalgia rheumatica.[97–99] The authors believe that the advent of total-body PET/CT imaging can benefit clinical diagnosis of these musculoskeletal disorders in addition to metabolic bone diseases.

GLOBAL DISEASE ASSESSMENT

Previous PET studies have reported SUVmax as a measure for osteoporosis severity.[100] This measurement, however, is easily influenced by random variations caused by noise, scatter, scanner differences, and differences in ROI delineation. As such, SUVmax may vary widely among subjects, as well as within a single subject. Therefore, the authors

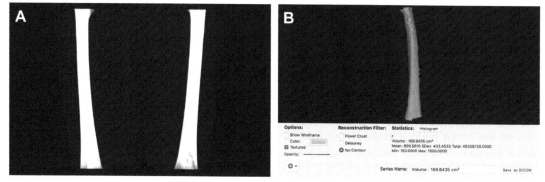

Fig. 2. Volumetric correction of the femur. A plain CT scan (A) followed by correction for volume (B) in a randomly selected patient. Such correction is needed due to variations in overall bone mass between different subjects, which can potentially skew overall SUVmean and SUVmax values..

believe that SUVmax is an oversimplification of the extent of osteoporosis.

In contrast, a global disease assessment offers a more sensitive and specific measurement of disease activity. In this methodology, the uptake measurements across an entire ROI, with ROIs along the entire length of an organ or lesion, are factored into a composite global disease score (GDS).[101] As such, an individual GDS as determined by PET imaging reproducible reflects the total disease burden. This methodology has been applied widely to pathologies from dementia to atherosclerosis.[102–104] More recently, the authors' laboratory has applied GDS toward degenerative bone pathologies using global SUVmean for NaF-PET/CT.[105] Combined with volumetric corrected SUV values, the authors believe that osteoporosis studies should employ NaF-PET/CT with global disease assessment to offer more robust insight into the total disease burden (Fig. 2).

SUMMARY

NaF-PET/CT is a sensitive and specific imaging modality to assess bone turnover in several skeletal regions. Preliminary research in age-related bone deterioration from the authors' laboratory has shown its efficacy in the assessment of a variety of regions, including the femoral neck, knee, hip, and spine in addition to musculoskeletal disorders. In large part due to the wide array of implicated skeletal structures, total-body imaging harbors significant advantages over whole-body or region-specific imaging in assessment of metabolic bone disorders, such as osteoporosis. Likewise, integrating metabolic and volumetric data to yield a single statistical, global disease assessment simply gives a more comprehensive view of actual uptake than alternative parameters, such as average SUVmax/SUVmean. Combining both,

prospective studies that measure osseous deposition with total-body NaF-PET/CT using global disease assessment are needed to further ascertain the true potential of this tool in quantification of osteoporotic burden.

DISCLOSURE

No conflicts of interest.

REFERENCES

1. Katsimbri P. The biology of normal bone remodelling. Eur J Cancer Care (Engl) 2017;26(6). https://doi.org/10.1111/ecc.12740.
2. Dimai HP. Use of dual-energy X-ray absorptiometry (DXA) for diagnosis and fracture risk assessment; WHO-criteria, T- and Z-score, and reference databases. Bone 2017;104:39–43.
3. Karaguzel G, Holick MF. Diagnosis and treatment of osteopenia. Rev Endocr Metab Disord 2010; 11(4):237–51.
4. Licata AA. Challenges of estimating fracture risk with DXA: changing concepts about bone strength and bone density. Aerosp Med Hum Perform 2015; 86(7):628–32.
5. Edwards M, Dennison E, Sayer AA, et al. Osteoporosis and sarcopenia in older age. Bone 2015;80: 126–30.
6. Morgan SL, Prater GL. Quality in dual-energy X-ray absorptiometry scans. Bone 2017;104:13–28.
7. Steller Wagner Martins C, Jorgetti V, Moysés RMA. Time to rethink the use of bone biopsy to prevent fractures in patients with chronic kidney disease. Curr Opin Nephrol Hypertens 2018;27(4):243–50.
8. Davila D, Antoniou A, Chaudhry MA. Evaluation of osseous metastasis in bone scintigraphy. Semin Nucl Med 2015;45(1):3–15.

9. Compston JE, Croucher PI. Histomorphometric assessment of trabecular bone remodelling in osteoporosis. Bone Mineral 1991;14(2):91–102.

10. Martin KJ, Olgaard K, Coburn JW, et al. Diagnosis, assessment, and treatment of bone turnover abnormalities in renal osteodystrophy. Am J Kidney Dis 2004;43(3):558–65.

11. Langsteger W, Rezaee A, Pirich C, et al. 18F-NaF-PET/CT and 99mTc-MDP bone scintigraphy in the detection of bone metastases in prostate cancer. Semin Nucl Med 2016;46(6):491–501.

12. Cherry SR, Badawi RD, Karp JS, et al. Total-body imaging: transforming the role of positron emission tomography. Sci Transl Med 2017;9(381). https://doi.org/10.1126/scitranslmed.aaf6169.

13. Abbasi J. Total-body PET scanner prototype due next year. JAMA 2017;318(2):116.

14. Jonnakuti VS, Raynor WY, Taratuta E, et al. A novel method to assess subchondral bone formation using [18F]NaF-PET in the evaluation of knee degeneration. Nucl Med Commun 2018;39(5):451–6.

15. Blake GM, Siddique M, Frost ML, et al. Imaging of site specific bone turnover in osteoporosis using positron emission tomography. Curr Osteoporos Rep 2014;12(4):475–85.

16. Blake GM, Siddique M, Frost ML, et al. Quantitative PET imaging using (18)F sodium fluoride in the assessment of metabolic bone diseases and the monitoring of their response to therapy. PET Clin 2012;7(3):275–91.

17. Blake GM, Puri T, Siddique M, et al. Site specific measurements of bone formation using [18F] sodium fluoride PET/CT. Quant Imaging Med Surg 2018;8(1):47–59.

18. Raijmakers P, Temmerman OPP, Saridin CP, et al. Quantification of 18F-fluoride kinetics: evaluation of simplified methods. J Nucl Med 2014;55(7):1122–7.

19. Siris ES, Adler R, Bilezikian J, et al. The clinical diagnosis of osteoporosis: a position statement from the National Bone Health Alliance Working Group. Osteoporos Int 2014;25(5):1439–43.

20. Frost ML, Fogelman I, Blake GM, et al. Dissociation between global markers of bone formation and direct measurement of spinal bone formation in osteoporosis. J Bone Miner Res 2004;19(11):1797–804.

21. Al-Beyatti Y, Siddique M, Frost ML, et al. Precision of 18F-fluoride PET skeletal kinetic studies in the assessment of bone metabolism. Osteoporos Int 2012;23(10):2535–41.

22. Installé J, Nzeusseu A, Bol A, et al. 18F-fluoride PET for monitoring therapeutic response in paget's disease of bone. J Nucl Med 2005;46(10):1650–8.

23. Tella SH, Gallagher JC. Prevention and treatment of postmenopausal osteoporosis. J Steroid Biochem Mol Biol 2014;142:155–70.

24. Frost ML, Siddique M, Blake GM, et al. Regional bone metabolism at the lumbar spine and hip following discontinuation of alendronate and risedronate treatment in postmenopausal women. Osteoporos Int 2012;23(8):2107–16.

25. LeBlanc KE, Muncie HL, LeBlanc LL. Hip fracture: diagnosis, treatment, and secondary prevention. Am Fam Physician 2014;89(12):945–51.

26. Veronese N, Maggi S. Epidemiology and social costs of hip fracture. Injury 2018;49(8):1458–60.

27. Reeve J, Loveridge N. The fragile elderly hip: mechanisms associated with age-related loss of strength and toughness. Bone 2014;61(100):138–48.

28. Puri T, Frost ML, Curran KM, et al. Differences in regional bone metabolism at the spine and hip: a quantitative study using 18F-fluoride positron emission tomography. Osteoporos Int 2013;24(2):633–9.

29. Pødenphant J, Engel U. Regional variations in histomorphometric bone dynamics from the skeleton of an osteoporotic woman. Calcif Tissue Int 1987;40(4):184–8.

30. Byers RJ, Denton J, Hoyland JA, et al. Differential patterns of altered bone formation in different bone compartments in established osteoporosis. J Clin Pathol 1999;52(1):23–8.

31. Frost ML, Siddique M, Blake GM, et al. Differential effects of teriparatide on regional bone formation using 18F-fluoride positron emission tomography. J Bone Miner Res 2011;26(5):1002–11.

32. Uchida K, Nakajima H, Miyazaki T, et al. Effects of alendronate on bone metabolism in glucocorticoid-induced osteoporosis measured by 18F-fluoride PET: a prospective study. J Nucl Med 2009;50(11):1808–14.

33. McClung MR, Martin JS, Miller PD, et al. Opposite bone remodeling effects of teriparatide and alendronate in increasing bone mass. Arch Intern Med 2005;165(15):1762–8.

34. Reilly CC, Raynor WY, Hong AL, et al. Diagnosis and monitoring of osteoporosis with 18F-sodium fluoride PET: an unavoidable path for the foreseeable future. Semin Nucl Med 2018;48(6):535–40.

35. Märdian S, Schwabe P, Schaser K-D. Fractures of the tibial shaft. Z Orthop Unfall 2015;153(1):99–117 [quiz: 118–9]. [in German].

36. Patel NK, Horstman J, Kuester V, et al. Pediatric tibial shaft fractures. Indian J Orthop 2018;52(5):522–8.

37. Schilcher J, Bernhardsson M, Aspenberg P. Chronic anterior tibial stress fractures in athletes: no crack but intense remodeling. Scand J Med Sci Sports 2019. https://doi.org/10.1111/sms.13466.

38. DeCoster TA, Nepola JV, el-Khoury GY. Cast brace treatment of proximal tibia fractures. A ten-year

follow-up study. Clin Orthop Relat Res 1988;231: 196–204.

39. Puno RM, Teynor JT, Nagano J, et al. Critical analysis of results of treatment of 201 tibial shaft fractures. Clin Orthop Relat Res 1986;(212): 113–21.

40. Bartl R, Bartl C. Immobilisation osteoporosis (disuse osteoporosis, disuse atrophy). In: Bone disorders. Cham (Switzerland): Springer International Publishing; 2017. p. 287–9. https://doi.org/10.1007/978-3-319-29182-6_43.

41. Gislason MK, Coupaud S, Sasagawa K, et al. Prediction of risk of fracture in the tibia due to altered bone mineral density distribution resulting from disuse: a finite element study. Proc Inst Mech Eng H 2014;228(2):165–74.

42. Wang P, Li Q-Z, Wang M-F. Biodistribution of (18)F-NaF as an imaging agent in osteoporotic rats for position emission tomography. Nan Fang Yi Ke Da Xue Xue Bao 2008;28(1):76–8 [in Chinese].

43. Lundblad H, Karlsson-Thur C, Maguire GQ, et al. Can spatiotemporal fluoride (18F−) uptake be used to assess bone formation in the tibia? A longitudinal study using PET/CT. Clin Orthop Relat Res 2017;475(5):1486–98.

44. Blache Y, Begon M, Michaud B, et al. Muscle function in glenohumeral joint stability during lifting task. PLoS One 2017;12(12):e0189406.

45. Spiguel AR, Steffner RJ. Humeral shaft fractures. Curr Rev Musculoskelet Med 2012;5(3):177–83.

46. Hertel R. Fractures of the proximal humerus in osteoporotic bone. Osteoporos Int 2005;16(Suppl 2): S65–72.

47. Jin J. Prevention of falls in older adults. JAMA 2018;319(16):1734.

48. Schumaier A, Grawe B. Proximal humerus fractures: evaluation and management in the elderly patient. Geriatr Orthop Surg Rehabil 2018;9. 215145851775051.

49. Khmelnitskaya E, Lamont LE, Taylor SA, et al. Evaluation and management of proximal humerus fractures. Adv Orthop 2012;2012:1–10.

50. Win AZ, Aparici CM. Normal SUV values measured from NaF18- PET/CT bone scan studies. PLoS One 2014;9(9):e108429.

51. Cheng S, Suominen H, Sakari-Rantala R, et al. Calcaneal bone mineral density predicts fracture occurrence: a five-year follow-up study in elderly people. J Bone Miner Res 1997;12(7): 1075–82.

52. Link TM, Majumdar S, Augat P, et al. In vivo high resolution MRI of the calcaneus: differences in trabecular structure in osteoporosis patients. J Bone Miner Res 1998;13(7):1175–82.

53. Rebuzzi M, Vinicola V, Taggi F, et al. Potential diagnostic role of the MRI-derived internal magnetic field gradient in calcaneus cancellous bone for evaluating postmenopausal osteoporosis at 3 T. Bone 2013;57(1):155–63.

54. Satoh Y, Imai M, Ikegawa C, et al. Dedicated breast PET versus whole-body PET/CT: a comparative study. J Nucl Med 2018;59(supplement 1):582.

55. Shortt CP, Gleeson TG, Breen KA, et al. Whole-body MRI versus PET in assessment of multiple myeloma disease activity. AJR Am J Roentgenol 2009;192(4):980–6.

56. Huang B, Law MW-M, Khong P-L. Whole-body PET/CT scanning: estimation of radiation dose and cancer risk. Radiology 2009;251(1):166–74.

57. Kaushik A, Jaimini A, Tripathi M, et al. Estimation of radiation dose to patients from (18) FDG whole body PET/CT investigations using dynamic PET scan protocol. Indian J Med Res 2015;142(6): 721–31.

58. Badawi RD, Shi H, Hu P, et al. First human imaging studies with the EXPLORER total-body PET scanner. J Nucl Med 2019;60(3):299–303.

59. Reardon S. Whole-body PET scanner produces 3D images in seconds. Nature 2019;570(7761):285–6.

60. Rupprecht M, Pogoda P, Barvencik F, et al. The calcaneus as the site of manifestation for osteoporosis-associated fractures: age- and sex-specific changes in calcaneal morphology correlate with the incidence and severity of intra-articular calcaneal fractures. Unfallchirurg 2007; 110(3):197–204 [in German].

61. Ito K, Hori K, Terashima Y, et al. Insufficiency fracture of the body of the calcaneus in elderly patients with osteoporosis: a report of two cases. Clin Orthop Relat Res 2004;422:190–4.

62. Cheng N, Raynor W, Werner T, et al. Assessment of degenerative joint disease with NaF PET. J Nucl Med 2016;57(supplement 2):375.

63. Savic D, Pedoia V, Seo Y, et al. Imaging bone-cartilage interactions in osteoarthritis using [18F]-NaF PET-MRI. Mol Imaging 2016;15:1–12.

64. Watanabe T, Takase-Minegishi K, Ihata A, et al. 18) F-FDG and (18)F-NaF PET/CT demonstrate coupling of inflammation and accelerated bone turnover in rheumatoid arthritis. Mod Rheumatol 2016;26(2):180–7.

65. Al-Zaghal A, Ayubcha C, Kothekar E, et al. Clinical applications of positron emission tomography in the evaluation of spine and joint disorders. PET Clin 2019;14(1):61–9.

66. Al-Zaghal A, Yellanki DP, Kothekar E, et al. Sacroiliac joint asymmetry regarding inflammation and bone turnover: assessment by FDG and NaF PET/CT. Asia Ocean J Nucl Med Biol 2019;7(2): 108–14.

67. Ayubcha C, Zirakchian Zadeh M, Stochkendahl MJ, et al. Quantitative evaluation of normal spinal osseous metabolism with 18F-NaF PET/CT. Nucl Med Commun 2018;39(10):945–50.

68. Al-Zaghal A, Yellanki DP, Ayubcha C, et al. CT-based tissue segmentation to assess knee joint inflammation and reactive bone formation assessed by 18F-FDG and 18F-NaF PET/CT: effects of age and BMI. Hell J Nucl Med 2018;21(2):102–7.

69. Kogan F, Fan AP, McWalter EJ, et al. PET/MRI of metabolic activity in osteoarthritis: a feasibility study. J Magn Reson Imaging 2017;45(6):1736–45.

70. Raynor W, Houshmand S, Gholami S, et al. Evolving role of molecular imaging with (18)F-sodium fluoride PET as a biomarker for calcium metabolism. Curr Osteoporos Rep 2016;14(4):115–25.

71. Lee S-G, Kim I-J, Kim K-Y, et al. Assessment of bone synthetic activity in inflammatory lesions and syndesmophytes in patients with ankylosing spondylitis: the potential role of 18F-fluoride positron emission tomography-magnetic resonance imaging. Clin Exp Rheumatol 2015;33(1):90–7.

72. Fischer DR, Pfirrmann CWA, Zubler V, et al. High bone turnover assessed by 18F-fluoride PET/CT in the spine and sacroiliac joints of patients with ankylosing spondylitis: comparison with inflammatory lesions detected by whole body MRI. EJNMMI Res 2012;2(1):38.

73. Bruijnen STG, van der Weijden MAC, Klein JP, et al. Bone formation rather than inflammation reflects ankylosing spondylitis activity on PET-CT: a pilot study. Arthritis Res Ther 2012;14(2):R71.

74. Guggenberger R, Fischer DR, Metzler P, et al. Bisphosphonate-induced osteonecrosis of the jaw: comparison of disease extent on contrast-enhanced MR imaging, [18F] fluoride PET/CT, and conebeam CT imaging. AJNR Am J Neuroradiol 2013;34(6):1242–7.

75. Wilde F, Steinhoff K, Frerich B, et al. Positron-emission tomography imaging in the diagnosis of bisphosphonate-related osteonecrosis of the jaw. Oral Surg Oral Med Oral Pathol Oral Radiol Endod 2009;107(3):412–9.

76. Raje N, Woo S-B, Hande K, et al. Clinical, radiographic, and biochemical characterization of multiple myeloma patients with osteonecrosis of the jaw. Clin Cancer Res 2008;14(8):2387–95.

77. Gamie S, El-Maghraby T. The role of PET/CT in evaluation of facet and disc abnormalities in patients with low back pain using (18)F-fluoride. Nucl Med Rev Cent East Eur 2008;11(1):17–21.

78. Lim R, Fahey FH, Drubach LA, et al. Early experience with fluorine-18 sodium fluoride bone PET in young patients with back pain. J Pediatr Orthop 2007;27(3):277–82.

79. Ovadia D, Metser U, Lievshitz G, et al. Back pain in adolescents: assessment with integrated 18F-fluoride positron-emission tomography-computed tomography. J Pediatr Orthop 2007. https://doi.org/10.1097/01.bpo.0000242438.11682.10.

80. Kothekar E, Raynor WY, Al-Zaghal A, et al. Evolving role of PET/CT-MRI in assessing muscle disorders. PET Clin 2019;14(1):71–9.

81. Sun L, Dong Y, Zhang N, et al. [18F]Fluorodeoxyglucose positron emission tomography/computed tomography for diagnosing polymyositis/dermatomyositis. Exp Ther Med 2018;15(6):5023–8.

82. Al-Nahhas A, Jawad ASM. PET/CT imaging in inflammatory myopathies. Ann N Y Acad Sci 2011;1228:39–45.

83. Ayubcha C, Zirakchian Zadeh M, Rajapakse C, et al. Effects of age and weight on the metabolic activities of the cervical, thoracic and lumbar spines as measured by fluorine-18 fluorodeoxyglucose-positron emission tomography in healthy males. Hell J Nucl Med 2018;21. https://doi.org/10.1967/s002449910700.

84. Saboury B, Parsons MA, Moghbel M, et al. Quantification of aging effects upon global knee inflammation by 18F-FDG-PET. Nucl Med Commun 2016;37(3):254–8.

85. Parsons MA, Moghbel M, Saboury B, et al. Increased 18F-FDG uptake suggests synovial inflammatory reaction with osteoarthritis: preliminary in-vivo results in humans. Nucl Med Commun 2015;36(12):1215–9.

86. Hong YH, Kong EJ. (18F)Fluoro-deoxy-D-glucose uptake of knee joints in the aspect of age-related osteoarthritis: a case-control study. BMC Musculoskelet Disord 2013;14:141.

87. Raynor WY, Jonnakuti VS, Zadeh MZ, et al. Comparison of methods of quantifying global synovial metabolic activity with FDG-PET/CT in rheumatoid arthritis. Int J Rheum Dis 2019;22(12):2191–8.

88. Lee SJ, Jeong JH, Lee C-H, et al. Development and validation of an 18 F-fluorodeoxyglucose-positron emission tomography with computed tomography-based tool for the evaluation of joint counts and disease activity in patients with rheumatoid arthritis. Arthritis Rheumatol 2019;71(8):1232–40.

89. Mountz JM, Alavi A, Mountz JD. Emerging optical and nuclear medicine imaging methods in rheumatoid arthritis. Nat Rev Rheumatol 2012;8(12):719–28.

90. Kwee TC, Basu S, Alavi A. The ongoing misperception that labeled leukocyte imaging is superior to 18F-FDG PET for diagnosing prosthetic joint infection. J Nucl Med 2017;58(1):182.

91. Basu S, Kwee TC, Saboury B, et al. FDG-PET for diagnosing infection in hip and knee prostheses: prospective study in 221 prostheses and subgroup comparison with combined 111In-labeled leukocyte/99mTc- sulfur colloid bone marrow imaging in 88 prostheses. Clin Nucl Med 2014;39(7):609–15.

92. Stumpe KDM, Nötzli HP, Zanetti M, et al. FDG PET for differentiation of infection and aseptic loosening in total hip replacements: comparison with conventional radiography and three-phase bone scintigraphy. Radiology 2004;231(2):333–41.

93. Al-Zaghal A, Raynor W, Khosravi M, et al. Applications of PET imaging in the evaluation of musculoskeletal diseases among the geriatric population. Semin Nucl Med 2018;48(6):525–34.

94. Kagna O, Srour S, Melamed E, et al. FDG PET/CT imaging in the diagnosis of osteomyelitis in the diabetic foot. Eur J Nucl Med Mol Imaging 2012; 39(10):1545–50.

95. Nawaz A, Torigian DA, Siegelman ES, et al. Diagnostic performance of FDG-PET, MRI, and plain film radiography (PFR) for the diagnosis of osteomyelitis in the diabetic foot. Mol Imaging Biol 2010;12(3):335–42.

96. Basu S, Chryssikos T, Houseni M, et al. Potential role of FDG PET in the setting of diabetic neuro-osteoarthropathy: can it differentiate uncomplicated Charcot's neuroarthropathy from osteomyelitis and soft-tissue infection? Nucl Med Commun 2007;28(6):465–72.

97. Palard-Novello X, Querellou S, Gouillou M, et al. Value of (18)F-FDG PET/CT for therapeutic assessment of patients with polymyalgia rheumatica receiving tocilizumab as first-line treatment. Eur J Nucl Med Mol Imaging 2016;43(4):773–9.

98. Takahashi H, Yamashita H, Kubota K, et al. Differences in fluorodeoxyglucose positron emission tomography/computed tomography findings between elderly onset rheumatoid arthritis and polymyalgia rheumatica. Mod Rheumatol 2015;25(4):546–51.

99. Rehak Z, Vasina J, Nemec P, et al. Various forms of (18)F-FDG PET and PET/CT findings in patients with polymyalgia rheumatica. Biomed Pap Med Fac Univ Palacky Olomouc Czech Repub 2015; 159(4):629–36.

100. Shin D-S, Shon O-J, Byun S-J, et al. Differentiation between malignant and benign pathologic fractures with F-18-fluoro-2-deoxy-D-glucose positron emission tomography/computed tomography. Skeletal Radiol 2008;37(5):415–21.

101. Høilund-Carlsen PF, Edenbrandt L, Alavi A. Global disease score (GDS) is the name of the game! Eur J Nucl Med Mol Imaging 2019;46(9):1768–72.

102. Alavi A, Newberg AB, Souder E, et al. Quantitative analysis of PET and MRI data in normal aging and Alzheimer's disease: atrophy weighted total brain metabolism and absolute whole brain metabolism as reliable discriminators. J Nucl Med 1993; 34(10):1681–7.

103. Blomberg BA, Thomassen A, de Jong PA, et al. Coronary fluorine-18-sodium fluoride uptake is increased in healthy adults with an unfavorable cardiovascular risk profile: results from the CAMONA study. Nucl Med Commun 2017;38(11):1007–14.

104. Borja AJ, Hancin EC, Zhang V, et al. Potential of PET/CT in assessing dementias with emphasis on cerebrovascular disorders. Eur J Nucl Med Mol Imaging 2020. https://doi.org/10.1007/s00259-020-04697-y.

105. Raynor W, Houshmand S, Gholami S, et al. Assessment of bone turnover by measuring global uptake of 18F-sodium fluoride in the femoral neck, a novel method for early detection of osteoporosis. J Nucl Med 2016;57(supplement 2):1769.

Applications of Hybrid PET/Magnetic Resonance Imaging in Central Nervous System Disorders

Austin J. Borja, BA[a,b,1], Emily C. Hancin, MS, BA[a,c,1], Mohsen Khosravi, MD[d], Rina Ghorpade, MD[a], Benjamin Koa, BS[a,e], Xuan Miao, BA[a], Thomas J. Werner, MS[a], Andrew B. Newberg, MD[d,f], Abass Alavi, MD[a,*]

KEYWORDS

- MR imaging • FDG • Alzheimer disease • Mini–mental State Examination • Amyloid-β protein
- Florbetapir • Mild cognitive impairment • PET

KEY POINTS

- Fused PET/magnetic resonance (MR) imaging may be used to diagnose and assess a wide array of central nervous system disorders.
- PET/MR imaging shows clear advantages compared with purely structural imaging modalities.
- Global disease assessment is a robust and reproducible quantitative 18F-fluorodeoxyglucose PET methodology.

INTRODUCTION

Disorders of the central nervous system (CNS) are among the most debilitating medical conditions, because they can affect people's ability to complete daily tasks, think critically, and direct the movement of their limbs.[1,2] The CNS directs neuronal transmission to and from the periphery and the brain, and therefore CNS disorders can diminish the function of the brain and other organ systems.[1,3,4] Purely structural imaging techniques, such as magnetic resonance (MR) imaging and computed tomography (CT), are widely used in the diagnosis of CNS disorders.[5,6] However, structural changes represent the final changes of neurodegenerative disease, at which point no therapies may be useful in reversing the damage (**Fig. 1**).[7–9] Recent literature shows that PET has excellent sensitivity and specificity in the early detection of neurodegenerative disorders on the molecular level.[10,11] The major advantage of PET compared with MR imaging is the ability to explore molecular tracers associated with various disease processes. Neurotransmitter tracers associated with molecules such as dopamine, serotonin, or glutamine, as well as disease-related tracers that bind to amyloid, tau, or various cellular messaging molecules, provide the ability of PET to evaluate the underlying pathophysiology of specific diseases. Combining this capability of PET imaging

[a] Department of Radiology, Hospital of the University of Pennsylvania, 3400 Spruce Street, Philadelphia, PA 19104, USA; [b] Perelman School of Medicine at the University of Pennsylvania, 3400 Civic Center Blvd, Philadelphia, PA 19104, USA; [c] Lewis Katz School of Medicine at Temple University, 3500 N Broad St, Philadelphia, PA 19140, USA; [d] Department of Radiology, Thomas Jefferson University, 901 Walnut St, Philadelphia, PA, USA; [e] Drexel University College of Medicine, 2900 West Queen Lane, Philadelphia, PA 19129, USA; [f] Department of Integrative Medicine and Nutritional Sciences, Thomas Jefferson University, 901 Walnut St, Philadelphia, PA, USA
[1] sharing co-first authorship.
* Corresponding author. Department of Radiology, Hospital of the University of Pennsylvania, 3400 Spruce Street, Philadelphia, PA 19104, USA.
E-mail address: abass.alavi@pennmedicine.upenn.edu

PET Clin 15 (2020) 497–508
https://doi.org/10.1016/j.cpet.2020.06.004
1556-8598/20/© 2020 Elsevier Inc. All rights reserved.

pet.theclinics.com

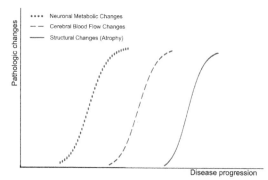

Fig. 1. The sequence of biological changes that occur during neurodegenerative diseases. Disease begins at the molecular and cellular level, including atherosclerotic plaques or protein accumulation. This stage gradually leads to changes in blood flow in the brain. In addition, structural alterations occur decades into the disease process. Therefore, molecular imaging techniques that detect early evidence for neurodegenerative disease, such as calcification and inflammation, are essential for diagnosis and treatment years before the presence of structural abnormalities.

with MR imaging can help better localize findings, as was shown more than a decade ago, using various data obtained from a joint PET measurement tool and 3-T MR imaging system.[12] In addition, functional MR imaging that evaluates functional connectivity or diffusion and fiber tracts can be combined with PET imaging in effective ways to delineate disease processes. Therefore, in this article, we show the superiority of PET/MR imaging compared with structural imaging modalities for the identification and treatment of CNS disorders.

CONVENTIONAL MAGNETIC RESONANCE IMAGING/STRUCTURAL IMAGING VERSUS FUSED PET/MAGNETIC RESONANCE IMAGING

MR imaging has greater spatial resolution than other structural imaging modalities, such as CT, in the delineation of most anatomic structures.[13] As a diagnostic tool, MR imaging has shown feasibility in a wide variety of disorders, from acute CNS diseases such as transient ischemic attacks to cancers, including small hepatocellular carcinoma.[14,15] For example, Poels and colleagues[16] used MR imaging alongside arterial pulse wave velocity to examine the association between arterial stiffness and small vessel disease. Increased arterial stiffness as detected by arterial pulse wave velocity was significantly associated with a larger volume of white matter lesions as detected by MR imaging, and this correlation was independent

of cardiovascular risk factors.[16] MR imaging has also been used in the identification and treatment of vascular cognitive impairment, and, when combined with MR angiography, has shown utility in identifying the location of symptomatic and asymptomatic strokes. Nonetheless, there have been many studies conducted to compare MR imaging and CT to identify the superior diagnostic tool. For example, Chen and colleagues[17] compared MR imaging and CT to determine which technique was better suited for identifying subsegmental artery pulmonary embolisms. They determined that MR imaging had significantly higher sensitivity and specificity in recognizing pulmonary embolisms, although CT still performed well in these areas. Wang and colleagues[14] compared CT with MR imaging in the diagnosis of small hepatocellular carcinoma, and they showed that MR imaging was superior to CT in diagnostic accuracy, sensitivity, and specificity, which suggests that MR imaging and its applications may have advantages compared with CT in radiologic imaging.

MR imaging and CT have been used to identify degenerative diseases, but structural changes represent the final pathologic stages of many of these diseases, at which point the damage present is irreversible.[9,12] Thus, although MR imaging is preferred to CT for nontraumatic, structural brain imaging, the incorporation of PET may prove superior in the assessment and quantification of brain function.[18] For example, an early study by Kubota and colleagues[19] determined that 18F-fluorodeoxyglucose (FDG) PET has a higher specificity, accuracy, and positive predictive value in detecting the recurrence of head and neck cancers following organ-sparing radiochemotherapy than MR imaging/CT. A related method, fused FDG-PET/CT, incorporates CT into the FDG-PET modality, and it is an established, cost-effective technology that is used worldwide in a wide range of oncologic and inflammatory disorders.[20] Additional research with PET/CT identified NaF as a superior tracer in examining the development of atherosclerosis and bone turnover.[21,22] Therefore, it is evident that PET/CT has great potential in the identification of a myriad of diseases.

In contrast with PET/CT, PET/MR imaging is an emerging technology that capitalizes on the distinct advantages of MR imaging compared with CT, including decreased radiation dose and improved motion correction.[22] Of note, PET/MR imaging offers superior soft tissue resolution compared with PET/CT, and PET/MR imaging has been applied to a variety of soft tissue malignancies. For example, Salamon and colleagues[23] showed the feasibility and superiority of PET/MR imaging in the detection and subsequent cortical dysplasia in a 45 patient cohort. In addition, Chandra and colleagues[24] used PET/MR imaging to assess the epileptogenic and nonepileptogenic brain lesions in 15 students with tuberous sclerosis. Although infectious and inflammatory processes have traditionally been assessed by PET/CT, PET/MR imaging may offer similar sensitivity and specificity with substantially decreased radiation dosage. Matthews and colleagues[25] showed the feasibility of PET/MR imaging in 7 diabetic patients. Zandieh and colleagues[26] used PET/MRI to examine cardiac sarcoidosis in 7 patients. Taken together, these studies suggest that PET/MR imaging is useful to evaluate inflammatory conditions. This finding is of particular importance in populations at increased sensitivity to radiation, such as pediatric patients. Therefore, additional research may be designed to show the feasibility of PET/MR imaging in these at-risk populations.

Carlbom and colleagues[27] determined that diffusion-weighted whole-body MR imaging could not compare with the diagnostic accuracy of 5-hydroxytryptophan (HTP) PET/CT, but they did confirm that MR imaging detected more liver metastases than 5-HTP PET/CT. This finding may indicate a place for a combined role of PET and MR imaging as a clinical diagnostic tool. Huang and colleagues[28] compared the efficacy of FDG-PET/MR imaging, FDG-PET/CT, MR imaging, and CT in determining the extent of the expansion of advanced buccal squamous cell carcinoma. FDG-PET/MR imaging had the highest likelihood ratio, sensitivity, and specificity compared with all the other techniques studied, which attests to the power of PET/MR imaging as a diagnostic imaging modality. Platzek and colleagues[29] used PET/MR imaging in 20 patients with head and neck malignancies. Fused PET/MR imaging was more sensitive in the detection of the main cancerous lesion and within seeded lymph nodes than either PET or MR alone. Other groups have applied PET/MR imaging to neoplasms of the lung parenchyma, gastrointestinal structures, and gynecologic organs.[30–33] Taken together, these studies suggest that PET/MR imaging has a wide range of potential diagnostic utility. More recently, PET/MR imaging has shown utility in the whole-body staging of recurrent breast cancer. As shown by Sawicki and colleagues,[34] FDG-PET/MR imaging correctly confirmed breast cancer in 17 out of 17 patients who presented with symptoms of suspected recurrence. Tate and colleagues[35] used PET-MR imaging to successfully identify both functional and morphologic bone marrow abnormalities in patients with plasma cell dyscrasias, to further understand the utility of PET-MR imaging in myeloma diagnostics. Recently, Freitag and colleagues[36] determined that PET/MR imaging significantly outperformed PET/CT in identifying bone and lymph node metastases in patients with prostate cancer.[37] Moving forward, future research is warranted to better show the superiority of PET/MR imaging compared with existing standard imaging modalities in the assessment of certain disease states.

ALZHEIMER DISEASE AND GLOBAL DISEASE ASSESSMENT

Alzheimer disease (AD) is an irreversible neurodegenerative disorder that leads to progressive memory and cognitive dysfunction.[38] An estimated 5.4 million Americans have AD, and the prevalence of this devastating disease is expected to increase incrementally.[39] AD is preceded for years to decades by mild cognitive impairment (MCI), in which patients first display memory loss and forgetfulness.[40] Although patients with MCI often develop dementia, MCI does not show the gross cerebral wasting of AD.[41] As such, purely structural and amyloid-based imaging modalities have shown limited efficacy in the assessment and quantification of MCI.[42] In contrast, fused PET imaging is greatly superior to purely structural modalities, because it can monitor the detriments to glucose uptake in various neurologic regions that have been associated with the progression of conditions such as AD.[43] Therefore, there exists a need for molecular imaging techniques such as PET/MR that can detect the metabolic changes in early MCI. Our group is currently examining PET images of the brain in patients with MCI and AD to confirm the utility of molecular imaging in the assessment of these disorders (**Fig. 2**).

On histology, AD is diagnosed by the stereotypical localization of beta-amyloid plaques, intraneuronal neurofibrillary tangles, and neuronal loss.[44] These pathologic changes are present in cortical regions in the early stages of the disease process and progressively move to subcortical structures.[45] The onset of these biomarkers has been shown to precede dementia by decades.[46] 18F-florbetapir, a radiopharmaceutical that binds beta-amyloid, was developed as a PET agent for use in AD pathology.[47,48] However, numerous studies indicate that florbetapir is inferior to FDG-PET.[49] In 2012, Newberg and colleagues[50] showed that florbetapir could not be correlated to the Mini–mental State Examination (MMSE) of patients with known AD. Similarly, Khosravi and colleagues[11] confirmed that FDG-PET is more strongly associated with cognitive function assessed by MMSE in MCI and AD than florbetapir (**Fig. 3**). Given these substantial pieces of

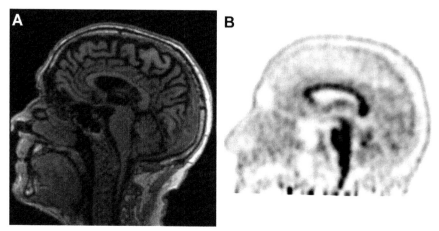

Fig. 2. Sagittal images of (A) MR and (B) PET in a patient with AD. For global disease assessment, it is planned to quantify FDG uptake across the entire cerebral cortex (global mean standardized uptake value) to measure the effect on brain metabolism and cognitive function.

evidence, the authors endorse the use of FDG imaging techniques such as PET-MR for the detection and management of MCI and AD.

Recently, the authors have challenged maximal standardized uptake value (SUVmax) as an oversimplified measure of brain function. Instead, we argue that global FDG-PET assessment is the most sensitive and reproducible methodology to measure brain function in patients with MCI/AD. Global disease assessment was first described by Alavi and colleagues[51] regarding FDG-PET/MR imaging analysis in MCI and AD. More recently, global disease score assessed by average SUVmean has been highlighted as an accurate and reproducible model for disease assessment moving forward.[52]

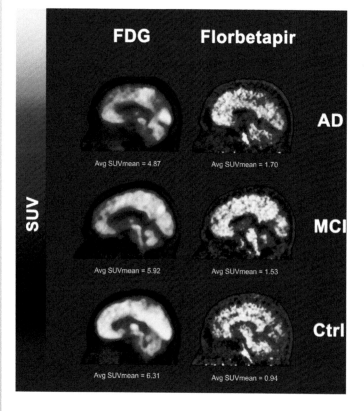

Fig. 3. Standardized uptake values (SUVs) in FDG-PET and 18F-florbetapir images of the brain in healthy controls (Ctrl), patients with MCI, and patients with AD, showing the superiority of FDG-PET/CT.

The authors believe that PET/MR imaging can be used in the evaluation of global disease assessment, and that it can have widespread impacts on patient health because of the development of comorbidities that may be morphologically unremarkable for an extended period. As such, we recommend the use of global FDG-PET/MR imaging to evaluate the extent of cognitive dysfunction in patients with MCI/AD.

CEREBROVASCULAR DISEASE

Progressive cardiovascular diseases may have a deleterious influence on the perfusion of cerebral blood vessels. This process is particularly harmful to the brain because it is one of the structures in the body that is least tolerant of ischemic conditions, because of its high metabolic demands.[53] For example, Pase Matthew and colleagues[54] used participants from the Framingham General Cardiovascular Risk Profile to assess blood velocity in both the common carotid and middle cerebral arteries using Doppler. They determined that patients with cardiovascular risk showed higher pulsatile and lower mean flow velocity in both vessels, effects that may contribute to cerebral dysfunction. Consequently, diagnostic technologies must continue to improve to hone the early identification of cardiovascular diseases to prevent progressive deterioration of global brain function. Because MR imaging can assess the morphologic features of plaque development, and several PET tracers, such as NaF and FDG, show increased uptake in atherosclerotic plaques, the 2 modalities should be used concurrently to better identify these calcifications.[55–57] Accordingly, PET/MR imaging may be a powerful candidate to understand the complex relationship between cardiovascular health and cognitive performance.

Cerebral blood flow is also particularly important to physicians looking to identify candidates for systemic thrombolysis outside of the standard 4.5-hour window following the development of ischemic stroke.[58] Thus, it is imperative to establish an effective imaging technique to accurately determine the level of detriment to cerebral perfusion in patients before the administration of particular therapies. Werner and colleagues[58] determined that PET/MR imaging using [15-O] H_2O as a tracer for cerebral perfusion may be a more powerful modality than MR imaging alone in prospectively identifying candidates for thrombolysis treatment. Furthermore, PET/MR imaging has been used to differentiate between ischemic and hemorrhagic strokes, which can help clinicians in deciding the correct course of action in resolving these pathologic developments. Because stroke recovery largely depends on the length of time required to resolve the infarct, using PET/MR imaging as a guide to monitor cerebral perfusion may have the potential to improve functional recovery in these patients.[59]

Age-related cognitive impairment is caused by a significant overlap between AD and vascular dementia. Preliminary evidence from our group has shown that patients with cardiovascular risk factors show decreased cerebral activity as assessed by FDG-PET (**Fig. 4**).[9] As such, we believe that drugs to treat the underlying vascular disruption offer a therapeutic opportunity to curb the cognitive dysfunction in patients with both cardiovascular risk factors and dementia.

SEIZURE DISORDERS

Although MR imaging has been used as the modality of choice for patients with epilepsy, it cannot always identify morphologic lesions that would otherwise aid in identifying the epileptogenic zone. In addition, existing standards of brain imaging, such as ictal-interictal single-photon emission computed tomography in epilepsy, rely on the presence of seizure activity to detect abnormal areas of brain function, whereas PET/MR imaging can identify these regions in the absence of seizure activity, which may be helpful in clinical diagnostics (**Fig. 5**).[12] Because FDG-PET can measure changes in glucose uptake, it can be used to reflect neuronal abnormalities such as hypometabolism, which can help to recognize epileptic lesions that would otherwise be untraceable on MR imaging alone to direct clinicians in identifying regions of the brain suitable for surgical resection.[60,61] Several studies have shown that PET/MR imaging as a combined technique provides additional specificity in achieving this goal. For example, Rubi and colleagues[62] examined the utility of FDG-PET/MR imaging in epileptogenic zone detection in 31 children with MR imaging nonlesional refractory epilepsy. They concluded that PET/MR imaging was at least as accurate as PET alone in detecting the epileptogenic zone in pediatric patients with nonappreciable morphologic differences on MR imaging. Shin and colleagues[63] used PET/MR imaging, PET/CT, and MR imaging alone to localize anatomic and functional lesions in patients undergoing epilepsy surgery evaluation.[64] They determined that PET/MR imaging had an increased yield in identifying potential epileptic abnormalities compared with MR imaging and PET/CT. In addition, Shang and colleagues[65] were successful in using PET/MR imaging and

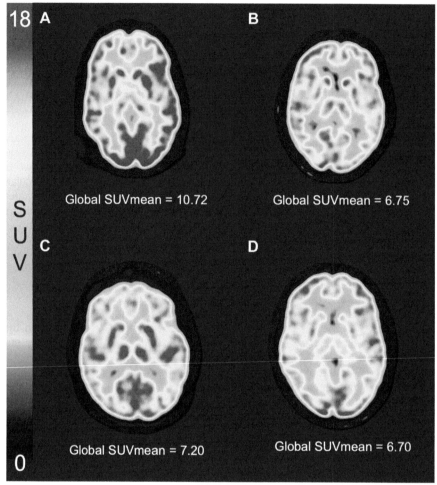

Fig. 4. FDG-PET/CT images and global SUVmean of the brain in (A) a young healthy control, (B) a young patient presenting with cardiovascular risk factors, (C) an old healthy control, and (D) an old patient presenting with cardiovascular risk factors. Green areas show decreased global brain metabolism, which is present in patients with cardiovascular risk factors. (Reproduced with permission from Borja et al.[9])

arterial spin labeling to localize the epileptogenic zone in patients with MR imaging negative for temporal lobe epilepsy. Taken together, these studies show the feasibility and advantages of PET/MR imaging in epilepsy and seizure disorders.

BRAIN TUMORS

PET/MR imaging has shown potential utility in the assessment of brain tumors, particularly in the setting of pediatric patients who are more vulnerable to harmful effects of radiation from CT imaging (**Fig. 6**).[66] Various tracers have been identified as being capable of crossing the blood-brain barrier to accomplish imaging in patients with these disorders. Schaarschmidt and colleagues[67] compared the efficacy of FDG-PET/

MR imaging with FDG-PET/CT and MR imaging in the staging of histopathologically confirmed head and neck squamous cell carcinoma, and they found no significant differences in diagnostic accuracy among the 3 techniques, which suggests that FDG-PET/MR imaging has the potential to match the power of existing imaging modalities. Diagnostic accuracy is also of critical importance in the therapeutic approach to brain tumors, and, because many types of brain cancer can appear similar on MR images, a modality such as fused PET/MR imaging that can identify both structural and functional abnormalities in disease regions can help clinicians in establishing suitable treatment plans for patients.[61] Filss and colleagues[68] determined that, in patients with cerebral glioma, 18F-fluoroethyl-L-tyrosinePET showed higher target-to-background ratios and larger tumor

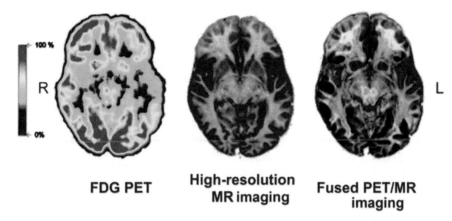

FDG PET **High-resolution MR imaging** **Fused PET/MR imaging**

Fig. 5. PET/MR imaging study in a patient with epilepsy. (*Left*) Axial PET scan obtained 60 to 75 minutes after injection of FDG. (*Center*) High-resolution MR imaging scan. (*Right*) Fused FDG-PET/MR imaging scan. These images reflect decreased metabolic activity in the polar region of the left temporal lobe. Data acquired on Biograph mMR scanner at Nuklearmedizinische Klinik und Poliklinik der Technischen Universität München. (Reproduced with permission from Catana et al.[12])

volumes than measurements of cerebral blood volume through perfusion-weighted MR imaging in a study of 56 patients with glioma. Sacconi and colleagues[69] used combined PET/MR imaging to establish tumor grades and determine treatment-induced changes to the brain tissue in patients with brain tumors. Perfusion-weighted imaging alone showed high diagnostic accuracy, whereas FDG-PET alone showed low diagnostic accuracy (90% vs 40% for low-grade tumors and 94.1% vs 55.6% for distinguishing treatment-induced effects from recurrent tumors). Deuschl and colleagues[70] also used PET/MR imaging, using 11C-methionine (MET) as a tracer, to determine its efficacy at distinguishing between treatment-induced effects and recurrent tumors in 50 patients with glioma. MET-PET/MR imaging showed higher diagnostic accuracy than MR imaging alone, as well as higher diagnostic confidence scales than in PET or MR imaging alone, in identifying glioma recurrence, which indicates

that PET/MR imaging may have great potential in this field. Taken together, these data suggest that FDG-PET and MR imaging have separate but clinically relevant strengths that, when combined, may establish a more effective method of classifying cancerous growths within brain tissue.

RADIOLABELED NEUROTRANSMITTERS

Radiolabeled neurotransmitter imaging is a powerful method that can be used in the diagnosis and surveillance of mood disorders. Although PET/MR imaging has not been extensively used as a modality by which to monitor the uptake of radiolabeled neurotransmitters, the existing data present an exciting potential avenue for the direction of future PET/MR imaging studies. For example, Tiger and colleagues[71] used PET alone to monitor serotonin-1B (5-HT1B) binding in the brains of patients with major depressive disorder. 5-HT1B binding in the anterior cingulate cortex, subgenual

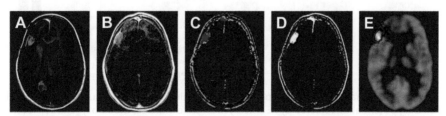

Fig. 6. Brain images from a 17-year-old girl with glioblastoma multiforme who relapsed during active treatment. (*A*) Baseline T1 contrast-enhanced MR imaging, (*B*) T1 permeability image, (*C*) T1 permeability map (Kpsmax, 27.539), (*D*) T1 permeability registered with FDG-PET study (registration grade, excellent), (*E*) and FDG-PET studies (T/Wmax, 8.788). (Reproduced with permission from Zukotynski et al.[66])

prefrontal cortex, and the hippocampus of individuals with major depressive disorder was significantly lower than the binding in these regions in healthy patients, which suggests that deficits in 5-HT1B binding may be associated with the clinical presentation of major depressive disorder. These findings may indicate a potential for fused PET/MR imaging, as opposed to PET alone, to be used to further understanding in this area of research. Wey and colleagues[72] used PET/functional MR (fMR) imaging and 11C-diprenorphine in a small study of 8 healthy volunteers to evaluate opioid neurotransmission and hemodynamic changes in response to painful stimuli. PET/fMR imaging successfully identified responses to pain in both the thalamus and the striatum (**Fig. 7**). Karjalainen and colleagues[73] also investigated the accuracy of PET/fMR imaging in identifying type 2 dopamine and mu-opioid receptor responses to visual observation of painful stimuli, using a cohort of 35 subjects. Availability of the type 2 dopamine receptor was not correlated with hemodynamic responses to visualizing painful stimuli, but the availability of the mu-opioid receptor was positively correlated with orbitofrontal hemodynamic responses and negatively correlated with hemodynamic responses in the anterior insulae, thalamus, and several other regions of the brain, which suggests a major role for the mu-opioid receptor in the neurologic response to vicarious pain. The success of PET and PET/fMR imaging in the aforementioned studies indicates that fused PET/MR imaging may have the potential to improve on existing imaging modalities to more accurately monitor the uptake of neurotransmitters to regions of the brain and detect pathologic abnormalities associated with several psychiatric disorders.

TRAUMATIC BRAIN INJURY

Traumatic brain injury (TBI) is associated with decreased glucose metabolism in brain tissue.[74,75] Therefore, PET can also be used to diagnose and monitor TBI in affected patients. Furthermore, although MR imaging and CT are the most widely used imaging techniques for evaluating the damage associated with these injuries, they are limited in that many TBIs present without any observable morphologic change, presenting instead with headaches, light sensitivity, forgetfulness, and difficulty adhering to tasks.[76,77] Although the potential for the combined molecular and morphologic powers of PET and MR imaging, respectively, to be used within this field is promising, few studies have used PET/MR imaging to investigate TBIs. Brabazon and colleagues[78] used FDG-PET/MR imaging and histologic examination to evaluate the effects of controlled cortical impact injuries on rats. They observed increased cytotoxic and vasogenic edema using MR imaging and increased FDG uptake in the corpus callosum, hippocampus, and amygdala. Importantly, they also determined that FDG-PET could identify glial cell activation but was confounded by cell damage, whereas MR imaging could identify cell damage but was confounded by glial cell activation; this suggests that combining these 2 imaging modalities may be a powerful step forward in the evaluation of TBIs. Furthermore, Fujita and colleagues[79] used PET to image translocator protein (TPSO), a common component involved in neuroinflammatory processes, in patients who presented with extra-axial hemorrhage, microhemorrhage, and contusion in the brain. They determined that PET can be used to identify an increased distribution of TPSO in damaged brain tissue, which is otherwise undetectable using MR

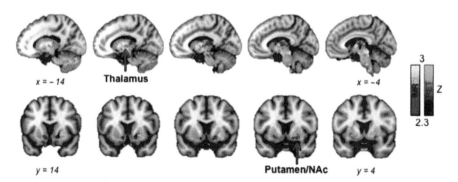

Fig. 7. fMR imaging–PET signals in response to painful and nonpainful pressure stimuli. Blue-green scale indicates radioligand binding potential as detected by PET. Red-yellow scale indicates blood oxygenation level–dependent (BOLD) fMR imaging data, representative of hemodynamic changes. Overlap of a decreased PET signal and an increased BOLD fMR imaging signal are seen in the regions of the thalamus and the striatum (putamen/nucleus accumbens [NAc]). fMR imaging signal for painful stimuli was greater than for nonpainful pressure stimuli. (Reproduced with permission from Wey et al.[72])

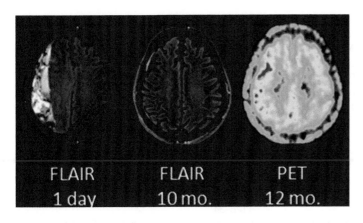

Fig. 8. Discrepancy between MR imaging and translocator protein (TSPO)–PET in brain lesion detection in a patient with a large extra-axial hemorrhage. (*Left*) Fluid-attenuated inversion recovery (FLAIR) MR imaging scan of patient's brain 1 day after hemorrhage. (*Middle*) FLAIR MR imaging scan of patient's brain 10 months after hemorrhage, showing no visible lesions. (*Right*) TSPO-PET image of patient's brain 12 months after hemorrhage, indicating a 20% increase in TSPO uptake in the region of the lesion. (Reproduced with permission from Fujita et al.[80])

imaging, a modality that can only identify areas of macroscopic morphologic damage (**Fig. 8**).[79,80] Lohmann and colleagues[81] used FET-PET combined with contrast-enhanced (CE) MR imaging to differentiate between patients presenting with brain metastasis recurrence and radiation injury, which is of critical clinical importance in oncology and neurology. Radiation injury to the brain following cancer treatments is a common complication, but it can appear similar to other brain disorders, which can subject patients to unnecessary surgeries or the discontinuation of beneficial therapies.[82] Lohmann and colleagues[81] determined that FET-PET/CE-MR imaging was 96% specific, 89% accurate, and 85% sensitive to the difference between these disorders, which is higher than the diagnostic performance of either FET-PET or CE-MR imaging alone. Taken together, this information shows a need for future prospective studies to be conducted, to investigate the utility of PET/MR imaging as a combined modality in the diagnosis and treatment of TBI in humans.

SUMMARY

This review of the current literature shows the expanded capacity of PET/MR imaging in the identification and monitoring of CNS disorders and injuries. In particular, it shows that PET/MR imaging has clear advantages compared with existing radiologic imaging tools in the early detection of certain disorders, as well as in the surveillance of progressive diseases, especially neurodegenerative disease. Because diagnosis is indispensable in the development of treatment plans, honing molecular imaging techniques to identify CNS conditions is critical to improving patient outcomes. PET/CT has notable advantages compared with PET/MR in terms of access, cost, and speed. However, in some cases, PET/MR imaging may offer notable benefits to PET/CT.

Because of the higher cost and operator proficiency demanded by PET/MR imaging, the authors, therefore, recommend that researchers carefully consider the disorders for which MR imaging offers notable advantages compared with CT. Future research is warranted to better show the superiority of PET/MR imaging in the assessment of certain disease states.

DISCLOSURE

No conflicts of interest.

REFERENCES

1. Reddy DS, Estes WA. Clinical potential of neurosteroids for CNS disorders. Trends Pharmacol Sci 2016;37:543–61.
2. Zhorne R, Dudley-Javoroski S, Shields RK. Skeletal muscle activity and CNS neuro-plasticity. Neural Regen Res 2016;11:69–70.
3. Parikh V, Tucci V, Galwankar S. Infections of the nervous system. Int J Crit Illn Inj Sci 2012;2:82–97.
4. Marcet P, Santos N, Borlongan CV. When friend turns foe: central and peripheral neuroinflammation in central nervous system injury. Neuroimmunol Neuroinflamm 2017;4:82–92.
5. Garden GA, Campbell BM. Glial biomarkers in human central nervous system disease. Glia 2016;64:1755–71.
6. Sharp AL, Nagaraj G, Rippberger EJ, et al. Computed tomography use for adults with head injury: describing likely avoidable emergency department imaging based on the canadian CT head rule. Acad Emerg Med 2017;24:22–30.
7. Borja A, Werner T, Alavi A. Role of PET/CT in vascular dementia. J Nucl Med 2019;60:1153.
8. Heiss W-D, Zimmermann-Meinzingen S. PET imaging in the differential diagnosis of vascular dementia. J Neurol Sci 2012;322:268–73.

9. Borja AJ, Hancin EC, Zhang V, et al. Potential of PET/CT in assessing dementias with emphasis on cerebrovascular disorders. Eur J Nucl Med Mol Imaging 2020. https://doi.org/10.1007/s00259-020-04697-y.

10. Peter J, Houshmand S, Werner T, et al. Potential role of global quantitative FDG-PET image analysis in assessing temporal lobe epilepsy. J Nucl Med 2016; 57:1232.

11. Khosravi M, Peter J, Wintering NA, et al. 18F-FDG is a superior indicator of cognitive performance compared to 18F-florbetapir in Alzheimer's disease and mild cognitive impairment evaluation: a global quantitative analysis. J Alzheimers Dis 2019;70(4): 1197–207.

12. Catana C, Drzezga A, Heiss W-D, et al. PET/MRI for neurologic applications. J Nucl Med 2012;53: 1916–25.

13. Herzog H, Lerche C. Advances in clinical PET/MRI instrumentation. PET Clin 2016;11:95–103.

14. Wang G, Zhu S, Li X. Comparison of values of CT and MRI imaging in the diagnosis of hepatocellular carcinoma and analysis of prognostic factors. Oncol Lett 2019;17:1184–8.

15. Chalela JA, Kidwell CS, Nentwich LM, et al. Magnetic resonance imaging and computed tomography in emergency assessment of patients with suspected acute stroke: a prospective comparison. Lancet 2007;369:293–8.

16. Poels Mariëlle MF, Kèren Z, Verwoert Germaine C, et al. Arterial stiffness and cerebral small vessel disease. Stroke 2012;43:2637–42.

17. Chen F, Shen Y-H, Zhu X-Q, et al. Comparison between CT and MRI in the assessment of pulmonary embolism: a meta-analysis. Medicine (Baltimore) 2017;96:e8935.

18. Bradley WG. Magnetic resonance imaging in the central nervous system: comparison with computed tomography. Magn Reson Annu 1986;6(2):81–122.

19. Kubota K, Yokoyama J, Yamaguchi K, et al. FDG-PET delayed imaging for the detection of head and neck cancer recurrence after radiochemotherapy: comparison with MRI/CT. Eur J Nucl Med Mol Imaging 2004;31:590–5.

20. Alavi A, Hess S, Werner TJ, et al. An update on the unparalleled impact of FDG-PET imaging on the day-to-day practice of medicine with emphasis on management of infectious/inflammatory disorders. Eur J Nucl Med Mol Imaging 2020;47:18–27.

21. Hoilund-Carlsen PF, Moghbel MC, Gerke O, et al. Evolving role of PET in detecting and characterizing atherosclerosis. PET Clin 2019;14:197–209.

22. Austin AG, Raynor WY, Reilly CC, et al. Evolving role of MR imaging and PET in assessing osteoporosis. PET Clin 2019;14:31–41.

23. Salamon N, Kung J, Shaw SJ, et al. FDG-PET/MRI coregistration improves detection of cortical dysplasia in patients with epilepsy. Neurology 2008;71:1594–601.

24. Chandra PS, Salamon N, Huang J, et al. FDG-PET/MRI coregistration and diffusion-tensor imaging distinguish epileptogenic tubers and cortex in patients with tuberous sclerosis complex: a preliminary report. Epilepsia 2006;47:1543–9.

25. Matthews R, Brunetti V, Martin B, et al. PET-MRI in diagnosing pedal osteomyelitis in diabetic patients. J Nucl Med 2015;56:307.

26. Zandieh S, Bernt R, Mirzaei S, et al. Image fusion between 18F-FDG PET and MRI in cardiac sarcoidosis: a case series. J Nucl Cardiol 2018;25: 1128–34.

27. Carlbom L, Caballero-Corbalán J, Granberg D, et al. Whole-body MRI including diffusion-weighted MRI compared with 5-HTP PET/CT in the detection of neuroendocrine tumors. Ups J Med Sci 2017;122: 43–50.

28. Huang S-H, Chien C-Y, Lin W-C, et al. A comparative study of fused FDG PET/MRI, PET/CT, MRI, and CT imaging for assessing surrounding tissue invasion of advanced buccal squamous cell carcinoma. Clin Nucl Med 2011;36:518–25.

29. Platzek I, Beuthien-Baumann B, Schneider M, et al. PET/MRI in head and neck cancer: initial experience. Eur J Nucl Med Mol Imaging 2013;40:6–11.

30. Heusch P, Buchbender C, Köhler J, et al. Correlation of the apparent diffusion coefficient (ADC) with the standardized uptake value (SUV) in hybrid 18F-FDG PET/MRI in non-small cell lung cancer (NSCLC) lesions: initial results. ROFO Fortschr Geb Rontgenstr Nuklearmed 2013;185:1056–62.

31. Lee J, Bijan B. Comparison of different functional imaging modalities including FDG PET/CT and DWI-MRI with respect to their value in TNM staging of cholangiocarcinoma. J Nucl Med 2016;57:1291.

32. Beiderwellen K, Grueneisen J, Ruhlmann V, et al. [(18)F]FDG PET/MRI vs. PET/CT for whole-body staging in patients with recurrent malignancies of the female pelvis: initial results. Eur J Nucl Med Mol Imaging 2015;42:56–65.

33. Nakajo K, Tatsumi M, Inoue A, et al. Diagnostic performance of fluorodeoxyglucose positron emission tomography/magnetic resonance imaging fusion images of gynecological malignant tumors: comparison with positron emission tomography/computed tomography. Jpn J Radiol 2010;28:95–100.

34. Sawicki LM, Grueneisen J, Schaarschmidt BM, et al. Evaluation of 18F-FDG PET/MRI, 18F-FDG PET/CT, MRI, and CT in whole-body staging of recurrent breast cancer. Eur J Radiol 2016;85:459–65.

35. Tate CJ, Mollee PN, Miles KA. Combination bone marrow imaging using positron emission tomography (PET)-MRI in plasma cell dyscrasias: correlation with prognostic laboratory values and clinicopathological diagnosis. BJR Open 2019;1:20180020.

36. Freitag MT, Radtke JP, Hadaschik BA, et al. Comparison of hybrid (68)Ga-PSMA PET/MRI and (68)Ga-PSMA PET/CT in the evaluation of lymph node and bone metastases of prostate cancer. Eur J Nucl Med Mol Imaging 2016;43:70–83.

37. Ehman EC, Johnson GB, Villanueva-Meyer JE, et al. PET/MRI: where might it replace PET/CT? J Magn Reson Imaging 2017;46:1247–62.

38. Bondi MW, Edmonds EC, Salmon DP. Alzheimer's disease: past, present, and future. J Int Neuropsychol Soc 2017;23:818–31.

39. Alzheimer's Association. 2016 Alzheimer's disease facts and figures. Alzheimers Dement 2016;12:459–509.

40. Sanford AM. Mild cognitive impairment. Clin Geriatr Med 2017;33:325–37.

41. Phelps ME. PET: molecular imaging and its biological applications. New York: Springer Science & Business Media; 2004.

42. Alavi A, Barrio JR, Werner TJ, et al. Suboptimal validity of amyloid imaging-based diagnosis and management of Alzheimer's disease: why it is time to abandon the approach. Eur J Nucl Med Mol Imaging 2019. https://doi.org/10.1007/s00259-019-04564-5.

43. Jena A, Renjen PN, Taneja S, et al. Integrated 18F-fluorodeoxyglucose positron emission tomography magnetic resonance imaging (18F-FDG PET/MRI), a multimodality approach for comprehensive evaluation of dementia patients: a pictorial essay. Indian J Radiol Imaging 2015;25:342–52.

44. Weller J, Budson A. Current understanding of Alzheimer's disease diagnosis and treatment. F1000Res 2018;7. https://doi.org/10.12688/f1000research.14506.1.

45. Braak H, Braak E. Neuropathological stageing of Alzheimer-related changes. Acta Neuropathol 1991;82:239–59.

46. Eliassen CF, Reinvang I, Selnes P, et al. Biomarkers in subtypes of mild cognitive impairment and subjective cognitive decline. Brain Behav 2017;7:e00776.

47. Bailly M, Ribeiro MJS, Vercouillie J, et al. 18F-FDG and 18F-florbetapir PET in clinical practice: regional analysis in mild cognitive impairment and alzheimer disease. Clin Nucl Med 2015;40:e111.

48. Kobylecki C, Langheinrich T, Hinz R, et al. 18F-Florbetapir PET in patients with frontotemporal dementia and alzheimer disease. J Nucl Med 2015;56:386–91.

49. Kepe V, Moghbel MC, Långström B, et al. Amyloid-β positron emission tomography imaging probes: a critical review. J Alzheimers Dis 2013;36:613–31.

50. Newberg AB, Arnold SE, Wintering N, et al. Initial clinical comparison of 18F-florbetapir and 18F-FDG PET in patients with Alzheimer disease and controls. J Nucl Med 2012;53:902–7.

51. Alavi A, Newberg AB, Souder E, et al. Quantitative analysis of PET and MRI data in normal aging and Alzheimer's disease: atrophy weighted total brain metabolism and absolute whole brain metabolism as reliable discriminators. J Nucl Med 1993;34:1681–7.

52. Høilund-Carlsen PF, Edenbrandt L, Alavi A. Global disease score (GDS) is the name of the game! Eur J Nucl Med Mol Imaging 2019;46:1768–72.

53. Shabir O, Berwick J, Francis SE. Neurovascular dysfunction in vascular dementia, Alzheimer's and atherosclerosis. BMC Neurosci 2018;19:62.

54. Pase Matthew P, Grima Natalie A, Stough Con K, et al. Cardiovascular disease risk and cerebral blood flow velocity. Stroke 2012;43:2803–5.

55. Rudd JHF, Warburton EA, Fryer TD, et al. Imaging atherosclerotic plaque inflammation with [18F]-fluorodeoxyglucose positron emission tomography. Circulation 2002;105:2708–11.

56. Rischpler C, Nekolla SG, Beer AJ. PET/MR imaging of atherosclerosis: initial experience and outlook. Am J Nucl Med Mol Imaging 2013;3:393–6.

57. McKenney-Drake ML, Moghbel MC, Paydary K, et al. 18F-NaF and 18F-FDG as molecular probes in the evaluation of atherosclerosis. Eur J Nucl Med Mol Imaging 2018;45:2190–200.

58. Werner P, Saur D, Zeisig V, et al. Simultaneous PET/mri in stroke: a case series. J Cereb Blood Flow Metab 2015;35:1421–5.

59. Marian M, Rodriguez-Luna D, Jorge P, et al. Impact of time to treatment on tissue-type plasminogen activator–induced recanalization in acute ischemic stroke. Stroke 2014;45:2734–8.

60. Kumar A, Chugani HT. The role of radionuclide imaging in epilepsy, part 1: sporadic temporal and extra-temporal lobe epilepsy. J Nucl Med Technol 2017;45:14–21.

61. Broski SM, Goenka AH, Kemp BJ, et al. Clinical PET/MRI: 2018 update. AJR Am J Roentgenol 2018;211:295–313.

62. Rubí S, Setoain X, Donaire A, et al. Validation of FDG-PET/MRI coregistration in nonlesional refractory childhood epilepsy. Epilepsia 2011;52:2216–24.

63. Shin HW, Jewells V, Sheikh A, et al. Initial experience in hybrid PET-MRI for evaluation of refractory focal onset epilepsy. Seizure 2015;31:1–4.

64. Oldan JD, Shin HW, Khandani AH, et al. Subsequent experience in hybrid PET-MRI for evaluation of refractory focal onset epilepsy. Seizure 2018;61:128–34.

65. Shang K, Wang J, Fan X, et al. Clinical Value of Hybrid TOF-PET/MR imaging–based multiparametric imaging in localizing seizure focus in patients with mri-negative temporal lobe epilepsy. Am J Neuroradiol 2018. https://doi.org/10.3174/ajnr.A5814.

66. Zukotynski KA, Fahey FH, Vajapeyam S, et al. Exploratory evaluation of MR permeability with

18F-FDG PET mapping in pediatric brain tumors: a report from the Pediatric Brain Tumor Consortium. J Nucl Med 2013;54:1237–43.

67. Schaarschmidt BM, Heusch P, Buchbender C, et al. Locoregional tumour evaluation of squamous cell carcinoma in the head and neck area: a comparison between MRI, PET/CT and integrated PET/MRI. Eur J Nucl Med Mol Imaging 2016;43:92–102.

68. Filss CP, Galldiks N, Stoffels G, et al. Comparison of 18F-FET PET and Perfusion-Weighted MR imaging: a PET/MR imaging hybrid study in patients with brain tumors. J Nucl Med 2014;55:540–5.

69. Sacconi B, Raad RA, Lee J, et al. Concurrent functional and metabolic assessment of brain tumors using hybrid PET/MR imaging. J Neurooncol 2016;127:287–93.

70. Deuschl C, Kirchner J, Poeppel TD, et al. 11C–MET PET/MRI for detection of recurrent glioma. Eur J Nucl Med Mol Imaging 2018;45:593–601.

71. Tiger M, Farde L, Rück C, et al. Low serotonin1B receptor binding potential in the anterior cingulate cortex in drug-free patients with recurrent major depressive disorder. Psychiatry Res Neuroimaging 2016;253:36–42.

72. Wey H-Y, Catana C, Hooker JM, et al. Simultaneous fMRI–PET of the opioidergic pain system in human brain. NeuroImage 2014;102:275–82.

73. Karjalainen T, Karlsson HK, Lahnakoski JM, et al. Dissociable roles of cerebral μ-opioid and type 2 dopamine receptors in vicarious pain: a combined PET-fMRI study. Cereb Cortex 2017;27:4257–66.

74. Giza CC, Hovda DA. The neurometabolic cascade of concussion. J Athl Train 2001;36:228–35.

75. Newberg AB, Alavi A. Neuroimaging in patients with head injury. Semin Nucl Med 2003;33:136–47.

76. Taylor HG, Dietrich A, Nuss K, et al. Post-concussive symptoms in children with mild traumatic brain injury. Neuropsychology 2010;24:148–59.

77. Byrnes KR, Wilson C, Brabazon F, et al. FDG-PET imaging in mild traumatic brain injury: a critical review. Front Neuroenergetics 2014;5. https://doi.org/10.3389/fnene.2013.00013.

78. Brabazon F, Wilson CM, Shukla DK, et al. [18F]FDG-PET combined with MRI elucidates the pathophysiology of traumatic brain injury in rats. J Neurotrauma 2016;34:1074–85.

79. Fujita M, Turtzo L, Fennell E, et al. PET imaging of translocator protein detects inflammation after traumatic brain injury in the areas with no MRI change. J Nucl Med 2017;58:205.

80. Fujita M, Turtzo L, Shenouda C, et al. PET imaging of translocator protein detects inflammation after traumatic brain injury. J Nucl Med 2016;57:214.

81. Lohmann P, Kocher M, Ceccon G, et al. Combined FET PET/MRI radiomics differentiates radiation injury from recurrent brain metastasis. Neuroimage Clin 2018;20:537–42.

82. Walker AJ, Ruzevick J, Malayeri AA, et al. Postradiation imaging changes in the CNS: how can we differentiate between treatment effect and disease progression? Future Oncol 2014;10:1277–97.

Applications of PET-MR Imaging in Cardiovascular Disorders

Rhanderson Cardoso, MD, Thorsten M. Leucker, MD, PhD*

KEYWORDS

- Cardiac PET • Cardiac MR imaging • Cardiac PET/MR imaging • Ischemic heart disease
- Myocardial viability • Sarcoidosis • Cardiac masses

KEY POINTS

- Integrated cardiac hybrid PET/MR imaging is an emerging imaging modality that combines anatomic and functional data from MR imaging and physiologic data from PET.
- This hybrid approach has the potential to improve diagnostic and prognostic imaging for several cardiovascular applications, such as ischemic heart disease, inflammatory disorders, infiltrative disease, and cardiac masses.
- Limitations to the expansion of PET/MR imaging use include cost, availability, and technical challenges in attenuation correction with MR imaging instead of computed tomography.
- Although there is enormous potential, thus far research in cardiac PET/MR imaging has been limited mostly to feasibility data. Next, studies should assess comparative effectiveness in relation to alternative imaging modalities.

INTRODUCTION

Over the last 15 to 20 years, there have been remarkable advancements in cardiovascular MR imaging and PET.[1] More recently, PET/MR imaging has been developed as an integrated imaging modality, using MR imaging data to provide attenuation correction for PET.[2] This technique uses the validated tools of MR imaging and PET to provide a complete morphologic, functional, and physiologic cardiac assessment, targeted at the specific cardiac condition by using specific MR imaging sequences and PET radiotracers.

This hybrid imaging approach has the potential to improve the diagnostic yield and assist in the management of a variety of cardiovascular disorders, such as ischemic heart disease, infiltrative diseases, and inflammatory conditions. In this report, the authors review the individual strengths of cardiovascular PET and MR imaging, as well as the current applications, limitations, and future potential of hybrid PET/MR imaging.

TECHNICAL ASPECTS
Attenuation Correction in PET/MR Imaging

The loss of photons owing to absorption in the body and/or hardware or scattering out of the detector field of view, also known as attenuation, is an important challenge in PET. Attenuation correction is technically challenging in PET/MR imaging because MR imaging is based on proton density and relaxation of magnetization, which are not directly correlated with tissue density (**Table 1**).[3]

One option for MR imaging-based attenuation correction is the atlas-based approach, whereby populational data are used to form a computational relationship between computed tomography (CT)-derived attenuation and MR imaging pairs. In this method, a patient scanned with PET/MR imaging is matched to a set of MR images within the atlas. Then, a pseudo-CT, generated from the atlas' MR imaging-CT pair, is used for attenuation data. This approach provides accurate attenuation correction for PET/MR imaging when there

Division of Cardiology, Johns Hopkins Hospital, 600 North Wolfe Street, Blalock 547, Baltimore, MD 21287, USA
* Corresponding author.
E-mail address: tleucke1@jhmi.edu

PET Clin 15 (2020) 509–520
https://doi.org/10.1016/j.cpet.2020.06.007

Table 1
Technical aspects of PET/MR imaging

Attenuation correction	• Atlas-based approach
	  ○ A patient's MR imaging is matched to a set of MR images within the atlas
	  ○ A "pseudo-CT" is created from the chosen MR imaging-CT pair in the atlas
	  ○ "Pseudo-CT" is used for attenuation correction
	• Direct methods
	  ○ Segments MR images into categories, such as air, lung, fat
	  ○ Voxels within the same category are given the same attenuation coefficient

Respiratory and cardiac motion	• Takes advantage of spatial and temporal resolution of MR imaging • MR imaging is used to create 3D motion fields • 3D motion fields provide motion correction for PET imaging
Cardiac devices	• Signal void in MR imaging leads to underestimation of attenuation and tracer uptake • Limited device data on safety of MR imaging scanning with 3-T field strength

is similarity between a patient's MR imaging and atlas images. When the patient's anatomy varies substantially from the populational average, this method can lead to significant error.[2,4]

Direct imaging methods, in contrast, use segmentation instead of an atlas-based approach. MR imaging voxels are segmented into categories, such as air, lung, soft tissue, and fat. All voxels within the same category are assigned the same attenuation coefficient. Direct methods are faster than atlas-based approaches, and they also account better for individual anatomic variability. However, assigning a constant attenuation coefficient to each "segment" may cause errors in the estimation of radiotracer uptake. Nevertheless, this method has been shown to have adequate correlation with standardized uptake values (SUVs) obtained by PET/CT.[2,5,6]

Respiratory and Cardiac Motion

The constant respiratory and cardiac motion is an important cause of image degradation in PET, causing dispersion of tracer activity and underestimation or overestimation of hot/cold spots.[7] Gating the images to periods of less motion in the cardiac cycle, as is done with CT, would dispose of valuable tracer counts, which can only be compensated by longer acquisition times or a higher dose of the radiotracer, none of which are desirable.[8,9] Also, a breath-hold is not possible because PET images are acquired over minutes, through many breathing cycles.[8,10]

To circumvent this problem, direct anatomic data from MR imaging is used to track the respiratory and cardiac motion during the scan, creating 3-dimensional (3D) motion fields. The PET data are then reconstructed with the MR imaging-based motion fields, generating motion-corrected images with improved tracer quantification.[8,10,11] In a study of 8 patients with suspected cardiac sarcoidosis who underwent ^{18}F-fluorodeoxyglucose (^{18}F-FDG) cardiac PET/MR imaging, motion-corrected images showed less blurring, better alignment of tracer activity and myocardial anatomy, and greater contrast-to-noise ratio as compared with no motion correction.[8]

Cardiac Devices

Artifacts owing to metallic cardiac implants constitute an important limitation in PET. In PET/MR imaging, nonmagnetic metallic cardiac devices lead to a signal void that falsely increases the object size which may result in an underestimation of attenuation and tracer uptake. Furthermore, there are safety concerns about PET/MR imaging scanning in patients with cardiac devices, specifically, device malfunction and heating. Because data on device compatibility are less available with 3-T field strength as compared with 1.5 T, many patients with cardiac devices are unsuitable for PET/MR imaging.[12]

MYOCARDIAL PERFUSION IMAGING
PET Perfusion

Historically, single photon-emission computed tomography (SPECT) has been the mainstay imaging for assessment of myocardial perfusion imaging (MPI). PET, however, has several advantages of SPECT, including improved spatial resolution, less radiation, better attenuation correction, and, more importantly, the potential for quantifying rest/stress regional blood flow with mathematical modeling of tracer uptake.[13–15] Assessment of the myocardial blood flow (MBF) and coronary flow reserve are valuable tools for identifying endothelial dysfunction, microvascular disease, and improved risk stratification in patients with ischemic heart disease.[6,14,16]

Radiotracers for Perfusion

Tracers used in PET perfusion, summarized in **Table 2**, include ^{15}O-water, ^{82}Rb-RbCl, and ^{13}N-NH$_3$. ^{15}O-water is a freely diffusible tracer; its accumulation and washout are independent of metabolic activity in the myocardium. As a result, it is the only tracer that has myocardial uptake in linear correlation with perfusion at all ranges of MBF. Myocardial uptake of ^{13}N-NH$_3$ and ^{82}Rb-RbCl plateaus at hyperemic flows greater than 2 to 4 mL/g/min ^{13}N-NH$_3$ is a nondiffusible tracer, retained in the myocardium as a function of blood flow and tissue metabolism. ^{82}Rb-RbCl is a potassium analogue, taken up by myocardial cells by a Na/K ATP transporter. It has a very short half-life (75 seconds); however, it is more easily obtained than other tracers because it is generator produced, obviating an on-site cyclotron. ^{18}F-Flurpiridaz is only available as a tracer for research. It has the longest half-life of PET perfusion tracers (110 minutes), which potentially allows for performance of exercise perfusion studies, as well as transport of the agent between sites.[13,14,17]

MR Imaging Perfusion

Stress MR imaging also has several advantages over SPECT, including no attenuation artifacts, significantly better spatial resolution, and no radiation. Stress MR imaging is typically done based on visual assessment, with gadolinium-based contrast agents (GBCA), with superior accuracy to SPECT.[18] Importantly, semiquantitative and quantitative methods to assess MPI are also available and increasingly being used with stress MR imaging. One option is to apply a model of left ventricular (LV) segmentation and analyze each segment's time-intensity curve, that is, the change in signal intensity over time after GBCA enhancement. The stress-to-rest ratio of the upslope or rate of increase in signal intensity can be used to calculate the myocardial perfusion reserve index.[19] Although this method can correctly identify obstructive coronary artery disease with sensitivity greater than 90% and specificity of 70% to 80%, it also has been shown to underestimate coronary flow reserve when compared with ^{13}N-PET.[20,21]

Exact quantification of MBF with MR imaging involves highly complex computations to deconvolute the time-intensity curve. The technique is limited by several challenges in the relationship between perfusion and change in signal intensity: (1) the extraction of GBCA is low and not exclusively dependent on blood flow; (2) the extraction of GBCA is nonlinear at higher flows; and (3) regional variation in magnetic or radiofrequency fields.[6,19] Despite its limitations, this method provides accurate estimates of myocardial perfusion reserve, with similar sensitivity and specificity as compared with ^{13}N-PET.[22] In a recent study, there was a strong correlation between absolute flow values by PET and MR imaging in 29 individuals.[23]

Hybrid PET/MR Imaging for Perfusion

Hybrid PET/MR imaging has the potential to combine the individual strengths of PET and MR imaging in the assessment of MPI, in particular, the accuracy of quantitative MBF with PET, the high spatial resolution of MR imaging, and the use of cine MR imaging to assess for regional wall motion abnormalities. PET/MR imaging also adds the benefit of motion correction and lower exposure to ionizing radiation as compared with PET/CT. Finally, hybrid imaging will allow for cross-modality validation, such as comparing MR imaging-derived quantitative blood flow assessments with PET results, which has the potential to improve both imaging modalities.[23–26] Despite these theoretic advantages, combined PET/MR imaging for perfusion imaging remains a research tool at this point.[23,26] As with other potential applications of PET/MR imaging, expansion into clinical use is hindered by high costs, low availability, and more importantly, the current lack of data supporting an incremental value over each imaging modality independently.

Table 2
Commonly used radiotracers in PET perfusion

Tracer	Molecule	Half-Life	Produced
^{82}Rb	RbCl	76 s	Cyclotron
^{13}N	NH$_3$	10 min	Cyclotron
^{15}O	H$_2$O	122 s	Generator
^{18}F	Flurpiridaz	110 min	Cyclotron

MYOCARDIAL VIABILITY

Viability assessment seeks to differentiate infarcted myocardial tissue from "hibernating" myocardium, a state of chronic hypoperfusion whereby the muscle is hypokinetic or akinetic, yet viable. Patients with viable myocardium have a greater improvement in systolic function following revascularization or medical therapy as compared with those without myocardial viability.[27] However, viability testing in the STICH trial did not significantly discriminate between patients who benefit versus those who do not benefit from revascularization in ischemic cardiomyopathy.[27,28]

Viability by PET

In PET, myocardial viability is examined with ^{18}F-FDG. This glucose analogue is taken up by the cardiomyocytes through transmembrane glucose transporters, where it is then trapped intracellularly. To standardize glucose uptake in the test, patients typically receive insulin and oral glucose loading before the test.[29] The ^{18}F-FDG tracer has a long half-life of approximately 110 minutes. If perfusion is impaired, the uptake of ^{18}F-FDG indicates hibernating myocardium, whereas the absence of ^{18}F-FDG uptake implies infarcted, nonviable tissue.[30,31] A metaanalysis of 24 studies and more than 750 patients found sensitivity of 92% and specificity of 63% of PET viability for prediction of regional contractile function recovery after revascularization, although these data are limited by heterogeneous definitions of viability and regional wall motion recovery.[32]

Viability by MR Imaging

MR imaging uses GBCA and delayed enhancement imaging to determine myocardial viability. Unlike PET radiotracers, GBCA are not taken up by myocytes. When there is tissue necrosis or fibrosis, the distribution volume and retention of GBCA in tissue increase.[31,33] The evaluation of viability by MR imaging is ultimately determined by the percentage of wall thickness with late-gadolinium enhancement (LGE).[34] This advantage is an important advantage of the MR imaging-based method, because the high spatial resolution of MR imaging with up to 1.5-mm in-plane resolution allows for precise localization of LGE in the subendocardium, midmyocardium, subepicardium, or transmurally.[34] In addition to being more available than PET for clinical use, MR imaging-based viability may be specifically preferred over PET in diabetic patients, because viability assessment with MR imaging is independent of glucose metabolism.

Hybrid PET-MR Imaging for Viability

PET/MR imaging has been shown to be feasible for assessment of viability, although it remains only investigational at this point. In a feasibility study, 20 patients with a history of myocardial infarction (MI) underwent PET/MR imaging; there was substantial agreement between PET and MR imaging-LGE images.[35] In a separate study, investigators found that nearly 20% of dysfunctional LV segments imaged with PET/MR imaging within 1 week after MI had discrepant viability findings between PET and MR imaging. These segments had worse functional recovery compared with segments viable by both PET and MR imaging.[36] Furthermore, PET/MR imaging not only provides information on myocardial viability but also characterizes infarct-related remodeling with insight into the infarct tissue microenvironment, for example, activation of metalloproteinases,[37] inflammatory and progenitor cell recruitment via chemokine receptor expression,[38] and stimulation of angiogenesis.[39]

Although it is conceivable that an improvement in the diagnostic assessment of myocardial viability with the hybrid PET/MR imaging approach may aid in the evaluation of challenging patients at high surgical risk and unclear benefit from revascularization, this remains to be proven in subsequent clinical studies.

INFLAMMATION

Following an acute MI, there is a proinflammatory response in the myocardial tissue, which is subsequently exacerbated by reperfusion injury and may contribute up to 50% of the final MI expansion.[40] The degree of inflammation within a few days of an acute MI has been linked to adverse LV remodeling and worse systolic function over time.[41,42]

^{18}F-FDG-PET/MR imaging has the potential to quantify the inflammatory response after MI with the PET portion, matched with the high spatial resolution of MR imaging-morphology and functional data. The uptake of ^{18}F-FDG predominantly by inflammatory cells, such as monocytes and macrophages, depends on adequate suppression of myocyte glucose uptake. Adequate suppression is accomplished by shifting myocardial metabolism from glucose to free fatty acids with a high-fat, no-carbohydrate diet followed by a fast of 4 to 12 hours and unfractionated heparin given 15 minutes before the study.[43] The intensity of ^{18}F-FDG uptake in the myocardium within the first 5 days following acute MI has been correlated with adverse LV functional outcomes assessed by MR imaging at 6 months, independently of infarct size.[44]

Animal models have shown feasibility of PET/MR imaging to assess monocyte response and inflammation after an acute MI.[45] Although the technique has been used in individual patients, there are no reported prospective studies or case series relating inflammation as assessed by PET/MR imaging to post-MI outcomes.[31] Future research is needed to uncover the relationship between PET/MR imaging results and scar formation versus functional recovery.

IMAGING OF ATHEROSCLEROTIC PLAQUE
MR Imaging in Atherosclerosis Imaging

PET/MR imaging has the potential to be used for anatomic and functional study of atherosclerotic plaque. With regards to anatomy, MR imaging angiography can adequately define the course of large epicardial vessels, being well suited to assess coronary artery anomalies and the course of surgical coronary bypass grafts.[46] MR imaging has also been studied to evaluate coronary stenosis. In a study of 12 individuals with known coronary plaques CT angiography, MR imaging with black blood sequence, designed to null signals (black) from blood, accurately identified plaques in the proximal and middle segments of coronary arteries.[47] Intracoronary thrombus in acute MI can also be identified with MR imaging, taking advantage of short T1 values of methemoglobin found in acute thrombus and plaque hemorrhage.[48]

PET in Atherosclerosis Imaging

PET, on the other hand, can offer molecular imaging to delineate biological processes in plaque. As previously described, ^{18}F-FDG can determine the inflammatory response, particularly after an acute MI. In stable plaque, however, a study with 8 patients found no correlation between ^{18}F-FDG uptake and CD68$^+$ macrophages in patients with plaque in the superficial femoral artery.[49]

Another tracer with applicability in plaque imaging is ^{18}F-sodium fluoride (NaF). ^{18}F-NaF is used most commonly in bone imaging. Most of the tracer is retained by bone after a single pass and added to the bone-forming matrix.[50] In fact, ^{18}F-NaF uptake identifies active tissue calcification in aortic stenosis, thereby predicting disease progression.[51] In coronary imaging, ^{18}F-NaF can detect subclinical calcification, and its uptake accurately identifies the culprit plaque in greater than 90% of patients with MI, more so than ^{18}F-FDG.[52] In carotid plaque, it is associated with active calcification, macrophage infiltration, and apoptosis.[52] In patients with stable angina, ^{18}F-NaF uptake correlates with high-risk features on intravascular ultrasound.[52]

PET/MR Imaging in Atherosclerosis Imaging

In the first report of coronary artery hybrid PET/MR imaging, Robson and colleagues[53] successfully imaged 23 patients with risk factors or diagnosed coronary artery disease using either ^{18}F-NaF or ^{18}F-FDG. The investigators demonstrated feasibility and also how to improve the technique based on their experience, by using a novel free-breathing attenuation correction approach and increasing the number of reconstruction iterations. One challenge of atherosclerotic plaque burden imaging is the rather low radiotracer uptake in addition to signal hampering by cardiac and respiratory motion. Gating MR imaging for motion correction potentially can overcome some of these limitations by improving the contrast and spatial resolution of vulnerable plaque composition.[39]

It remains to be proven whether hybrid PET/MR imaging can effectively combine anatomic with physiologic data to identify high-risk plaques beyond the risk prediction granted by total atherosclerotic burden (eg, CT angiography). Similarly, the technology might be studied to predict recurrence of events after an acute coronary syndrome, and potentially guide prevention strategies.

SARCOIDOSIS

Sarcoidosis is a multisystem inflammatory condition, of unknown cause, characterized by the presence of noncaseating granulomas. The diagnosis of cardiac sarcoidosis is particularly challenging because of the wide spectrum of clinical manifestations and lack of a "gold-standard" testing strategy. The low yield and invasive nature of endomyocardial biopsy underscore the importance of imaging for the diagnosis of cardiac sarcoid.[54,55] The disease is patchy and multifocal and progresses from edema and inflammation to fibrosis and scarring.[55]

MR Imaging in Sarcoidosis

Cardiac MR imaging can evaluate for cardiac sarcoidosis in all these stages. Scar can be identified by ventricular wall thinning and, more importantly, LGE. As previously described, the spatial resolution of MR imaging allows for precise localization of LGE. Classically, cardiac sarcoidosis follows a noncoronary distribution, with subepicardial and midmyocardium LGE involving the basal septal and inferolateral walls, although various patterns can be seen.[56] The extent of LGE is a strong, independent predictor of major adverse cardiac events in sarcoidosis.[57] Edema and acute inflammatory changes can be identified with T2 mapping, an important sequence in complement to LGE.[58] Finally, cine MR imaging can accurately assess the extent of right ventricular and LV systolic dysfunction, also important prognostic markers in cardiac sarcoidosis.[55]

PET in Sarcoidosis

Similarly, PET is also a valuable tool in the diagnosis and staging (inflammation vs fibrosis) of cardiac sarcoidosis, which is done with perfusion (^{13}N-NH_3 or ^{82}Rb-$RbCl$) and metabolic (^{18}F-FDG) imaging. In the presence of active inflammation, macrophages have an increased metabolic rate and glucose uptake. As previously discussed, special care with dietary suppression of myocardial glucose uptake is needed for optimal image quality. The presence of increased ^{18}F-FDG uptake in the presence of normal (early disease) or reduced perfusion (progressive disease) indicates active inflammation. In contrast, a severe perfusion defect with minimal or no ^{18}F-FDG uptake implies fibrosis and scarring.[56] Repeated ^{18}F-FDG PET studies have a role in the serial examination of patients with cardiac sarcoidosis, guiding immunosuppressive therapy, and monitoring the response to treatment.[56,59]

Hybrid PET/MR Imaging in Sarcoidosis

Comparing the efficacy of ^{18}F-FDG PET and MR imaging in the diagnosis of sarcoidosis is limited by the lack of a gold-standard diagnostic tool. In a study with 21 patients suspected of having cardiac sarcoid, including 8 confirmed by the Japanese Ministry of Health (JMH) criteria, ^{18}F-FDG PET had higher sensitivity as compared with MR imaging (88% vs 75%), albeit with lower specificity (39% vs 77%).[60] However, the often-quoted JMH criteria for cardiac sarcoidosis may perform inferiorly to the diagnostic yield of MR imaging and ^{18}F-FDG PET.[56]

Rather than choosing 1 modality over the other, however, sarcoidosis is a condition in which PET and MR imaging are truly complementary to each other (**Fig. 1**). Hybrid PET/MR imaging may evolve to play a larger role in the diagnosis and assessment of the immunosuppressive treatment response of cardiac sarcoidosis. A pioneer study by Wicks and colleagues[61] showed improved sensitivity of combined PET/MR imaging (94%) as compared with PET (85%) or MR imaging (82%) alone in 51 patients with suspected cardiac sarcoid. There was also poor agreement between modalities in the location of cardiac abnormalities,

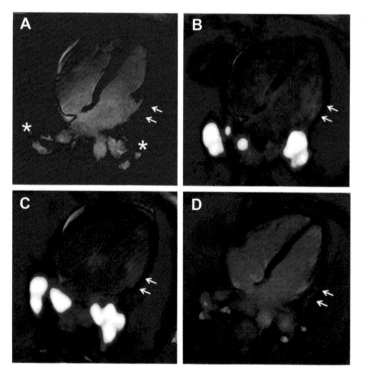

Fig. 1. A case of a 32-year-old man who presented with acute chest pain, general malaise, recurring fevers, and palpitations. Further workup revealed an electrocardiogram (ECG) demonstrating an incomplete right bundle branch block, persistent precordial S waves, and a flattened T wave in lead III. In the initial PET/MR imaging scan, bihilar lymphadenopathy (A, asterisks) and patchy LGE in lateral left-ventricular wall were found (A, arrows), which was in excellent agreement with the increased ^{18}F-FDG uptake found in PET images (B, arrows). Based on the imaging findings, sarcoidosis with cardiac involvement was diagnosed, and treatment with a corticosteroid pulse therapy and sequential dose tapering was initiated. Although LGE in the lateral LV wall remained constant in follow-up scans, FDG uptake was slightly reduced after 4 weeks (C) and significantly reduced after 4 months (D). The decreasing FDG uptake correlated with the improvement of clinical symptoms. PET/MR imaging is an emerging imaging modality in the diagnosis, monitoring of disease activity, and assessment of the immunosuppressive treatment response of cardiac sarcoidosis. (Reproduced with permission from: Eur Heart J. 2015 Mar 1;36(9):550.)

suggesting that they offer complementary information about the disease process.

AMYLOIDOSIS

Cardiac amyloidosis is an infiltrative cardiomyopathy caused by the deposit of amyloid, an abnormally folded protein, in the myocardium. The source of amyloid when there is cardiac involvement is either transthyretin (TTR), in TTR-amyloidosis, or monoclonal immunoglobulin light chains in amyloid light-chain (AL) amyloid.

In patients with suspected amyloidosis, cardiac MR imaging can identify a phenotype of restrictive cardiomyopathy (biatrial enlargement, increased wall thickness) and evaluate LV function with cine imaging. LGE in a noncoronary distribution can be absent, subendocardial, or transmural according to an increasing burden of amyloid.[62] A metaanalysis including 257 patients reported sensitivity and specificity of 85% and 92%, respectively, of MR imaging in the diagnosis of amyloidosis. Importantly, however, MR imaging is unable to differentiate amyloid types.[63]

There is ongoing research with PET in the field of cardiac amyloidosis. Thus far, ^{11}C-Pittsburgh B and ^{18}F-florbetapir have demonstrated some success in early studies in differentiating patients with versus patients without cardiac amyloid.[64,65] It should be noted that PET and MR imaging cannot yet reliably differentiate TTR versus AL amyloid. SPECT with technetium-99m remains the most validated imaging tool for such assessment.

In a pioneer study of hybrid PET/MR imaging for the evaluation of cardiac amyloid, investigators compared 4 TTR-amyloid, 3 AL-amyloid, and 7 control individuals with ^{18}F-sodium fluoride PET/MR imaging. Results showed low uptake of ^{18}F-sodium fluoride in controls and those with AL amyloid, as compared with an increased uptake in patients with TTR amyloid, which correlated with regions of LGE on MR imaging. Although these results are encouraging, further studies are warranted to validate these findings in a larger sample size and compare PET/MR imaging to other imaging alternatives in cardiac amyloidosis.[66]

MYOCARDITIS

MR imaging is recommended by guidelines in the diagnostic and prognostic evaluation of patients with suspected myocarditis.[67,68] Myocardial inflammation, capillary leak, edema, myocyte injury, and ultimately, scar can be identified with special sequences in MR imaging. Tissue edema prolongs both T1 and T2 relaxation times and is best assessed by T2-weighted images. T1-weighted spin-echo images and early GBCA enhancement can identify capillary leak. LGE identifies myocyte necrosis and fibrosis. These sequences are part of the revised Lake Louise criteria for the diagnosis of myocarditis.[69] Classically, myocarditis causes patchy disease in the

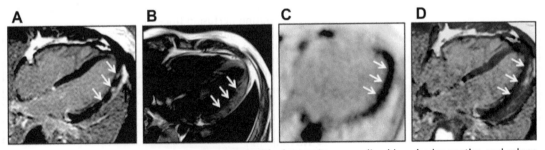

Fig. 2. A case of a 21-year-old man who presented with chest pain, generalized lymphadenopathy, and splenomegaly. Further workup revealed diffuse repolarization abnormalities on ECG, elevated troponin T, impaired LV systolic function, and no evidence of coronary artery disease on angiography. Polymerase chain reaction showed Epstein-Barr virus DNA in the peripheral blood. Acute myocarditis was confirmed on cardiac MRI in the presence of focal intramyocardial nodules (A, white arrows) as well as diffuse subepicardial enhancement (blue arrow) of the lateral wall with an inversion-recovery sequence acquired 10 minutes after injection of gadolinium chelate (0.2 mmol/L of gadopentetate dimeglumine; Bayer Healthcare, Leverkusen, Germany). However, on T2-weighted images, only a weak focal intramyocardial as well as diffuse subepicardial signal of the lateral wall compatible with local edema could be identified (B, white arrows). One hour after injection of ^{18}F-FDG (4 MBq/kg), the PET scan revealed an intense radiotracer in the lateral wall only, suggestive of active inflammation in this territory (C, white arrows). Fused PET/MR images of the heart (D, white arrows) confirmed the colocalization of FDG uptake within the areas of late gadolinium enhancement on MR imaging. PET/MR imaging in detection of acute myocarditis offers the combination of high spatial resolution of MR imaging for the identification of lesions and the high sensitivity of FDG for the detection of acute inflammatory processes. (Reproduced with permission from: Circulation. 2014;130:925–926.)

subepicardium of basal and mid inferolateral walls, although it can present heterogeneously, much like sarcoidosis.[69]

Assessment and differentiation between acute and chronic inflammation by ^{18}F-FDG PET, as previously described, can also be used to evaluate for myocarditis (Fig. 2). A study of hybrid PET/MR imaging in 65 patients with suspected myocarditis showed good agreement between PET and T2-weighted imaging (κ = 0.75). PET had near-perfect specificity; however, because PET focuses exclusively on macrophage uptake of ^{18}F-FDG, without properly evaluating capillary leak and edema, it has low sensitivity (74%) when compared with MR imaging.[70] ^{18}F-FDG-PET/MR imaging is well suited to differentiate between acute and chronic myocarditis and possibly guide treatment options; however, at this time, it is still unknown if combined PET/MR imaging can enhance the endomyocardial biopsy in cases of suspected myocarditis and add potential value in clinical decision making any better than either imaging modality alone.

CARDIAC MASSES

Cardiac MR imaging is perhaps the best imaging modality to characterize cardiac masses because of its many attributes in structural and functional assessment; tissue characterization (T1- and T2-weighted imaging); and evaluation of perfusion (tumor vascularity).[71] In a study of 55 individuals with cardiac masses, cardiac MR imaging differentiated malignant versus benign lesions with an area under the curve (receiver-operating characteristics) of nearly 0.9.[72] Because of the increased metabolic activity of malignant tumors, ^{18}F-FDG PET also has the potential to differentiate malignant versus benign cardiac masses, with an accuracy reported as high as 95% in 1 study.[73]

In an elegant study, Nensa and colleagues[74] evaluated the diagnostic yield of hybrid PET/MR imaging as compared with each individual modality in 20 patients with various benign and malignant masses. Using all available features in MR imaging and a maximum SUV cutoff of $\geq$5.2 in ^{18}F-FDG PET, both modalities had 100% sensitivity and 92% specificity for the diagnosis of malignant cases. By combining both modalities, specificity improved to 100%. A separate study also reported the utility of hybrid PET/MR imaging in the evaluation of 6 patients with cardiac masses.[75] Finally, ^{18}F-FDG-PET/MR imaging adds further clinical value in the planning stage of surgical resection, particularly in patients with complex infiltration of

Table 3 Summary of advantages and limitations of PET, MR imaging, and hybrid PET/MR imaging		
PET	Advantages	• Less radiation compared with SPECT
		• Quantitative assessment of rest/stress regional blood flow by computing perfusion tracer uptake
		• Molecular imaging with specific PET tracers for each condition
	Disadvantages	• Poor spatial resolution
		• Attenuation correction with CT adds radiation
MR imaging	Advantages	• Excellent spatial and temporal resolution
		• Use of cine MR imaging for gold-standard evaluation of ventricular function and regional wall motion abnormalities
		• No radiation
		• Gadolinium-based contrast agents allow for perfusion and delayed enhancement imaging
	Disadvantages	• Limited quantification of MBF
PET/MR imaging	Advantages	• High spatial resolution of MR imaging
		• Quantitative MBF assessment with PET
		• Molecular imaging can target different diseases with specific PET tracers
		• Lower radiation compared with PET/CT
	Disadvantages	• Limited availability
		• Increased cost
		• Few studies showing incremental benefit over nonhybrid imaging modalities
		• Technical challenges with the use of MR imaging data for attenuation correction

cardiac structures as well as during the follow-up period to assess for potential recurrence after surgical intervention.[76]

SUMMARY

Integrated cardiac PET/MR imaging is a powerful imaging modality that combines the strengths of MR imaging in morphology, function, and tissue characterization, with the physiologic data from PET (Table 3). Combined PET/MR imaging has the potential to assist in the diagnosis and management of many cardiovascular conditions, such as ischemic heart disease, infiltrative cardiomyopathies, inflammatory disorders, and cardiac tumors. Current barriers to the growth of PET/MR imaging include cost, availability, challenges with attenuation correction, and limited data, demonstrating improved diagnostic efficacy or clinical outcomes over competing methods. Nevertheless, PET/MR imaging is emerging as an advancement to PET/CT, with less radiation and improved imaging quality in selected indications. The superior molecular and multiparametric imaging potential of PET/MR imaging is emerging and likely will change the future field of cardiovascular imaging.

ACKNOWLEDGMENTS

Dr T.M. Leucker is supported by an American Heart Association Career Development Award (19CDA34760040) and a pilot project award from the National Institutes of Health, National Institute on Aging, Johns Hopkins Older Americans Independence Center (P30AG021334). Dr R. Cardoso is the Pollin Cardiovascular Prevention Fellow at Johns Hopkins Hospital, supported by the Ciccarone Center for the Prevention of Cardiovascular Disease.

DISCLOSURE

The authors have nothing to disclose.

REFERENCES

1. Wintersperger BJ, Bamberg F, De Cecco CN. Cardiovascular imaging: the past and the future, perspectives in computed tomography and magnetic resonance imaging. Invest Radiol 2015;50(9):557–70.
2. Chen Y, An H. Attenuation correction of PET/MR imaging. Magn Reson Imaging Clin N Am 2017;25(2):245–55.
3. Akbarzadeh A, Ay MR, Ahmadian A, et al. MRI-guided attenuation correction in whole-body PET/MR: assessment of the effect of bone attenuation. Ann Nucl Med 2013;27(2):152–62.
4. Hofmann M, Bezrukov I, Mantlik F, et al. MRI-based attenuation correction for whole-body PET/MRI: quantitative evaluation of segmentation- and atlas-based methods. J Nucl Med 2011;52(9):1392–9.
5. Lau JMC, Laforest R, Sotoudeh H, et al. Evaluation of attenuation correction in cardiac PET using PET/MR. J Nucl Cardiol 2017;24(3):839–46.
6. Rischpler C, Woodard PK. PET/MR imaging in cardiovascular imaging. PET Clin 2019;14(2):233–44.
7. Ouyang J, Li Q, El Fakhri G. Magnetic resonance-based motion correction for positron emission tomography imaging. Semin Nucl Med 2013;43(1):60–7.
8. Robson PM, Trivieri M, Karakatsanis NA, et al. Correction of respiratory and cardiac motion in cardiac PET/MR using MR-based motion modeling. Phys Med Biol 2018;63(22):225011.
9. Qiao F, Pan T, Clark JW Jr, et al. A motion-incorporated reconstruction method for gated PET studies. Phys Med Biol 2006;51(15):3769–83.
10. Munoz C, Kolbitsch C, Reader AJ, et al. MR-based cardiac and respiratory motion-compensation techniques for PET-MR imaging. PET Clin 2016;11(2):179–91.
11. Munoz C, Kunze KP, Neji R, et al. Motion-corrected whole-heart PET-MR for the simultaneous visualisation of coronary artery integrity and myocardial viability: an initial clinical validation. Eur J Nucl Med Mol Imaging 2018;45(11):1975–86.
12. Marinskis G, Bongiorni MG, Dagres N, et al. Performing magnetic resonance imaging in patients with implantable pacemakers and defibrillators: results of a European Heart Rhythm Association survey. Europace 2012;14(12):1807–9.
13. Dilsizian V, Bacharach SL, Beanlands RS, et al. ASNC imaging guidelines/SNMMI procedure standard for positron emission tomography (PET) nuclear cardiology procedures. J Nucl Cardiol 2016;23(5):1187–226.
14. Driessen RS, Raijmakers PG, Stuijfzand WJ, et al. Myocardial perfusion imaging with PET. Int J Cardiovasc Imaging 2017;33(7):1021–31.
15. Flotats A, Bravo PE, Fukushima K, et al. (8)(2)Rb PET myocardial perfusion imaging is superior to (9)(9)mTc-labelled agent SPECT in patients with known or suspected coronary artery disease. Eur J Nucl Med Mol Imaging 2012;39(8):1233–9.
16. Kajander SA, Joutsiniemi E, Saraste M, et al. Clinical value of absolute quantification of myocardial perfusion with (15)O-water in coronary artery disease. Circ Cardiovasc Imaging 2011;4(6):678–84.
17. Berman DS, Maddahi J, Tamarappoo BK, et al. Phase II safety and clinical comparison with single-photon emission computed tomography myocardial perfusion imaging for detection of coronary artery disease: flurpiridaz F 18 positron emission tomography. J Am Coll Cardiol 2013;61(4):469–77.

18. de Jong MC, Genders TS, van Geuns RJ, et al. Diagnostic performance of stress myocardial perfusion imaging for coronary artery disease: a systematic review and meta-analysis. Eur Radiol 2012; 22(9):1881–95.

19. Daly C, Kwong RY. Cardiac MRI for myocardial ischemia. Methodist Debakey Cardiovasc J 2013; 9(3):123–31.

20. Ibrahim T, Nekolla SG, Schreiber K, et al. Assessment of coronary flow reserve: comparison between contrast-enhanced magnetic resonance imaging and positron emission tomography. J Am Coll Cardiol 2002;39(5):864–70.

21. Giang TH, Nanz D, Coulden R, et al. Detection of coronary artery disease by magnetic resonance myocardial perfusion imaging with various contrast medium doses: first European multi-centre experience. Eur Heart J 2004;25(18):1657–65.

22. Morton G, Chiribiri A, Ishida M, et al. Quantification of absolute myocardial perfusion in patients with coronary artery disease: comparison between cardiovascular magnetic resonance and positron emission tomography. J Am Coll Cardiol 2012;60(16): 1546–55.

23. Kunze KP, Nekolla SG, Rischpler C, et al. Myocardial perfusion quantification using simultaneously acquired (13) NH3 -ammonia PET and dynamic contrast-enhanced MRI in patients at rest and stress. Magn Reson Med 2018;80(6):2641–54.

24. Krumm P, Mangold S, Gatidis S, et al. Clinical use of cardiac PET/MRI: current state-of-the-art and potential future applications. Jpn J Radiol 2018;36(5): 313–23.

25. Robson PM, Dey D, Newby DE, et al. MR/PET imaging of the cardiovascular system. JACC Cardiovasc Imaging 2017;10(10 Pt A):1165–79.

26. O'Doherty J, Sammut E, Schleyer P, et al. Feasibility of simultaneous PET-MR perfusion using a novel cardiac perfusion phantom. Eur J Hybrid Imaging 2017; 1(1):4.

27. Panza JA, Ellis AM, Al-Khalidi HR, et al. Myocardial viability and long-term outcomes in ischemic cardiomyopathy. N Engl J Med 2019;381(8):739–48.

28. Panza JA, Bonow RO. Ischemia and viability testing in ischemic heart disease: the available evidence and how we interpret it. JACC Cardiovasc Imaging 2017;10(3):365–7.

29. Sarikaya I, Elgazzar AH, Alfeeli MA, et al. Status of F-18 fluorodeoxyglucose uptake in normal and hibernating myocardium after glucose and insulin loading. J Saudi Heart Assoc 2018;30(2): 75–85.

30. Schinkel AF, Poldermans D, Elhendy A, et al. Assessment of myocardial viability in patients with heart failure. J Nucl Med 2007;48(7):1135–46.

31. Rischpler C, Nekolla SG, Kunze KP, et al. PET/MRI of the heart. Semin Nucl Med 2015;45(3):234–47.

32. Schinkel AF, Bax JJ, Poldermans D, et al. Hibernating myocardium: diagnosis and patient outcomes. Curr Probl Cardiol 2007;32(7):375–410.

33. Klein C, Nekolla SG, Balbach T, et al. The influence of myocardial blood flow and volume of distribution on late Gd-DTPA kinetics in ischemic heart failure. J Magn Reson Imaging 2004;20(4):588–93.

34. Kim RJ, Wu E, Rafael A, et al. The use of contrast-enhanced magnetic resonance imaging to identify reversible myocardial dysfunction. N Engl J Med 2000;343(20):1445–53.

35. Nensa F, Poeppel TD, Beiderwellen K, et al. Hybrid PET/MR imaging of the heart: feasibility and initial results. Radiology 2013;268(2):366–73.

36. Rischpler C, Langwieser N, Souvatzoglou M, et al. PET/MRI early after myocardial infarction: evaluation of viability with late gadolinium enhancement transmurality vs. 18F-FDG uptake. Eur Heart J Cardiovasc Imaging 2015;16(6):661–9.

37. Sahul ZH, Mukherjee R, Song J, et al. Targeted imaging of the spatial and temporal variation of matrix metalloproteinase activity in a porcine model of postinfarct remodeling: relationship to myocardial dysfunction. Circ Cardiovasc Imaging 2011;4(4): 381–91.

38. Thackeray JT, Derlin T, Haghikia A, et al. Molecular imaging of the chemokine receptor CXCR4 after acute myocardial infarction. JACC Cardiovasc Imaging 2015;8(12):1417–26.

39. Sinusas AJ, Thomas JD, Mills G. The future of molecular imaging. JACC Cardiovasc Imaging 2011; 4(7):799–806.

40. Yellon DM, Hausenloy DJ. Myocardial reperfusion injury. N Engl J Med 2007;357(11):1121–35.

41. van der Laan AM, Hirsch A, Robbers LF, et al. A proinflammatory monocyte response is associated with myocardial injury and impaired functional outcome in patients with ST-segment elevation myocardial infarction: monocytes and myocardial infarction. Am Heart J 2012;163(1):57–65.e52.

42. Orn S, Ueland T, Manhenke C, et al. Increased interleukin-1beta levels are associated with left ventricular hypertrophy and remodelling following acute ST segment elevation myocardial infarction treated by primary percutaneous coronary intervention. J Intern Med 2012;272(3):267–76.

43. Osborne MT, Hulten EA, Murthy VL, et al. Patient preparation for cardiac fluorine-18 fluorodeoxyglucose positron emission tomography imaging of inflammation. J Nucl Cardiol 2017;24(1):86–99.

44. Rischpler C, Dirschinger RJ, Nekolla SG, et al. Prospective evaluation of 18F-fluorodeoxyglucose uptake in postischemic myocardium by simultaneous positron emission tomography/magnetic resonance imaging as a prognostic marker of functional outcome. Circ Cardiovasc Imaging 2016;9(4): e004316.

45. Lee WW, Marinelli B, van der Laan AM, et al. PET/ MRI of inflammation in myocardial infarction. J Am Coll Cardiol 2012;59(2):153–63.

46. American College of Cardiology Foundation Task Force on Expert Consensus D, Hundley WG, Bluemke DA, et al. ACCF/ACR/AHA/NASCI/SCMR 2010 expert consensus document on cardiovascular magnetic resonance: a report of the American College of Cardiology Foundation Task Force on Expert Consensus Documents. J Am Coll Cardiol 2010;55(23):2614–62.

47. He Y, Da QY, An J, et al. Coronary artery plaque imaging: comparison of black-blood MRI and 64-multidetector computed tomography. Chronic Dis Transl Med 2016;2(3):159–65.

48. Jansen CH, Perera D, Makowski MR, et al. Detection of intracoronary thrombus by magnetic resonance imaging in patients with acute myocardial infarction. Circulation 2011;124(4):416–24.

49. Dregely I, Koppara T, Nekolla SG, et al. Observations with simultaneous 18F-FDG PET and MR imaging in peripheral artery disease. JACC Cardiovasc Imaging 2017;10(6):709–11.

50. Jadvar H, Desai B, Conti PS. Sodium 18F-fluoride PET/CT of bone, joint, and other disorders. Semin Nucl Med 2015;45(1):58–65.

51. Dweck MR, Jenkins WS, Vesey AT, et al. 18F-sodium fluoride uptake is a marker of active calcification and disease progression in patients with aortic stenosis. Circ Cardiovasc Imaging 2014;7(2):371–8.

52. Joshi NV, Vesey AT, Williams MC, et al. 18F-fluoride positron emission tomography for identification of ruptured and high-risk coronary atherosclerotic plaques: a prospective clinical trial. Lancet 2014; 383(9918):705–13.

53. Robson PM, Dweck MR, Trivieri MG, et al. Coronary artery PET/MR imaging: feasibility, limitations, and solutions. JACC Cardiovasc Imaging 2017;10(10 Pt A):1103–12.

54. Uemura A, Morimoto S, Hiramitsu S, et al. Histologic diagnostic rate of cardiac sarcoidosis: evaluation of endomyocardial biopsies. Am Heart J 1999;138(2 Pt 1):299–302.

55. Birnie DH, Nery PB, Ha AC, et al. Cardiac sarcoidosis. J Am Coll Cardiol 2016;68(4):411–21.

56. Hulten E, Aslam S, Osborne M, et al. Cardiac sarcoidosis-state of the art review. Cardiovasc Diagn Ther 2016;6(1):50–63.

57. Greulich S, Deluigi CC, Gloekler S, et al. CMR imaging predicts death and other adverse events in suspected cardiac sarcoidosis. JACC Cardiovasc Imaging 2013;6(4):501–11.

58. Crouser ED, Ono C, Tran T, et al. Improved detection of cardiac sarcoidosis using magnetic resonance with myocardial T2 mapping. Am J Respir Crit Care Med 2014;189(1):109–12.

59. Osborne MT, Hulten EA, Singh A, et al. Reduction in (1)(8)F-fluorodeoxyglucose uptake on serial cardiac positron emission tomography is associated with improved left ventricular ejection fraction in patients with cardiac sarcoidosis. J Nucl Cardiol 2014;21(1): 166–74.

60. Ohira H, Tsujino I, Ishimaru S, et al. Myocardial imaging with 18F-fluoro-2-deoxyglucose positron emission tomography and magnetic resonance imaging in sarcoidosis. Eur J Nucl Med Mol Imaging 2008;35(5):933–41.

61. Wicks EC, Menezes LJ, Barnes A, et al. Diagnostic accuracy and prognostic value of simultaneous hybrid 18F-fluorodeoxyglucose positron emission tomography/magnetic resonance imaging in cardiac sarcoidosis. Eur Heart J Cardiovasc Imaging 2018; 19(7):757–67.

62. Fontana M, Pica S, Reant P, et al. Prognostic value of late gadolinium enhancement cardiovascular magnetic resonance in cardiac amyloidosis. Circulation 2015;132(16):1570–9.

63. Zhao L, Tian Z, Fang Q. Diagnostic accuracy of cardiovascular magnetic resonance for patients with suspected cardiac amyloidosis: a systematic review and meta-analysis. BMC Cardiovasc Disord 2016; 16:129.

64. Lee SP, Lee ES, Choi H, et al. 11C-Pittsburgh B PET imaging in cardiac amyloidosis. JACC Cardiovasc Imaging 2015;8(1):50–9.

65. Dorbala S, Vangala D, Semer J, et al. Imaging cardiac amyloidosis: a pilot study using (1)(8)F-florbetapir positron emission tomography. Eur J Nucl Med Mol Imaging 2014;41(9):1652–62.

66. Trivieri MG, Dweck MR, Abgral R, et al. (18)F-sodium fluoride PET/MR for the assessment of cardiac amyloidosis. J Am Coll Cardiol 2016;68(24):2712–4.

67. Bozkurt B, Colvin M, Cook J, et al. Current diagnostic and treatment strategies for specific dilated cardiomyopathies: a scientific statement from the American Heart Association. Circulation 2016; 134(23):e579–646.

68. Ponikowski P, Voors AA, Anker SD, et al. 2016 ESC Guidelines for the diagnosis and treatment of acute and chronic heart failure: the Task Force for the Diagnosis and Treatment of Acute and Chronic Heart Failure of the European Society of Cardiology (ESC) developed with the special contribution of the Heart Failure Association (HFA) of the ESC. Eur Heart J 2016;37(27):2129–200.

69. Ferreira VM, Schulz-Menger J, Holmvang G, et al. Cardiovascular magnetic resonance in nonischemic myocardial inflammation: expert recommendations. J Am Coll Cardiol 2018;72(24):3158–76.

70. Nensa F, Kloth J, Tezgah E, et al. Feasibility of FDG-PET in myocarditis: comparison to CMR using integrated PET/MRI. J Nucl Cardiol 2018;25(3):785–94.

71. Hoey ET, Shahid M, Ganeshan A, et al. MRI assessment of cardiac tumours: part 1, multiparametric imaging protocols and spectrum of appearances of

histologically benign lesions. Quant Imaging Med Surg 2014;4(6):478–88.

72. Hoffmann U, Globits S, Schima W, et al. Usefulness of magnetic resonance imaging of cardiac and paracardiac masses. Am J Cardiol 2003; 92(7):890–5.

73. Shao D, Wang SX, Liang CH, et al. Differentiation of malignant from benign heart and pericardial lesions using positron emission tomography and computed tomography. J Nucl Cardiol 2011;18(4): 668–77.

74. Nensa F, Tezgah E, Poeppel TD, et al. Integrated 18F-FDG PET/MR imaging in the assessment of cardiac masses: a pilot study. J Nucl Med 2015;56(2): 255–60.

75. Yaddanapudi K, Brunken R, Tan CD, et al. PET-MR imaging in evaluation of cardiac and paracardiac masses with histopathologic correlation. JACC Cardiovasc Imaging 2016;9(1):82–5.

76. Nensa F, Beiderwellen K, Heusch P, et al. Clinical applications of PET/MRI: current status and future perspectives. Diagn Interv Radiol 2014;20(5):438–47.

PET/MR Imaging in Musculoskeletal Precision Imaging - Third wave after X-Ray and MR

Emily C. Hancin, MS, BA[a,1], Austin J. Borja, BA[b,1],
Moozhan Nikpanah, MD[c,1], William Y. Raynor, BS[b], Debanjan Haldar, BS[b],
Thomas J. Werner, MS[b], Michael A. Morris, MD, MS[c],
Babak Saboury, MD, MPH[b,c], Abass Alavi, MD[b],
Ali Gholamrezanezhad, MD[d,*]

KEYWORDS

- MR imaging • PET • Musculoskeletal disease • Inflammation • Infection • Osteoradiomics
- PET/MR • Arthritis • Osteoarthrosis • Bone Tumor

KEY POINTS

- Fused PET/MR imaging demonstrates distinct advantages over structural imaging modalities.
- PET/MR imaging may be used to detect, diagnose, and quantify disease severity for several musculoskeletal pathologies.
- ^{18}F-NaF-PET has demonstrated effectiveness compared with existing imaging modalities in identifying the progression of degenerative musculoskeletal diseases, osteoarthrosis, and inflammatory arthropathies.

INTRODUCTION

Bone appears as a rigid and static structure that makes up the skeleton. Contrary to this appearance, bone is a dynamic organ, and the fine balance between active osseous production and resorption keeps the framework stable while repairing microdamages.[1] The fascinating tango of osteoblasts and osteoclasts produces a brilliant, dynamic network that combines continuous renewal at the microlevel with the preserved shape at the macrolevel.[2] However, bone dynamism is a multifaceted process with numerous mechanical and metabolic regulators, so there exist many opportunities for dysregulation, resulting in skeletal pathologies.[3] Consequently, there is a need for sensitive and specific imaging biomarkers to quantify various aspects of this system to study anabolic and catabolic activities (turnover rate) while also assessing the net result (trabecular and cortical bone architecture and mineralization).

Historically, structural imaging modalities including plain radiograph and computed tomography (CT) have been used in the assessment of

[a] Department of Radiology, Hospital of the University of Pennsylvania, Lewis Katz School of Medicine at Temple University, Philadelphia, PA, USA; [b] Department of Radiology, Hospital of the University of Pennsylvania, 3400 Spruce Street, Philadelphia, PA 19104, USA; [c.] Department of Radiology and Imaging Sciences, Clinical Center, National Institutes of Health, 9000 Rockville Pike, Bethesda, MD 20892, USA; [d] Department of Radiology, Keck School of Medicine, University of Southern California (USC), Health Sciences Campus, 1500 San Pablo Street, Los Angeles, CA 90033, USA
[1] Indicates cofirst author.
* Corresponding author.
E-mail address: gholamre@usc.edu

PET Clin 15 (2020) 521–534
https://doi.org/10.1016/j.cpet.2020.06.001

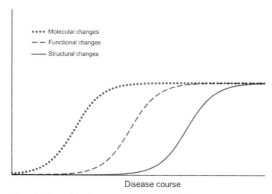

Fig. 1. Graphical representation of the sequence of changes in bone density with age. Molecular changes refer to physiologic alterations in bone matrix, which precede structural changes. As such, molecular imaging with PET may provide earlier evidence of disease progression.

musculoskeletal diseases (first wave). Subsequently, MR imaging provides invaluable information by its great soft tissue contrast-resolution and characterization of bone marrow and soft tissue edema (second wave). It is now understood that structural changes represent the final changes in pathogenesis (**Fig. 1**).[4,5] In contrast to purely structural imaging modalities, PET offers insight into the molecular processes underlying many disease pathologies. ^{18}F-Fluorodeoxyglucose (FDG), a radiolabeled glucose analogue, has emerged as the powerhouse of molecular imaging in inflammatory, infectious, and neoplastic pathologies.[6,7] More recently, ^{18}F-sodium fluoride (^{18}F-NaF) has been applied toward the evaluation of calcium and bone remodeling processes.[8] Furthermore, many other tracers, such as 68-gadolinium-citrate and 68-gadolinium-transferrin, have also been used in the detection of inflammation and infection, particularly within the musculoskeletal system.[9,10]

Fused PET/CT hybrid imaging was introduced to optimize the benefits of molecular imaging with the anatomic correlation of CT. More recently, researchers have begun investigating PET/MR imaging, which demonstrates improved motion correction over PET/CT.[11] Based on the importance of the simultaneous integrated data acquisition, we hope to apply PET/MR imaging to pathologies that would benefit the best from its unique advantages. Of note, FDG-PET/MR imaging has demonstrated particular advantages in vascular diseases, chiefly the dynamic process of vasculitis.[12,13] In addition, PET/MR imaging demonstrates decreased radiation dose, which is a great advantage, particularly in the pediatric population.[14] Based on this evidence, we propose

that PET/MR imaging offers an opportunity to capitalize on the unique advantages of this modality in musculoskeletal pathologies. In this review, we discuss the current research regarding PET/MR imaging in musculoskeletal diseases (third wave). We focus on the benefits of FDG-PET/MR imaging, especially in inflammatory, infectious, and neoplastic conditions of bone marrow and soft tissue. Then, we briefly consider the potential of ^{18}F-NaF-PET in conjunction with MR imaging.

BONE MARROW

Unlike the dense cortical bone, trabecular bone is flush with marrow, a semisolid mixture of adipose tissue and hematopoietic cells.[15] In adults, the red bone marrow exists primarily within the central skeleton and represents the major site of blood cell production.[16] Hematopoietic stem cells in the marrow differentiate into red blood cells (erythrocytes), white blood cells (leukocytes), and platelets (thrombocytes), and pathology in any combination of these developmental pathways may be a major source for morbidity and mortality.[17] Although PET/CT has traditionally been used in the evaluation of bone marrow, PET/MR imaging may demonstrate better potential in the detection and characterization of various bone marrow pathologies, such as inflammation (eg, spondyloarthropathies), radiation toxicity, malignancies and marrow infiltrative processes (lymphoma, leukemia, multiple myeloma), or infections (osteomyelitis and spondylodiscitis [SD]).

Schraml and colleagues[18] retrospectively examined FDG-PET/MR imaging scans of 110 patients to investigate the relationship between bone marrow composition and metabolic activity. They determined that the metabolic activity in bone marrow adipose tissue is inversely correlated with FDG uptake as measured by standardized uptake value (SUV), which suggests that bone marrow adipose tissue does not exhibit a high degree of metabolic activity. Similarly, Fukada and colleagues[19] used PET/MR imaging to evaluate the metabolic activity of yellow marrow. They determined that bone marrow cellularity was the primary determinant of metabolic activity and vascularity. Baratto and colleagues[20] also investigated bone marrow in the context of systemic amyloid deposition. Using whole-body PET/MR imaging and 18F-florbetaben as a tracer, they found that, in seven of their nine patients with suspected cardiac amyloidosis, abnormally increased uptake levels were detected in bone marrow, which suggests that PET/MR imaging can be used to identify bone marrow as a deposition site for amyloid aggregates.

Bone marrow neoplastic pathologies is studied in three categories: (1) primary malignant tumors originating from the bone marrow, such as multiple myeloma and primary bone lymphoma; (2) benign tumors derived from bone marrow, such as hemangiomas; and (3) metastatic tumors that secondarily involve bone marrow. FDG uptake is increased in highly metabolic cells, so neoplasia represents a major pathology grouping for FDG-PET. Several FDG-PET studies have examined primary bone malignancies, including osteosarcoma and multiple myeloma (**Fig. 2**).[21,22] An early study by Ghanem and colleagues[23] determined that whole-body MR imaging was superior to radiologic skeletal surveys in evaluating patients with plasma cell neoplasms, which presents a possibility for the power of MR imaging in serving as a detection tool in bone marrow abnormalities, and

sets the stage for PET/MR imaging to improve the existing standard of care for bone marrow imaging. Because of the addition of an attenuation correction (AC) factor and the difficulty involved in using PET/MR imaging on areas nearby osseous structures, PET/MR imaging tends to underestimate SUV measurements in bone marrow compared with PET/CT.[24,25] Nonetheless, several studies have demonstrated the efficacy of PET/MR imaging in bone marrow imaging. Sachpekidis and colleagues[26] compared the performance of 18F-FDG PET/CT and PET/MR imaging in patients with multiple myeloma. The authors reported an equivalent efficacy of PET/MR imaging compared with PET/CT. In addition, although statistically significant differences in SUVs were reported between PET/CT and PET/MR imaging, the authors noted a statistically significant correlation between

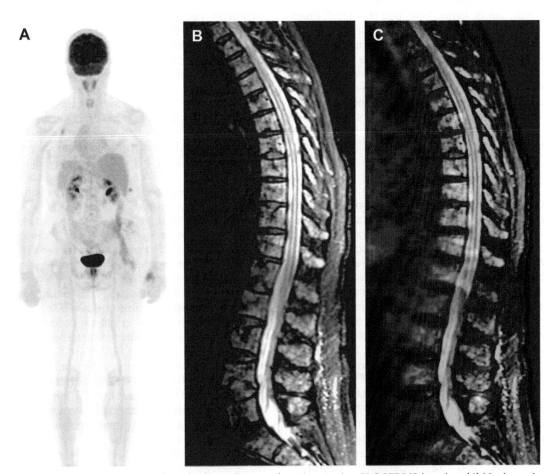

Fig. 2. A 54-year-old woman with multiple myeloma undergoing staging FDG PET/MR imaging. (*A*) Maximum intensity projection PET image shows normal FDG biodistribution throughout the skeletal bone marrow. (*B*) Sagittal T2-weighted FS MR image of the thoracolumbar spine shows diffuse heterogeneous T2-hyperintense marrow infiltration, consistent with diffuse involvement by multiple myeloma. (*C*) Corresponding fused T2-weighted FS PET/MR image shows only normal low-grade marrow activity throughout the spine. Subsequent bone marrow biopsy demonstrated involvement by 80% to 90% clonal plasma cells. FS, fat saturation. (Reproduced with permission from Kogan et al.[22])

the two techniques for SUVs derived from multiple myeloma lesions and reference bone marrow. Shah and Oldan[27] highlighted the role of PET/MR imaging in multiple myeloma and other plasma cell dyscrasias, not only in the evaluation of lesion distribution and activity but also in monitoring the progression, assessing disease burden, and determining therapeutic response and recurrence. However, Zambello and colleagues[28] determined that FDG-PET/MR imaging alone was not successful in identifying patterns of lytic lesions in multiple myeloma that are indicative of symptomatic disease, whereas whole-body low-dose CT could differentiate two different patterns of lytic lesions. This suggests that FDG-PET/MR imaging may not yet be the gold standard in the imaging of this pathology. Primary bone lymphoma, a rare type of extranodal lymphoma, mainly affects sites of constant bone marrow formation, such as humerus, pelvis, femur, tibia, and fibula.[29,30] Promising results have been reported in the assessment of primary bone lymphomas with PET/MR imaging, with comparable sensitivity to PET/CT in the evaluation of disease burden.[31,32] Additionally, MR imaging sequences, particularly diffusion-weighted imaging sequences and MR imaging spectroscopy, have been shown to add more value to the characterization of cellular content variations of this pathology.[31,33]

BONE METASTASES

Osseous metastases represent a special case of bone marrow lesions. Bone metastases are most likely from highly vascularized malignancies, and, of note, prostate, breast, and lung carcinomas are among the most likely to metastasize to bone.[34] The CXCL12/CXCR4 pathway has been shown to play a central role in the metastatic spread of tumor cells to the osseous tissue.[35] Organs with high levels of CXCL12, such as bone marrow, tend to attract cancer cells with high expression of CXCR4 receptors. This pathway has been extensively studied previously in metastatic prostate and breast cancers.[36–38]

Multiple groups have used PET/MR imaging to investigate bone metastases. In MR imaging, bone metastases manifest as marrow-replacing lesions with or without an associated soft tissue component. The lesions typically demonstrate T1 hyposignal and T2 hypersignal intensity.[39] Samarin and colleagues[40] compared FDG-PET/MR imaging with FDG-PET/CT in the assessment of osseous metastatic lesions in 24 patients. They found that, although the overall detection rate of bone metastases between the two imaging modalities was similar, the MR imaging

component of FDG-PET/MR imaging offered a higher degree of confidence in identifying mean lesion conspicuity than did CT. This suggests that PET/MR imaging may offer distinct advantages compared with PET/CT as a metastatic diagnostic tool. Additionally, Ringheim and colleagues[41] used 68Ga-PMSA-11 as a tracer in PET/CT and PET/MR imaging to determine the reproducibility of scans in 30 patients with prostate cancer. They determined that the SUVmax values from PET/CT and PET/MR imaging are linearly correlated, but because SUVmax values in PET/CT were 20% higher than those obtained in PET/MR imaging, the results from the two imaging modalities should be differentiated and consistency should be maintained in longitudinal patient care. Meanwhile, Amorim and colleagues[42] used ^{18}F-fluciclovine as a tracer in PET/MR imaging in the evaluation of osseous metastases from castration-resistant prostate cancer. They found that, of seven lesions, PET/MR imaging detected 100% of them, compared with lower success rates with MR imaging alone, PET alone, or radionuclide bone scan. Similarly, Riola-Parada and colleagues[43] used ^{18}F-choline as a tracer in PET/MR imaging to identify bone metastases from prostate cancer, and they found that this method was effective even though the prostate-specific antigen levels, which are usually elevated in prostate cancer, obtained from the patients were low. These findings confirm that PET/MR imaging may be a strong addition to the detection of osseous metastases from prostate cancer.

Using PET/MR imaging to evaluate breast cancer in rats, Doré-Savard and colleagues[44] demonstrated that PET/MR imaging was successful in evaluating tumor progression and bone damage from surgically implanted cancer cells in the femurs of these animals. Catalano and colleagues[45] compared the effectiveness of FDG-PET/CT with FDG-PET/MR imaging in identifying osseous metastases in 109 patients with metastatic breast cancer. They determined that FDG-PET/MR imaging identified a significantly higher number of osseous metastases than did FDG-PET/CT, which demonstrates the multifaceted power of PET/MR imaging in the recognition of bone abnormalities at the intersection of musculoskeletal disease and oncology. A more recent study conducted by Çelebi[46] compared whole-body FDG-PET/MR imaging with whole-body contrast-enhanced fused MR imaging and CT alone in the assessment of bone metastases in 23 patients with invasive breast cancer. He found that, although there was no significant difference in the success of whole-body contrast-enhanced fused MR imaging and FDG-PET/MR imaging in identifying bone metastases, whole-body

FDG-PET/MR imaging was superior to PET alone. These studies demonstrate the feasibility of FDG-PET/MR imaging in the assessment of metastasis within osseous structures.

INFLAMMATION

Functional imaging of inflammatory processes was primarily limited to planar imaging and single-photon emission CT until recent years. The emergence of rising numbers of PET radiotracers has led to improved identification and quantification of biologic processes involved in inflammation. The hallmark of acute inflammation is edema, and MR imaging excels at imaging the buildup of liquid within soft tissues. The use of combined PET and MR imaging provides more accurate quantitative functional data in addition to the proper evaluation of the exact anatomic localization and extent of involvement of the inflammatory lesions in various regions of the body. For example, Padoan and colleagues,[47] in a retrospective study of 23 patients with large vessel vasculitis using PET/MR imaging with FDG as a tracer, successfully identified increased SUVmax values for patients with various vasculitis-related diseases, such as giant cell arteritis, Takayasu arteritis, and isolated aortitis. Similarly, Einspieler and colleagues[48] determined that PET/MR imaging and PET/CT SUVmax values in patients with large-vessel vasculitis were well-correlated. This points to its potential as a tool to survey inflammatory processes in vessels, which is important for the development of disease in the musculoskeletal system.

Many musculoskeletal disorders also have an underlying immunologic component, which complicates their diagnosis and approach to treatment. However, this is another area of study in which PET/MR imaging may improve existing imaging modalities for early detection, guiding toward the proper therapeutic strategies, and enhancing patient outcomes.

Rheumatoid arthritis (RA) has also been extensively studied using radiologic approaches, because it is characterized by chronic autoimmune-driven inflammation of the synovial joints that is detected using PET radiotracers. This is a particularly important avenue of study, because many patients with RA are diagnosed using radiographs, although this method is not effective in assessing early disease burden or response to treatment.[49,50] Dhawan and colleagues[51] used FDG-PET to examine the extent of RA damage to the joints in the hands and feet of five patients. Increased FDG uptake was noted in several areas of pain or stiffness. This demonstrates that FDG-

PET can be used to identify the development of this pathology, and it sets the stage for the potential of PET/MR imaging to be an effective tool in this area of study. An early study by Miese and colleagues[52] established that FDG-PET/MR imaging successfully identified areas of synovitis and tenosynovitis in the hand of a patient with early RA. Fuchs and colleagues[53] used 3'-deoxy-3'-^{18}F-fluorothymidine as a tracer to identify the effects of induced arthritic joint disease in mice, which is similar in presentation to RA. They found that PET/MR imaging was successful in identifying inflamed regions surrounding the subtalar joints, although they acknowledged that PET/CT may be a preferable method for identifying RA progression in cases where severe bone destruction is present.

PET/MR imaging may have utility in the diagnosis of several other immune-mediated musculoskeletal diseases, such as polymyalgia rheumatica (PMR) and ankylosing spondylitis (AS), although studies involving PET/MR imaging are scarce and PET/CT has been the primary imaging modality used in these analyses. PMR is a rheumatologic disorder that presents with bilateral shoulder and hip girdle pain, increased morning stiffness, and augmented levels of inflammatory markers in patients older than age 50.[54] Because RA and PMR are addressed using different treatment plans and pharmacologic approaches, improvement of the existing diagnostic criteria used to differentiate between these two conditions is critical. It has also been demonstrated that PET/MR imaging can be used to successfully image the metabolic changes associated with fasciitis and antisynthetase syndrome, which is related to dermatomyositis and polymyositis.[55] The results of this study point to a need to refine existing diagnostic imaging techniques based on the systemic effects associated with PMR, and it demonstrates that FDG-PET/CT may be an efficacious imaging modality in the identification of these associated pathologic developments.

AS is another immune-mediated musculoskeletal disorder characterized by inflammation of the axial skeleton, peripheral joints, and the sacroiliac joints.[56] Several studies have determined that PET has the potential to serve as a powerful imaging technique in the diagnosis of this pathology. Bruijnen and colleagues[57] compared FDG and [^{11}C](R)PK11195 PET/CT scans with MR imaging to evaluate their utility in imaging disease activity in five patients with high and five patients with low AS activity. They also conducted ^{18}F-NaF-PET/CT scans on two additional patients to assess ^{18}F-NaF as a tracer. They determined that, whereas there was no significant increase in uptake in either FDG or [^{11}C](R)PK11195 in patients with either low or high AS activity, there was significantly increased uptake of ^{18}F-NaF in the two additional patients in 17 regions in the vertebral column and sacroiliac joints. This suggests that ^{18}F-NaF may be a more powerful tracer than either FDG or [^{11}C](R)PK11195 in identifying AS activity, because of variations in bone remodeling as opposed to increases in inflammation, although this study was limited by the lack of patients receiving the ^{18}F-NaF scans. Strobel and colleagues[58] used ^{18}F-NaF-PET/CT to assess the progression of AS in a cohort of 15 patients, compared with a cohort of 13 patients with mechanical low back pain, to determine if ^{18}F-NaF-PET could differentiate between the two pathologies. They determined that ^{18}F-NaF-PET/CT was most sensitive in identifying grade 3 sacroiliitis, which supports the idea that ^{18}F-NaF-PET can be used as an alternative modality in assessing the progression of AS. Lee and colleagues[59] used the idea that ^{18}F-NaF-PET/CT can be used to monitor active bone synthesis in the spines of patients with AS and concluded that inflammatory lesions and syndesmophytes exhibited increased ^{18}F-NaF uptake. This suggests that active bone synthesis in AS is associated with the presence of inflammation and syndesmophyte formation, which may help clinicians in properly distinguishing AS from other diseases through imaging. Similarly, Fischer and colleagues[60] assessed ^{18}F-NaF-PET/CT uptake in the sacroiliac joints and spine in 10 patients with AS to determine if bone marrow edema, as observed on whole-body MR imaging and associated with AS progression, was correlated with higher uptake values in these regions. They found that ^{18}F-NaF uptake was not highly associated with bone marrow edema that was observed on MR imaging scans. This suggests that ^{18}F-NaF-PET/CT can be used to identify regions of pathologic bone formation that may or may not be associated with inflammatory processes, whereas traditional modalities, such as MR imaging, may only be able to identify regions of pathologic bone formation if inflammation is present.

OSTEOARTHRITIS

Osteoarthritis (OA) is the most common form of joint disease.[61] This chronic disorder is represented by degeneration of all tissues surrounding the joint including bone and soft tissues. Inflammatory mechanisms have been proposed as a probable mechanism of tissue degeneration in OA.[62] MR imaging provides exquisite high-resolution structural information of the joint. However, previous studies on OA have shown that despite being able to

identify early biochemical changes of the soft tissue surrounding the joint, MR imaging cannot directly quantify bone metabolism especially in the subchondral bone.[63,64] Kogan and colleagues[62] used PET/MR imaging in both knees of 22 patients with OA to assess its performance in identifying and characterizing bone metabolic abnormalities and relating them to joint pathologies seen on MR imaging. The authors reported the utility of PET/MR imaging in the evaluation of early morphologic and functional osseous changes in OA. Particularly, they suggested that this modality could detect metabolic abnormalities of the bone in the subchondral region, which appears unremarkable on MR imaging alone.

INFECTION

Like inflammatory pathologies, infectious diseases may also present with soft tissue edema and may be imaged best by MR imaging. PET/MR imaging has previously shown success in non-musculoskeletal infections, such as those caused by *Echinococcus multilocularis*. Lotsch and colleagues[65] determined that PET/MR imaging was comparable with PET/CT in identifying liver lesions associated with this infection. This may be of critical importance in patients looking to reduce their exposure to radiation because PET/MR imaging doses needed to identify these lesions are much less than those used in PET/CT.[66]

Thomas and colleagues[67] compared the strengths of PET/CT and PET/MR imaging using FDG as a tracer in the examination of 10 patients with pulmonary tuberculosis. They determined that, whereas SUVmean and SUVmax were significantly lower in PET/MR imaging, likely caused by underestimation error from AC, PET/MR imaging identified 108 lesions, and PET/CT identified 112, suggesting that the two modalities are comparable in the detection of this pathology.

Previous studies have also shown the utility of PET/MR imaging for diagnosis and assessment of musculoskeletal infectious processes. SD, a form of osteomyelitis that particularly affects the intervertebral disks, is associated with surgical procedures of the spine or hematogenous spread from distant infectious foci. Even though MR imaging has shown high sensitivity, its limited specificity has made the diagnosis of SD challenging.[68] Fahnert and colleagues[69] used PET/MR imaging to assess SD in 30 patients with suspected SD and previously inconclusive MR imaging results (**Fig. 3**). They found that fused PET/MR imaging offered significantly greater sensitivity, specificity, positive predictive value, and negative predictive value than MR imaging

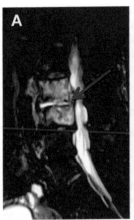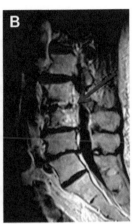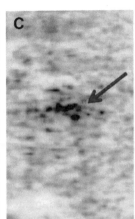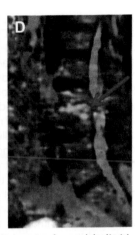

Fig. 3. Simultaneous 18F-FDG PET/MR imaging in a 71-year-old woman with final diagnosis of spondylodiscitis. MR imaging alone was inconclusive. (*A*) TIRM with typical hyperintense signal alterations at intervertebral disk level L4–L5 (*arrow*). (*B*) Moderate postcontrast signal (*arrow*) on T1-weighted MR imaging. (*C, D*) 18F-FDG PET (*C*) and combined 18F-FDG PET/MR imaging (*D*) show focally elevated uptake in affected disk (*arrow*; SUVmax, 8.14; SUVmean, 3.99) as sign of active inflammation. TRIM, turbo inversion recovery magnitude. (Reprinted with permission from Fahnert et al.[69])

alone. In the setting of SD, MR imaging is superior to CT as the cross-sectional component of PET imaging, because it may provide more information about epidural or prevertebral soft tissue abscess formation and the extension of the inflammatory response to the central canal.[70,71]

Rao and colleagues[72] reported the application of PET/MR imaging in simultaneous quantification of PET-detectable functional changes and magnetic resonance spectroscopy measurable metabolites in diabetic neuropathy. Additionally, Basu and colleagues[73] investigated the utility of PET/MR imaging in the evaluation of diabetic foot infections. The authors proposed the role of this imaging modality in differentiating soft tissue infection from osteomyelitis, distinguishing Charcot arthropathy from osteomyelitis, and assessing the ischemia/atherogenesis component in specific cases. Several other groups have suggested that FDG threshold values can be used as a mark of differentiation between various diseases, and stages among diseases; however, there is not consensus regarding ideal threshold values.[74,75]

Moving forward, we envision a greater role for FDG-PET in preliminary detection and assessment of infectious musculoskeletal disease, potentially in conjunction with MR imaging. Of note, Basu and colleagues[76] demonstrated the feasibility of FDG-PET for imaging prosthetic joints and periprosthetic infections. Zhuang and colleagues[77] previously demonstrated persistently increased FDG uptake in the setting of noninfected prostheses. Taken together, these results suggest a possible role for FDG-PET in screening for suspected infection after orthopedic procedures.

SOFT TISSUE CANCERS

In contrast to cortical bone, soft tissues, such as muscle and fat, readily take up FDG.[78,79] Moreover, these types of tissue do not attenuate radiograph significantly. Therefore, MR imaging demonstrates a distinct advantage over CT in soft tissue imaging. Because FDG uptake is increased in hypermetabolic cells, neoplasia represents a major pathology grouping for FDG-PET. In turn, FDG-PET/MR imaging may represent the strongest imaging modality for soft tissue malignancies. This is specifically important for preoperative planning, including but not limited to the evaluation of neurovascular bundle involvement.[80]

There have been several studies comparing PET/MR imaging with PET/CT in the evaluation of various cancer pathologies. For example, Probst and colleagues[81] used New Zealand white rabbits to test the efficacy of PET/MR imaging in detecting human papillomavirus-induced tumors. They determined that FDG and 11C-choline are successful tracers in detecting these tumors up to 2 months postinfection, although FDG was more effective than 11C-choline. Xin and colleagues[82] determined that FDG-PET/CT and FDG-PET/MR imaging are successful in obtaining clear images of various abdominal and pelvic lesions associated with cancer.

More specifically, PET/MR imaging has been used to investigate patients with lymphoma. Heacock and colleagues used residual FDG from PET/CT scans to obtain PET/MR imaging from 28 lymphoma patients. They found that both modalities were successful in appropriately staging patients, and that, in one case, PET/MR imaging properly staged a patient when PET/CT did not.[83] Afaq and colleagues[84] compared PET/CT and PET/MR imaging in the study of Hodgkin or non-Hodgkin lymphoma and found that PET/MR imaging is a comparable modality to PET/CT in the radiologic identification of nodal and extranodal lesions. Atkinson and colleagues[85] used whole-body PET/MR imaging and PET/CT scans from a cohort of 18 adult patients with either Hodgkin or non-Hodgkin lymphoma to draw similar conclusions. Kirchner and colleagues[86] incorporated diffusion-weighted and contrast-enhanced imaging to PET/MR imaging and determined that it improved the staging of patients with lymphoma. A different study from the same laboratory also found that FDG-PET/MR imaging was superior to whole-body diffusion-weighted MR imaging in the staging of pediatric lymphoma patients.[87] Furthermore, Ponisio and colleagues[88] performed whole-body PET/MR imaging scans on eight pediatric patients and found that PET/MR imaging was comparable with PET/CT in detecting lesions. This is particularly of importance to pediatric patients, because MR imaging carries a much smaller radiation dose than CT, and it is thus safer to use on developing children.[89]

PET/MR imaging has been used in several studies to monitor soft tissue sarcoma progression and response to treatment. Partovi and colleagues[90] studied the use of PET/MR imaging in two patients with sarcoma and concluded that PET/MR imaging is a powerful modality to monitor treatment progress in this kind of cancer, and it also may be better at staging the extent of metastases of these tumors. Loft and colleagues[91] used FDG-PET/MR imaging to examine the tumor volumes in two patients with soft tissue sarcomas, and they concluded that this technique improved the identification of tumor cell invasion into adjacent tissues, and the delineation of tumor edges when compared with gadolinium-enhanced MR imaging. Grueneisen and colleagues[92] determined that FDG-PET data were superior over MR imaging data in the evaluation of soft tissue sarcomas in 45 patients undergoing isolated limb perfusion therapy, but they acknowledged that combining the two modalities could be beneficial in monitoring the efficacy of this treatment. Furthermore, Erfanian and colleagues[93] found that, in a study of 41 patients with suspected recurrence of soft tissue sarcoma following surgical removal of a primary tumor, FDG-PET/MR imaging was a superior modality compared with MR imaging in lesion identification. Armeanu-Ebinger and colleagues[94] used a metastatic rhabdomyosarcoma mouse model to evaluate the efficacy of PET/MR imaging in this neoplasm. They used FDG-PET/MR imaging to successfully monitor the effects of vincristine on tumor growth, and they determined that ^{18}F-fluorothymidine was a more efficient tracer than FDG in correlating tracer uptake with tumor weight. Taken together, these data point toward the feasibility of PET/MR imaging in soft tissue malignancies.

CARTILAGE

Cartilage is a dense connective tissue composed primarily of glycosaminoglycans, proteoglycans, and collagen. Cartilage is present within the joints of long bones, ribs, and vertebrae, and within the ears, nose, and airways. Cartilage is avascular and aneural, and, like other soft tissues, it does not absorb X-rays well. As such, MR imaging is the standard of imaging for structural chondropathies. In turn, PET/MR imaging may offer some clinical benefits to imaging infectious and inflammatory pathologies of the cartilage.

Cartilage degeneration is a major contributor to pain in a myriad of degenerative joint conditions.[95] Although PET/MR imaging has not been tested extensively in the study of cartilage, the available studies demonstrate promising avenues for the use of this imaging modality in surveilling cartilage destruction in various pathologic developments. For example, Kogan and colleagues[62] used NaF-PET/MR imaging to scan the knees of individuals presenting with knee pain and potential OA to examine cartilage degeneration, and nearby bone abnormalities. Using the Outerbridge system, they graded cartilage that was adjacent to areas of osseous dysfunction, which ranks cartilage on a scale of 0 to 4, 0 being a normal knee and 4 being cartilage damaged to the extent that the subchondral bone is completely exposed, as in severe OA.[96,97] The authors determined that PET SUVmax in subchondral bone adjacent to grade 0 cartilage was significantly lower compared with subchondral bone adjacent to cartilage of grades 1, 2, 3, or 4. This result suggests that ^{18}F-NaF uptake is higher in regions where cartilage has been damaged, which demonstrates the utility of this modality in evaluating cartilaginous and osseous dysfunction. Tibrewala and colleagues[98] used ^{18}F-NaF-PET/MR imaging and blood flow surveillance to the femur and acetabulum in patents with hip OA, of which 80% presented with cartilage abnormalities in these joints. The authors did individual case examinations to determine that several patients exhibited increased uptake in areas surrounding cartilaginous lesions, which may suggest the presence of bone remodeling in these regions. However, the authors also observed increased ^{18}F-NaF uptake values in regions where cartilage damage was not visible on MR imaging, which may suggest the presence of early bone remodeling before the appearance of large-scale structural changes, further demonstrating a need for the use of molecular tracers to monitor functional changes occurring in the joints. Future studies should focus on the integration of new MR imaging sequences (eg, ultrashort-TE MR imaging) to PET imaging to evaluate early changes related to cartilage pathologies.

CORTICAL BONE

Bone scintigraphy with ^{99m}Tc-methylene diphosphonate has been commonly used to assess bone formation.[99] However, this methodology is limited by its slow systemic clearance and poor spatial resolution.[100] ^{18}F-NaF-PET is gaining increasing traction in musculoskeletal diseases, from osteoporosis to multiple myeloma.[101,102] As such, we believe that, in addition to shorter study times, ^{18}F-NaF-PET allows for greater sensitivity and specificity for musculoskeletal pathologies.

Cortical bone is difficult to image in MR imaging because of the lack of strong proton signal in these regions, because water or air, which is not detectable on MR imaging, often sits within lacunae.[103] Samarin and colleagues[104] used modified CT AC maps, based on electron density, to replace bone with soft tissue and measured the error resulting from this alteration.[105] They found that, in making this replacement, FDG uptake was significantly underestimated in bone lesions, which presents a need for an accurate AC to be established for the evaluation of cortical bone in PET/MR imaging. However, Eiber and

colleagues[106] found that, even with differences in AC, full-body FDG-PET/MR imaging was more clinically robust than FDG-PET/CT in the evaluation of bone malignancies. Schramm and colleagues[107] recently introduced a new algorithm involving bone segmentation to reduce bias in the identification of spinal and pelvic lesions using PET/MR imaging, which was shown to improve the accuracy of uptake measurements in these regions. This study indicates that it is possible to establish new methods of attaining uptake values, which indicates a shift toward improved accuracy in PET/MR imaging measurements in bone structures.

POTENTIAL FOR SODIUM FLUORIDE (^{18}F-NaF) PET MR IMAGING

[18]F-NaF-PET has demonstrated effectiveness compared with existing imaging modalities in identifying the progression of degenerative musculoskeletal diseases, namely OA.[108–110] ^{18}F-NaF-PET/MR imaging was also applied to this pathology in the aforementioned studies by Kogan and colleagues[62] and Tibrewala and colleagues[98] **(Fig. 4)**.

In addition, ^{18}F-NaF has demonstrated some utility in metabolic bone diseases.[3,8] However, few studies use PET/MR imaging in conjunction with ^{18}F-NaF in the study of metabolic bone diseases. Most of the existing literature used ^{18}F-NaF-PET alone or in conjunction with CT. In osteoporosis, ^{18}F-NaF-PET and PET/CT have been used to characterize the dysfunctional osteogenesis via decreased ^{18}F-NaF uptake.[14,101,111] Additionally, ^{18}F-NaF-PET alone has been used to track the response of patients with osteoporosis to treatments, including bisphosphonates and

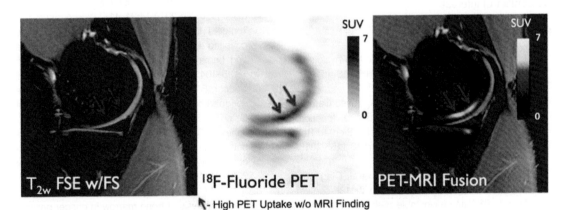

↖- High PET Uptake w/o MRI Finding

Fig. 4. 18F-Fluoride PET (SUV) and MR images of a 27-year-old woman with early stage OA. High uptake on PET (*arrows*) is seen in subchondral bone, which does not correlate with MR imaging findings. This may suggest that metabolic abnormalities in the bone occur before structural changes seen on MR imaging. (Reprinted with permission from Kogan et al.[62])

chimeric antibody.[112–115] Additionally, ^{18}F-NaF-PET has been used to examine osteoclastic and osteoblastic disarray, which are characteristic of Paget disease of bone.[116–119] Finally, no ^{18}F-NaF-PET studies have been performed investigating osteomalacia, rickets, or osteogenesis imperfecta; rather, techniques, such as bone densitometry or radiographs, are widely used for the identification and research of these diseases.[120–122] No studies have been performed in metabolic bone pathologies using PET/MR imaging. Although bony imaging may not be a strong suit for PET/MR imaging, we can envision this modality being used in pathologies with a characteristic absence of bone. Future studies are warranted to determine the feasibility of such an approach.

SUMMARY

This review of the current literature has demonstrated that combined structural and functional modalities have a powerful potential in the diagnosis, surveillance, and treatment of a myriad of musculoskeletal disorders. Specifically, we have demonstrated that FDG-PET/MR imaging has a wide range of clinical applications, from degenerative joint pathologies to bone marrow metastasis. This may be of particular importance to pediatric patients, who are at higher risk for organ damage associated with the higher radiation levels of other existing musculoskeletal imaging modalities, such as PET/CT.[123–127] Moving forward, additional research is warranted to further elucidate the role of ^{18}F-NaF-PET/MR imaging in musculoskeletal disorders.

DISCLOSURE

No conflict of interest.

REFERENCES

1. El Sayed SA, Nezwek TA, Varacallo M. Physiology, bone. StatPearls. Treasure Island (FL): StatPearls Publishing; 2020.
2. Florencio-Silva R, Sasso GR da S, Sasso-Cerri E, et al. Biology of bone tissue: structure, function, and factors that influence bone cells. Biomed Res Int 2015;2015. https://doi.org/10.1155/2015/421746.
3. Reilly CC, Raynor WY, Hong AL, et al. Diagnosis and monitoring of osteoporosis with 18F-sodium fluoride PET: an unavoidable path for the foreseeable future. Semin Nucl Med 2018;48:535–40.
4. Palmer AJR, Brown CP, McNally EG, et al. Noninvasive imaging of cartilage in early osteoarthritis. Bone Joint J 2013;95-B:738–46.
5. Korb-Pap A, Stratis A, Mühlenberg K, et al. Early structural changes in cartilage and bone are required for the attachment and invasion of inflamed synovial tissue during destructive inflammatory arthritis. Ann Rheum Dis 2012;71:1004–11.
6. Peppicelli S, Andreucci E, Ruzzolini J, et al. FDG uptake in cancer: a continuing debate. Theranostics 2020;10:2944–8.
7. Feng H, Wang X, Chen J, et al. Nuclear imaging of glucose metabolism: beyond 18F-FDG. Contrast Media Mol Imaging 2019. https://doi.org/10.1155/2019/7954854.
8. Raynor W, Houshmand S, Gholami S, et al. Evolving role of molecular imaging with 18F-sodium fluoride PET as a biomarker for calcium metabolism. Curr Osteoporos Rep 2016;14:115–25.
9. Gholamrezanezhad A, Basques K, Batouli A, et al. Clinical nononcologic applications of PET/CT and PET/MRI in musculoskeletal, orthopedic, and rheumatologic imaging. Am J Roentgenol 2018;210:W245–63.
10. Gholamrezanezhad A, Basques K, Batouli A, et al. Non-oncologic applications of PET/CT and PET/MR in musculoskeletal, orthopedic, and rheumatologic imaging: general considerations, techniques, and radiopharmaceuticals. J Nucl Med Technol 2017. https://doi.org/10.2967/jnmt.117.198663.
11. Rakvongthai Y, Fakhri GE. MR-based motion correction for quantitative PET in simultaneous PET-MR imaging. PET Clin 2017;12:321–7.
12. Laurent C, Ricard L, Fain O, et al. PET/MRI in large-vessel vasculitis: clinical value for diagnosis and assessment of disease activity. Sci Rep 2019;9:1–7.
13. Sgard B, Brillet P-Y, Bouvry D, et al. Evaluation of FDG PET combined with cardiac MRI for the diagnosis and therapeutic monitoring of cardiac sarcoidosis. Clin Radiol 2019;74:81.e9-18.
14. Austin AG, Raynor WY, Reilly CC, et al. Evolving role of MR imaging and PET in assessing osteoporosis. PET Clin 2019;14:31–41.
15. Turner RT, Martin SA, Iwaniec UT. Metabolic coupling between bone marrow adipose tissue and hematopoiesis. Curr Osteoporos Rep 2018;16:95–104.
16. Cooper B. The origins of bone marrow as the seedbed of our blood: from antiquity to the time of Osler. Proc (Bayl Univ Med Cent) 2011;24:115–8.
17. Janeway CA Jr, Travers P, Walport M, et al. Immunobiology: the immune system in health and disease. 5th edition. New York: Garland Science; 2001. The components of the immune system.
18. Schraml C, Schmid M, Gatidis S, et al. Multiparametric analysis of bone marrow in cancer patients using simultaneous PET/MR imaging: correlation of fat fraction, diffusivity, metabolic activity, and anthropometric data. J Magn Reson Imaging 2015;42:1048–56.

19. Fukuda T, Huang M, Janardhanan A, et al. Correlation of bone marrow cellularity and metabolic activity in healthy volunteers with simultaneous PET/MR imaging. Skeletal Radiol 2019;48:527–34.

20. Baratto L, Park SY, Hatami N, et al. 18F-florbetaben whole-body PET/MRI for evaluation of systemic amyloid deposition. EJNMMI Res 2018;8. https://doi.org/10.1186/s13550-018-0425-1.

21. Zadeh MZ, Raynor WY, Seraj SM, et al. Evolving roles of fluorodeoxyglucose and sodium fluoride in assessment of multiple myeloma patients: introducing a novel method of PET quantification to overcome shortcomings of the existing approaches. PET Clin 2019;14:341–52.

22. Kogan F, Broski SM, Yoon D, et al. Applications of PET-MRI in musculoskeletal disease. J Magn Reson Imaging 2018;48:27–47.

23. Ghanem N, Lohrmann C, Engelhardt M, et al. Whole-body MRI in the detection of bone marrow infiltration in patients with plasma cell neoplasms in comparison to the radiological skeletal survey. Eur Radiol 2006;16:1005–14.

24. Varoquaux A, Rager O, Poncet A, et al. Detection and quantification of focal uptake in head and neck tumours: 18F-FDG PET/MR versus PET/CT. Eur J Nucl Med Mol Imaging 2014;41:462–75.

25. Schäfer JF, Gatidis S, Schmidt H, et al. Simultaneous whole-body PET/MR imaging in comparison to PET/CT in pediatric oncology: initial results. Radiology 2014;273:220–31.

26. Sachpekidis C, Hillengass J, Goldschmidt H, et al. Comparison of 18F-FDG PET/CT and PET/MRI in patients with multiple myeloma. Am J Nucl Med Mol Imaging 2015;5:469–78.

27. Shah SN, Oldan JD. PET/MR imaging of multiple myeloma. Magn Reson Imaging Clin 2017;25:351–65.

28. Zambello R, Crimì F, Lico A, et al. Whole-body low-dose CT recognizes two distinct patterns of lytic lesions in multiple myeloma patients with different disease metabolism at PET/MRI. Ann Hematol 2019;98:679–89.

29. Singh. Primary bone lymphoma: a report of two cases and review of the literature n.d. Available at: http://www.cancerjournal.net/article.asp?issn=0973-1482;year=2010;volume=6;issue=3;spage=296;epage=298;aulast=Singh. Accessed April 14, 2020.

30. Kitsoulis P, Vlychou M, Papoudou-Bai A, et al. Primary lymphomas of bone. Anticancer Res 2006; 26:325–37.

31. Rakheja R, Chandarana H, DeMello L, et al. Correlation between standardized uptake value and apparent diffusion coefficient of neoplastic lesions evaluated with whole-body simultaneous hybrid PET/MRI. Am J Roentgenol 2013;201:1115–9.

32. Wu X, Korkola P, Pertovaara H, et al. No correlation between glucose metabolism and apparent diffusion coefficient in diffuse large B-cell lymphoma: a PET/CT and DW-MRI study. Eur J Radiol 2011;79:e117–21.

33. Behzadi AH, Raza SI, Carrino JA, et al. Applications of PET/CT and PET/MR imaging in primary bone malignancies. PET Clin 2018;13:623–34.

34. Virk MS, Lieberman JR. Tumor metastasis to bone. Arthritis Res Ther 2007;9(Suppl 1):S5.

35. Wang J, Loberg R, Taichman RS. The pivotal role of CXCL12 (SDF-1)/CXCR4 axis in bone metastasis. Cancer Metastasis Rev 2006;25:573–87.

36. Sun Y-X, Schneider A, Jung Y, et al. Skeletal localization and neutralization of the SDF-1(CXCL12)/CXCR4 axis blocks prostate cancer metastasis and growth in osseous sites in vivo. J Bone Miner Res 2005;20:318–29.

37. Taichman RS, Cooper C, Keller ET, et al. Use of the stromal cell-derived factor-1/CXCR4 pathway in prostate cancer metastasis to bone. Cancer Res 2002;62:1832–7.

38. Müller A, Homey B, Soto H, et al. Involvement of chemokine receptors in breast cancer metastasis. Nature 2001;410:50–6.

39. O'Sullivan GJ, Carty FL, Cronin CG. Imaging of bone metastasis: an update. World J Radiol 2015; 7:202–11.

40. Samarin A, Hüllner M, Queiroz M, et al. 18F-FDG-PET/MR increases diagnostic confidence in detection of bone metastases compared with 18F-FDG-PET/CT. Nucl Med Commun 2015;36:1165–73.

41. Ringheim A, Campos Neto G de C, Martins KM, et al. Reproducibility of standardized uptake values of same-day randomized 68Ga-PSMA-11 PET/CT and PET/MR scans in recurrent prostate cancer patients. Ann Nucl Med 2018;32:523–31.

42. Amorim BJ, Prabhu V, Marco SS, et al. Performance of 18F-fluciclovine PET/MR in the evaluation of osseous metastases from castration-resistant prostate cancer. Eur J Nucl Med Mol Imaging 2020;47:105–14.

43. Riola-Parada C, Carreras-Delgado JL, Pérez-Dueñas V, et al. 18F-choline PET/MRI in suspected recurrence of prostate carcinoma. Rev Esp Med Nucl Imagen Mol 2018;37:296–301.

44. Doré-Savard L, Barrière DA, Midavaine É, et al. Mammary cancer bone metastasis follow-up using multimodal small-animal MR and PET imaging. J Nucl Med 2013;54:944–52.

45. Catalano OA, Nicolai E, Rosen BR, et al. Comparison of CE-FDG-PET/CT with CE-FDG-PET/MR in the evaluation of osseous metastases in breast cancer patients. Br J Cancer 2015;112:1452–60.

46. Çelebi F. What is the diagnostic performance of 18F-FDG-PET/MRI in the detection of bone metastasis in patients with breast cancer? Eur J Breast Health 2019;15:213–6.

47. Padoan R, Crimì F, Felicetti M, et al. Fully integrated 18F-FDG PET/MR in large vessel vasculitis. Q J Nucl Med Mol Imaging 2019. https://doi.org/10.23736/S1824-4785.19.03184-4.

48. Einspieler I, Thürmel K, Pyka T, et al. Imaging large vessel vasculitis with fully integrated PET/MRI: a pilot study. Eur J Nucl Med Mol Imaging 2015;42:1012–24.

49. Kgoebane K, Ally MMTM, Duim-Beytell MC, et al. The role of imaging in rheumatoid arthritis. SA J Radiol 2018;22. https://doi.org/10.4102/sajr.v22i1.1316.

50. Tins BJ, Butler R. Imaging in rheumatology: reconciling radiology and rheumatology. Insights Imaging 2013;4:799–810.

51. Dhawan R, Lokitz K, Lokitz S, et al. FDG PET imaging of extremities in rheumatoid arthritis. J La State Med Soc 2016;168:156–61.

52. Miese F, Scherer A, Ostendorf B, et al. Hybrid 18F-FDG PET-MRI of the hand in rheumatoid arthritis: initial results. Clin Rheumatol 2011;30:1247–50.

53. Fuchs K, Kohlhofer U, Quintanilla-Martinez L, et al. In vivo imaging of cell proliferation enables the detection of the extent of experimental rheumatoid arthritis by 3′-deoxy-3′-18F-fluorothymidine and small-animal PET. J Nucl Med 2013;54:151–8.

54. Helliwell T, Hider SL, Barraclough K, et al. Diagnosis and management of polymyalgia rheumatica. Br J Gen Pract 2012;62:275–6.

55. Wehrl HF, Sauter AW, Divine MR, et al. Combined PET/MR: a technology becomes mature. J Nucl Med 2015;56:165–8.

56. Garcia-Montoya L, Gul H, Emery P. Recent advances in ankylosing spondylitis: understanding the disease and management. F1000Res 2018;7. https://doi.org/10.12688/f1000research.14956.1.

57. Bruijnen STG, van der Weijden MAC, Klein JP, et al. Bone formation rather than inflammation reflects ankylosing spondylitis activity on PET-CT: a pilot study. Arthritis Res Ther 2012;14:R71.

58. Strobel K, Fischer DR, Tamborrini G, et al. 18F-fluoride PET/CT for detection of sacroiliitis in ankylosing spondylitis. Eur J Nucl Med Mol Imaging 2010;37:1760–5.

59. Lee S-G, Kim I-J, Kim K-Y, et al. Assessment of bone synthetic activity in inflammatory lesions and syndesmophytes in patients with ankylosing spondylitis: the potential role of 18F-fluoride positron emission tomography-magnetic resonance imaging. Clin Exp Rheumatol 2015;33:90–7.

60. Fischer DR, Pfirrmann CWA, Zubler V, et al. High bone turnover assessed by 18F-fluoride PET/CT in the spine and sacroiliac joints of patients with ankylosing spondylitis: comparison with inflammatory lesions detected by whole body MRI. EJNMMI Res 2012;2:38.

61. Glyn-Jones S, Palmer AJR, Agricola R, et al. Osteoarthritis. Lancet 2015;386:376–87.

62. Kogan F, Fan AP, McWalter EJ, et al. PET/MRI of metabolic activity in osteoarthritis: a feasibility study. J Magn Reson Imaging 2017;45:1736–45.

63. Guermazi A, Alizai H, Crema MD, et al. Compositional MRI techniques for evaluation of cartilage degeneration in osteoarthritis. Osteoarthr Cartil 2015;23:1639–53.

64. Matzat SJ, Kogan F, Fong GW, et al. Imaging strategies for assessing cartilage composition in osteoarthritis. Curr Rheumatol Rep 2014;16:462.

65. Lötsch F, Waneck F, Groger M, et al. FDG-PET/MRI imaging for the management of alveolar echinococcosis: initial clinical experience at a reference centre in Austria. Trop Med Int Health 2019;24(6):663–70.

66. Oldan JD, Shin HW, Khandani AH, et al. Subsequent experience in hybrid PET-MRI for evaluation of refractory focal onset epilepsy. Seizure 2018;61:128–34.

67. Thomas BA, Molton JS, Leek F, et al. A comparison of 18F-FDG PET/MR with PET/CT in pulmonary tuberculosis. Nucl Med Commun 2017;38:971–8.

68. Sollini M, Berchiolli R, Kirienko M, et al. PET/MRI in infection and inflammation. Semin Nucl Med 2018;48:225–41.

69. Fahnert J, Purz S, Jarvers J-S, et al. Use of simultaneous 18F-FDG PET/MRI for the detection of spondylodiskitis. J Nucl Med 2016;57:1396–401.

70. Gala FB, Aswani Y. Imaging in spinal posterior epidural space lesions: a pictorial essay. Indian J Radiol Imaging 2016;26:299–315.

71. Yeom JA, Lee IS, Suh HB, et al. Magnetic resonance imaging findings of early spondylodiscitis: interpretive challenges and atypical findings. Korean J Radiol 2016;17:565–80.

72. Rao H, Gaur N, Tipre D. Assessment of diabetic neuropathy with emission tomography and magnetic resonance spectroscopy. Nucl Med Commun 2017;38:275–84.

73. Basu S, Zhuang H, Alavi A. FDG PET and PET/CT imaging in complicated diabetic foot. PET Clin 2012;7:151–60.

74. Kim S-J, Kim I-J, Suh KT, et al. Prediction of residual disease of spine infection using F-18 FDG PET/CT. Spine 2009;34:2424–30.

75. Guhlmann A, Brecht-Krauss D, Suger G, et al. Fluorine-18-FDG PET and technetium-99m antigranulocyte antibody scintigraphy in chronic osteomyelitis. J Nucl Med 1998;39:2145–52.

76. Basu S, Chryssikos T, Moghadam-Kia S, et al. Positron emission tomography as a diagnostic tool in infection: present role and future possibilities. Semin Nucl Med 2009;39:36–51.

77. Zhuang H, Chacko TK, Hickeson M, et al. Persistent non-specific FDG uptake on PET imaging following hip arthroplasty. Eur J Nucl Med Mol Imaging 2002;29:1328–33.

78. Kothekar E, Yellanki D, Borja AJ, et al. 18F-FDG-PET/CT in measuring volume and global metabolic activity of thigh muscles: a novel CT-based tissue segmentation methodology. Nucl Med Commun 2020;41:162–8.

79. Kothekar E, Borja AJ, Gerke O, et al. Assessing respiratory muscle activity with 18F-FDG-PET/CT in patients with COPD. Am J Nucl Med Mol Imaging 2019;9:309–15.

80. Lee J, Lee S, Kim S-J, et al. Clinical utility of fluoride-18 positron emission tomography/CT in temporomandibular disorder with osteoarthritis: comparisons with 99mTc-MDP bone scan. Dentomaxillofac Radiol 2013;42:29292350.

81. Probst S, Wiehr S, Mantlik F, et al. Evaluation of positron emission tomographic tracers for imaging of papillomavirus-induced tumors in rabbits. Mol Imaging 2014;13. 10.2310/7290.2013.00070.

82. Xin J, Ma Q, Guo Q, et al. PET/MRI with diagnostic MR sequences vs PET/CT in the detection of abdominal and pelvic cancer. Eur J Radiol 2016;85(4):751–9.

83. Heacock L, Weissbrot J, Raad R, et al. PET/MRI for the evaluation of patients with lymphoma: initial observations. AJR Am J Roentgenol 2015;204:842–8.

84. Afaq A, Fraioli F, Sidhu H, et al. Comparison of PET/MRI with PET/CT in the evaluation of disease status in lymphoma. Clin Nucl Med 2017;42. https://doi.org/10.1097/RLU.0000000000001344.

85. Atkinson W, Catana C, Abramson JS, et al. Hybrid FDG-PET/MR compared to FDG-PET/CT in adult lymphoma patients. Abdom Radiol (NY) 2016;41:1338–48.

86. Kirchner J, Deuschl C, Grueneisen J, et al. 18F-FDG PET/MRI in patients suffering from lymphoma: how much MRI information is really needed? Eur J Nucl Med Mol Imaging 2017;44:1005–13.

87. Kirchner J, Deuschl C, Schweiger B, et al. Imaging children suffering from lymphoma: an evaluation of different 18F-FDG PET/MRI protocols compared to whole-body DW-MRI. Eur J Nucl Med Mol Imaging 2017;44:1742–50.

88. Ponisio MR, McConathy J, Laforest R, et al. Evaluation of diagnostic performance of whole-body simultaneous PET/MRI in pediatric lymphoma. Pediatr Radiol 2016;46:1258–68.

89. Cho IH, Han EO, Kim ST. Very different external radiation doses in patients undergoing PET/CT or PET/MRI scans and factors affecting them. Hell J Nucl Med 2014;17:13–8.

90. Partovi S, Kohan AA, Zipp L, et al. Hybrid PET/MR imaging in two sarcoma patients: clinical benefits and implications for future trials. Int J Clin Exp Med 2014;7:640–8.

91. Loft A, Jensen KE, Löfgren J, et al. PET/MRI for preoperative planning in patients with soft tissue sarcoma: a technical report of two patients. Case Rep Med 2013. https://doi.org/10.1155/2013/791078.

92. Grueneisen J, Schaarschmidt B, Demircioglu A, et al. 18F-FDG PET/MRI for therapy response assessment of isolated limb perfusion in patients with soft-tissue sarcomas. J Nucl Med 2019;60:1537–42.

93. Erfanian Y, Grueneisen J, Kirchner J, et al. Integrated 18F-FDG PET/MRI compared to MRI alone for identification of local recurrences of soft tissue sarcomas: a comparison trial. Eur J Nucl Med Mol Imaging 2017;44:1823–31.

94. Armeanu-Ebinger S, Griessinger CM, Herrmann D, et al. PET/MR imaging and optical imaging of metastatic rhabdomyosarcoma in mice. J Nucl Med 2014;55:1545–51.

95. Medvedeva EV, Grebenik EA, Gornostaeva SN, et al. Repair of damaged articular cartilage: current approaches and future directions. Int J Mol Sci 2018;19. https://doi.org/10.3390/ijms19082366.

96. Slattery C, Kweon CY. Classifications in brief: Outerbridge classification of chondral lesions. Clin Orthop 2018;476:2101–4.

97. Wright RW, Ross JR, Haas AK, et al. Osteoarthritis classification scales: interobserver reliability and arthroscopic correlation. J Bone Joint Surg Am 2014;96:1145–51.

98. Tibrewala R, Bahroos E, Mehrabian H, et al. [18F]-sodium fluoride PET/MR imaging for bone–cartilage interactions in hip osteoarthritis: a feasibility study. J Orthop Res 2019;37:2671–80.

99. Bartel TB, Kuruva M, Gnanasegaran G, et al. SNMMI procedure standard for bone scintigraphy 4.0. J Nucl Med Technol 2018;46:398–404.

100. Grant FD, Fahey FH, Packard AB, et al. Skeletal PET with 18F-fluoride: applying new technology to an old tracer. J Nucl Med Off Publ Soc Nucl Med 2008;49:68–78.

101. Ayubcha C, Raynor W, Werner T, et al. Evolving role of NaF-PET in the diagnosis and treatment of osteoporosis. J Nucl Med 2017;58:1007.

102. Raynor WY, Zadeh MZ, Kothekar E, et al. Evolving role of PET-based novel quantitative techniques in the management of hematological malignancies. PET Clin 2019;14:331–40.

103. Techawiboonwong A, Song HK, Wehrli FW. In vivo MRI of submillisecond T2 species with two-dimensional and three-dimensional radial sequences and applications to the measurement of cortical bone water. NMR Biomed 2008;21:59–70.

104. Samarin A, Burger C, Wollenweber SD, et al. PET/MR imaging of bone lesions: implications for PET quantification from imperfect attenuation

correction. Eur J Nucl Med Mol Imaging 2012;39: 1154–60.

105. Ciarmiello A, Mansi L. PET-CT and PET-MRI in neurology: SWOT analysis applied to hybrid imaging. Switzerland: Springer; 2016.

106. Eiber M, Takei T, Souvatzoglou M, et al. Performance of whole-body integrated 18F-FDG PET/MR in comparison to PET/CT for evaluation of malignant bone lesions. J Nucl Med 2014;55: 191–7.

107. Schramm G, Maus J, Hofheinz F, et al. Correction of quantification errors in pelvic and spinal lesions caused by ignoring higher photon attenuation of bone in [18F]NaF PET/MR. Med Phys 2015;42: 6468–76.

108. Kobayashi N, Inaba Y, Tateishi U, et al. New application of 18F-fluoride PET for the detection of bone remodeling in early-stage osteoarthritis of the hip. Clin Nucl Med 2013;38. https://doi.org/10.1097/RLU.0b013e31828d30c0.

109. Kobayashi N, Inaba Y, Tateishi U, et al. Comparison of 18F-fluoride positron emission tomography and magnetic resonance imaging in evaluating early-stage osteoarthritis of the hip. Nucl Med Commun 2015;36:84–9.

110. Hirata Y, Inaba Y, Kobayashi N, et al. Correlation between mechanical stress by finite element analysis and 18F-fluoride PET uptake in hip osteoarthritis patients. J Orthop Res 2015;33:78–83.

111. Schmitz A, Risse JH, Textor J, et al. FDG-PET findings of vertebral compression fractures in osteoporosis: preliminary results. Osteoporos Int 2002;13: 755–61.

112. Uchida K, Nakajima H, Miyazaki T, et al. Effects of alendronate on bone metabolism in glucocorticoid-induced osteoporosis measured by 18F-fluoride PET: a prospective study. J Nucl Med 2009;50: 1808–14.

113. Frost ML, Siddique M, Blake GM, et al. Differential effects of teriparatide on regional bone formation using 18F-fluoride positron emission tomography. J Bone Miner Res 2011;26:1002–11.

114. Frost ML, Moore AE, Siddique M, et al. 18F-fluoride PET as a noninvasive imaging biomarker for determining treatment efficacy of bone active agents at the hip: a prospective, randomized, controlled clinical study. J Bone Miner Res 2013;28:1337–47.

115. Hao K, Wang Q. 18F-FDG PET/CT imaging in evaluation the efficacy of denosumab for giant cell tumor of bone. J Nucl Med 2019;60:1279.

116. Cook GJR, Blake GM, Marsden PK, et al. Quantification of skeletal kinetic indices in Paget's disease using dynamic18f-fluoride positron emission tomography. J Bone Miner Res 2002;17:854–9.

117. Cucchi F, Simonsen L, Abild-Nielsen AG, et al. 18F-sodium fluoride PET/CT in Paget disease. Clin Nucl Med 2017;42:553–4.

118. Installé J, Nzeusseu A, Bol A, et al. 18F-Fluoride PET for monitoring therapeutic response in Paget's disease of bone. J Nucl Med 2005;46:1650–8.

119. Nebot Valenzuela E, Pietschmann P. Epidemiology and pathology of Paget's disease of bone: a review. Wien Med Wochenschr 2017;167:2–8.

120. Thorby-Lister A, Högler W, Hodgson K, et al. Cumulative radiation exposure from medical imaging and associated lifetime cancer risk in children with osteogenesis imperfecta. Bone 2018;114: 252–6.

121. Dipaola CP, Bible JE, Biswas D, et al. Survey of spine surgeons on attitudes regarding osteoporosis and osteomalacia screening and treatment for fractures, fusion surgery, and pseudoarthrosis. Spine J 2009;9:537–44.

122. Bondioni MP, Pazzaglia UE, Izzi C, et al. Comparative X-ray morphometry of prenatal osteogenesis imperfecta type 2 and thanatophoric dysplasia: a contribution to prenatal differential diagnosis. Radiol Med 2017;122:880–91.

123. Ehman EC, Johnson GB, Villanueva-Meyer JE, et al. PET/MRI: where might it replace PET/CT? J Magn Reson Imaging 2017;46:1247–62.

124. Gholamrezanejhad A, Mirpour S, Mariani G. Future of nuclear medicine: SPECT versus PET. J Nucl Med 2009;50(7):16N–8N.

125. Katal S, Gholamrezanezhad A, Kessler M, et al. PET in the diagnostic management of soft tissue sarcomas of musculoskeletal origin. PET Clin 2018;13(4):609–21.

126. Batouli A, Gholamrezanezhad A, Petrov D, et al. Management of primary osseous spinal tumors with PET. PET Clin 2019;14(1):91–101.

127. Batouli A, Braun J, Singh K, et al. Diagnosis of non-osseous spinal metastatic disease: the role of PET/CT and PET/MRI. J Neurooncol 2018;138(2): 221–30.

PET/Computed Tomography Scans and PET/MR Imaging in the Diagnosis and Management of Musculoskeletal Diseases

Navdeep Singh Manhas, BS[a], Sana Salehi, MD[b],*, Peter Joyce, MD[b],
Ali Guermazi, MD, PhD[c], Hojjat Ahmadzadehfar, MD, MSc[d],
Ali Gholamrezanezhad, MD, FEBNM, DABR[b]

KEYWORDS

- Positron-emission tomography • Tomography • X-ray computed • Magnetic resonance imaging
- Musculoskeletal system • Arthritis • Rheumatoid • Osteoporosis • Multiple Myeloma
- Osteosarcoma

KEY POINTS

- PET has been used for more than 4 decades as a powerful tool for most oncologic disorders.
- Within the last decade, significant advances have been made through the use of hybrid imaging in PET/computed tomography scans and PET/MR imaging.
- Applications of PET/computed tomography scans and PET/MR imaging are now being extended to nononcologic musculoskeletal pathologies, such as osteoarthritis, rheumatoid arthritis, and osteoporosis.

INTRODUCTION

For years, several standard imaging modalities such as computed tomography (CT) scanning, MR imaging, and ultrasound examination have been used in the assessment of oncologic diseases involving the musculoskeletal system.[1–3] Although these traditional modalities provide incredible specificity in regards to anatomic features of a specific pathology, there is a lack of qualitative measurements, such as lesional metabolic activity. These modalities are at a further

disadvantage owing to image degradation secondary to metallic implant artifact.[4,5] PET scanning has been used for more than 4 decades as a powerful tool for most oncologic disorders because it can determine tissue metabolic activity through the use of specific radiotracers, with malignant tissues often demonstrating greater metabolic activity.[5–7] Owing to low or minimal reimbursement, limited spatial resolution, and restricted anatomic localization, PET imaging has historically been underused in musculoskeletal imaging.[4,6] Additionally, the synthetization of

Conflict of Interest: The authors declare no conflict of interest related to the material discussed in this article.
[a] California University of Science and Medicine, 1501 Violet St, Colton, CA 92324, USA; [b] Department of Radiology, Keck School of Medicine, University of Southern California, 1500 San Pablo Street, Los Angeles, CA 90033, USA; [c] Department of Radiology, Boston University School of Medicine, 1400 VFW Parkway, Suite 1B105 West Roxbury, MA 02132, USA; [d] Department of Nuclear Medicine, Klinikum Westfalen, Dortmund, Germany
* Corresponding author.
E-mail address: ss_633@usc.edu

radiotracers necessary for PET use is a time-consuming process, further limiting its acceptance in practice.[8] Within the last decade, significant advances have been made through the use of hybrid imaging in PET/CT scans and PET/MR imaging. These fused techniques provide a complete and thorough depiction of pathology by providing detailed information on both anatomic position and lesional metabolic activity.[9,10] For this reason, these hybrid tools have garnered heightened interest in several applications, particularly within the field of musculoskeletal disease. This review briefly compares and contrasts PET/CT scans and PET/MR imaging with a primary focus on PET/CT scanning and PET/MR imaging in the current management of various musculoskeletal processes, both oncologic and nononcologic.

PET/COMPUTED TOMOGRAPHY SCANS VERSUS PET/MR IMAGING

Whereas conventional imaging (eg, radiography, ultrasonography, CT, MR imaging) demonstrates strength in the depiction of late-stage anatomic changes in infective and inflammatory processes such as osteomyelitis, molecular imaging can depict acute physiologic and pathophysiologic changes in earlier stages, yielding potential for earlier diagnosis and improved outcomes.[11–15] PET/CT scanning and PET/MR imaging provide several advantages over conventional imaging, most significantly the simultaneous view of anatomic positioning and spatial resolution of disease alongside information regarding radiotracer labeled metabolic activity.[4,9,10,16] In recent years, hybrid imaging has produced heightened interest in their use in the diagnostic management of musculoskeletal diseases. PET/MR imaging provides specific advantages over PET/CT. Eiber and colleagues[17] juxtaposed the performance of PET with fludeoxyglucose F 18 with MR imaging with PET with fludeoxyglucose F 18 with CT scanning determining that both modalities performed equally in the detection of bone pathologies, with PET/MR imaging demonstrating superior lesional description and allocation of PET-positive findings.[18] Samarin and colleagues[19] confirmed these findings in a study of 24 patients with malignant tumors, finding no significant difference in the detection rate between modalities with PET/MR imaging providing "higher reading confidence and improved conspicuity compared to PET/CT." The results of these 2 studies show that although both imaging modalities provide similar views of cancer activity, PET/MR imaging may provide a more refined view, which can be beneficial for therapy management. Additional advantages of

PET/MR imaging over PET/CT scanning include decreased radiation exposure and increased soft tissue contrast, specifically aiding in the evaluation of pathologies involving ligaments and tendons. Of note, PET/MR imaging also provides superior coregistration of PET data and MR imaging–based motion correction.[10,13] The advantages of PET/CT scanning, when compared with PET MR imaging, include lower cost and improved attenuation correction. An additional limitation of PET/MR imaging includes its contraindication in patients with hardware (eg, pacemaker, aneurysm clips).[9]

ROLE OF HYBRID IMAGING IN COMMON MUSCULOSKELETAL PROCESSES
Osteoarthritis

Osteoarthritis (OA) is the most common joint disease attributed to multiple factors including but not limited to altered weight bearing, chronic inflammation, aging, obesity, trauma, surgery, and genetic predisposition. OA is the primary musculoskeletal cause of compromised mobility in the elderly, with prevalence and incidence anticipated to increase owing to medical advances resulting in longevity.[10,20–22]

Conventional radiographic features of OA include asymmetric joint space narrowing, osteophytosis, subchondral sclerosis, and subchondral cyst formation. However, these features alone do not provide a definitive diagnosis of OA. Rather, diagnosis of "radiographic OA" can be made with the use of the Kellgren and Lawrence grading scale where grades 0 through 4 are applied to a particular radiographic study; grade 0 defined as normal with grade 4 defined as complete ("bone-on-bone") joint space loss.[23] In this grading system, diagnosis occurs well after the initiation of damage, when the threshold for visualization on conventional radiography is reached.

Hybrid imaging provides an opportunity for earlier diagnosis of OA owing to metabolic changes that can be visualized before radiographic changes (**Figs. 1** and **2**). OA demonstrates increased metabolic activity in osteophytes and subchondral lesions such as bone marrow lesions and sclerosis.[24] PET scanning alone with sodium fluoride (NaF) tracer can identify early osteoblastic activity before the development of morphologic changes on MR imaging.[10] Specifically, in the setting of synovitis, PET scans demonstrate increased radiotracer uptake by knee synovium, which correlates with symptomatic knee pain in patients with OA, before the visualization of structural changes.[25] Nakamura and colleagues[26] looked at 15 patients with OA using FDG-PET/CT scans, demonstrating increased lesional

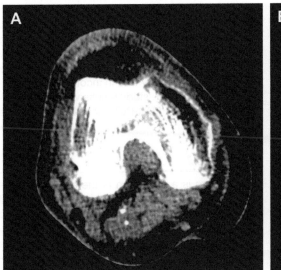 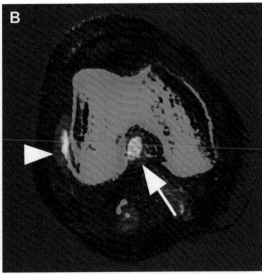

Fig. 1. OA. A 2-18F-fluoro-2-deoxy-ᴅ-glucose (FDG) PET scan. Reconstructed axial low-resolution coronal CT image (*A*) shows no relevant features of OA. Corresponding axial fusion image of PET and CT (*B*) exhibits marked pathologic glucose accumulation in the parapatellar medial recess (*arrowhead*) representing active synovitis. There is additional synovitis around the cruciate ligaments in the femoral notch (*arrow*), the anatomic location where synovitis is most frequently seen in knee OA. Note high sensitivity of PET for hypermetabolism but low specificity and poor spatial localization without correlation with additional cross-sectional imaging (as CT scanning or MR imaging).

radiotracer uptake, particularly within the periarticular region.

A study completed by Draper and colleagues[27] compared MR imaging with NaF PET/CT scans in 22 patients who presented with knee pain.

This study determined that metabolically active lesions that were visible on NaF PET imaging did not match with MR imaging patellofemoral structural changes. Furthermore, the team performed a "lesion-based analysis," discovering that "12%

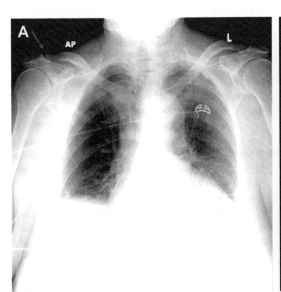 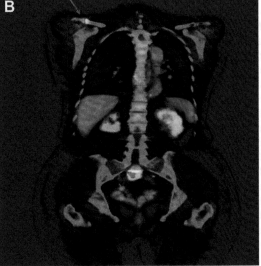

Fig. 2. OA. Anteroposterior (AP) radiograph of the chest (*A*) demonstrates asymmetric joint space loss and osteophytosis of the right acromioclavicular joint (*arrow*), compatible with OA. Coronal fused PET/CT scanning (*B*) again demonstrates joint space loss and osteophytosis of the right acromioclavicular joint, with superimposed hypermetabolic activity (*arrow*). These findings are compatible with OA.

of all abnormal areas were identified by MRI alone" whereas 49% were detected by increased uptake of NaF on PET. The remaining 39% were detected by combined PET/MR imaging.[27] This analysis demonstrates the strength of hybrid imaging techniques in the evaluation of abnormal pathology that would have otherwise missed identification.

Rheumatoid Arthritis

Rheumatoid arthritis (RA) is the most frequent type of inflammatory arthritis, involving an estimated 1% of the population.[28] RA is a systemic disorder defined by chronic autoimmune inflammation, resulting in synovitis and pannus formation. Over time, these features result in the degradation of both osseous and cartilaginous structures.[11,13]

The current gold standard for the evaluation of RA involves conventional radiographs. This modality details a "snapshot" of the cumulative effect of RA. Radiographs serve as the first line of imaging evaluation in arthritic diseases such as RA, psoriatic arthritis, and others.[29] In the early stages of RA, associated erosions are only present in a minority with a prevalence ranging between 8% and 40% at 6 months of disease progression.[30–34]

Inflammatory synovitis and pannus formation are mediated by leukocytes. These white blood cells take up FDG to a greater extent when compared with other cell types, allowing this radiotracer in combination with a PET scan (FDG PET scans) to reveal important information regarding inflammatory states associated with RA, before the appearance of chronic or late-stage changes, such as erosions.[35–37] The usefulness of FDG PET scans, coupled with the ability of MR imaging to delineate synovial inflammation and high anatomic resolution, has helped to garner increased interest in the study of RA with hybrid imaging modalities, such as PET/MR imaging.[38] One study that reviewed the use of PET/MR imaging in patients with early RA of the hand concluded that areas with greater FDG radiotracer uptake corresponded with sites of synovitis and tenosynovitis.[39] Another study that reviewed the use of FDG PET/CT in diagnostic management established an association between large joint lesions in RA patients with areas of inflammatory metabolic activity. Furthermore, this study determined that FDG PET/CT accurately represented the level of large joint inflammatory activity, which was reportedly helpful in the assessment of early RA extent.[40]

There is an increasing trend in studies that explore the use of hybrid imaging in the evaluation of RA treatments. Kumar and colleagues[41] used FDG PET/CT scans to evaluate treatment response to antirheumatic drugs, observing that the inflammatory activity found in joints affected by RA with "quantitative parameters" is promising for entire body assessment of disease activity along with treatment response assessment. This finding was especially true in inconclusive clinical scenarios, however, study results were indeterminate in support of FDG/PET scans in more routine cases of RA.

Osteoporosis

When there is a disruption in the equilibrium between bone-building osteoblastic activity and bone-resorptive osteoclastic activity, metabolic disease occurs.[42] Osteopenia occurs when new bone is unable to be formed as fast as it is resorbed. This condition serves as a bridge between normal bone and more severely deteriorated bone, known as osteoporosis. In osteoporosis, such severe microstructural deterioration occurs that patients are left with decreased bone mass and increased risk of fracture.[43,44] Currently, the gold standard for diagnosis of osteoporosis is through a special form of x-ray imaging termed dual-energy x-ray absorptiometry. A dual-energy x-ray absorptiometry scan assesses mineralized bone mass for a particular bone volume, typically in the lumbar spine or proximal femur, and reports a bone mineral density. A T value is generated, which provides a comparison of the patient's bone mass to a population of 30-year-old individuals' of the same race and gender. If the patient has a bone mineral density that is 2.5 standard deviations below the mean, a diagnosis of osteoporosis is made. A major weakness of this diagnostic test is its inability to provide a detailed assessment of osseous integrity and mechanical competence; its limited resolution, and 2-dimensional/planar imaging (in comparison with 3-dimensional imaging) fails to account for complex distribution and geometry, and of certain bone constituents. Additionally, there are inconsistencies between bone mineral density values obtained by dual-energy x-ray absorptiometry and fracture incidence, particularly in areas with a greater amount of trabecular bone.[44,45]

NaF PET/CT scanning provides a unique usefulness in the assessment of patients at risk for osteoporosis. NaF has a high affinity for sites of osteoblastic new bone formation, which is an intrinsic finding in an osteoporotic state.[44] In 18F-NaF PET scans, lumbar spine standardized uptake value quantities are considerably decreased in patients with osteoporosis in comparison with healthy individuals and possess a significant statistical relationship with mineral density of the bone before treatment.[46] Calculation of fluoride bone plasma clearance (kinetic influx constant) has been used to quantify regional bone formation. In this method, a static scan is performed subsequent to injection of the fluorine–18-NaF radiotracer. After 30 to 60 minutes, a blood sample is collected, and the kinetic influx constant is calculated for different regions. This technique has been used in combination with other conventional assessments such as biopsy and biochemical markers.[47] The data acquired from this method are helpful in observing the response to treatment in patients with osteoporosis.[48] The use of PET/CT scans and PET/MR imaging along with NaF is advantageous owing to their ability to demonstrate these molecular changes before the development of structural changes, such as bone deformity and fracture.[13]

ROLE OF HYBRID IMAGING IN PRIMARY MUSCULOSKELETAL MALIGNANCIES
Osteosarcoma and Other Malignant Bone Tumors

Osteosarcoma is the most frequent primary malignancy of bone, with a survival rate that strongly depends on the metastatic spread of the disease. For example, the 5-year survival rate for localized osteosarcoma is about 70.1%, whereas the 5-year survival in metastatic osteosarcoma is 31.6%.[49–55]

Conventional radiography and MR imaging play an important role in management, with initial diagnosis performed by the former and staging by the latter. MR imaging specifically provides critical information regarding soft tissue extension, infiltration of bone marrow and the existence of bone skip lesions.[51,52]

Most malignant tumors demonstrate increased metabolic activity, with osteosarcoma being no exception. These tumors demonstrate greater glucose uptake and perform increased rates of glycolysis than an average cell, which results in the increased FDG uptake as seen on hybrid imaging modalities. Therefore, FDG PET scanning is a very helpful modality in the evaluation of local diseases, as well as the staging of the cancer by detection of metastatic diseases. Studies show that when FDG PET scanning is combined in a hybrid modality, there is high sensitivity for not only initial staging studies but also in the

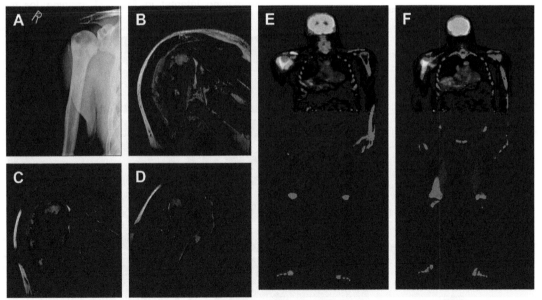

Fig. 3. Osteosarcoma. (*A*) Anteroposterior radiograph of the right shoulder demonstrates an aggressive sclerotic lesion within the right proximal humerus with osteoid mineralization and soft tissue component laterally, concerning for osteosarcoma. Coronal proton density (PD) (*B*), T2 fast spin (*C*), and sagittal T2 fast spin (*D*) sequences of the right shoulder show abnormal signal within the right proximal humerus with a large surrounding soft tissue mass compatible with biopsy-proven osteosarcoma. The mass demonstrates heterogeneous enhancement, with some multiloculated collections of nonenhancing fluid within the mass which may represent superimposed infection. There is extensive surrounding cellulitis and myositis. Coronal PET/CT images (*E*, *F*) demonstrate fragmentation and destructive changes involving the proximal right humerus with soft tissue component, sparing the right glenohumeral joint and right scapula, maximum standardized uptake values of 10.9, compatible with biopsy-proven osteosarcoma.

determination of recurrent disease and metastasis[56,57] (**Fig. 3**). Although the role of PET/MR imaging is not as well-established as PET/CT scanning, it has shown great accuracy in the detection of metastatic osteosarcomas.[58] An added benefit of PET/MR imaging is its ability to perform full TNM staging in one session, with minimization of patient radiation exposure. One can see the benefit of this, for example, in a patient undergoing therapy. The same mechanism can be applied to other tumors, like chondrosarcoma and Ewing's sarcoma.

FDG PET scanning can determine treatment response at a high standard, because metabolic activity will decrease as the osteosarcoma regresses. This activity is mainly assessed via standardized uptake values, with a decrease in standardized uptake values correlating well with the degree of tumor necrosis and positive patient outcomes.[59,60]

Multiple Myeloma

Multiple myeloma (MM) is a primary bone tumor of hematopoietic derivation, most common in the elderly population. Conventional radiographs are commonly used in the new diagnosis of MM or relapse via a "myeloma series," which demonstrates focal osteolytic lesions. However, as

osseous involvement increases, sensitivity decreases.[1,61] As mentioned repeatedly, this imaging method provides only a "snapshot" of lesional activity, which may not be visible until the disease has progressed substantially along its natural course. Additional conventional imaging modalities also suffer from this major drawback.

FDG PET/CT scanning has been shown not only high sensitivity but also high specificity and prognostic value (**Figs. 4** and **5**). According to Bartel and colleagues,[62] the information provided by FDG PET/CT scanning is superior to conventional radiographs, and comparable with results from MR imaging. In their study, FDG PET/CT scanning was performed on 239 patients with MM at baseline and again following neoadjuvant therapy. Complete normalization of FDG PET/CT scanning correlated well with event-free survival and better overall outcomes.[62] A study by Zamagni and colleagues[63] compared FDG PET/CT, PET/MR imaging, and whole-body planar images in 23 patients with new-onset MM, determining that PET/CT scanning was superior to radiographs alone and demonstrated higher sensitivity for lesions outside of MR imaging field of view.

Although PET/CT scanning has shown superiority in the previously described studies, there is increasing interest in PET/MR imaging for the

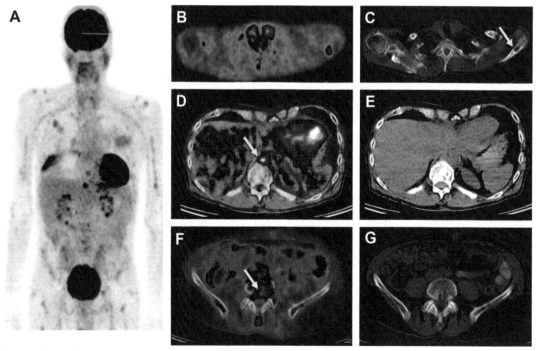

Fig. 4. MM. FDG PET/CT scan in 64-year-old patient with MM and history of stem cell transplantation whole body MIP PET/CT scan (*A*) shows multiple bony and extramedullary lesions. (*B, C*) Osteolytic lesion with FDG uptake. (*D, E*) Lymph node involvement retrocrural. (*F, G*) Osteolytic lesions in lumbar vertebra with mild to moderate FDG uptake.

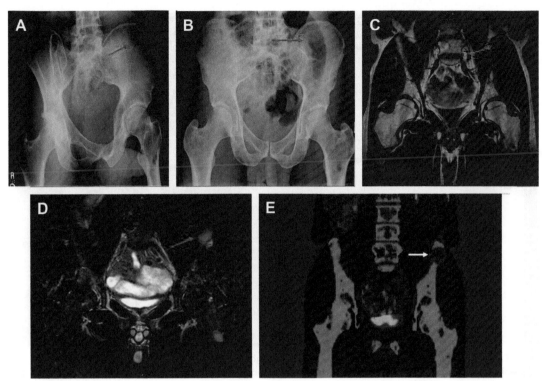

Fig. 5. MM. Anteroposterior (*A*) and Judet view (*B*) radiographs of the pelvis demonstrate innumerable osteolytic lesions, with largest identified within the left iliac wing (*arrows*). Coronal T1 (*C*) and short T1 inversion recovery (*D*) images of the pelvis demonstrate an aggressive lesion within the left iliac wing, with demonstrates isointense signal on T1 and mild hyperintensive short T1 inversion recovery signal (*arrows*), with associated periosteal reaction, cortical breakthrough and soft tissue extension. Coronal PET/CT scan (*E*) demonstrates a lytic lesion with cortical disruption within the left iliac wing (*arrow*), with associated hypermetabolic activity peripherally, suggestive of peripheral osteoclastic activity, and most suggestive of a myeloma lesion.

diagnostic management of MM, specifically in the monitoring of disease progression and assessment of treatment response. Behzadi and colleagues[1] mention that this form of hybrid imaging can serve as a baseline in the assessment of both response to treatment and disease relapse.

ROLE OF HYBRID IMAGING FOR BENIGN PRIMARY SPINAL TUMORS: ANOTHER PERSPECTIVE

Spinal tumors can be either primary (originating within the spine) or secondary/metastatic (arising from an extraspinal origin), which require different treatment plans. Determination of origin is critical to provide the appropriate treatment plan and stop preventable consequences (eg, mass effect that can lead to an irreversible neurologic complication). There are demographic features that help to delineate these masses, with patient age the most important factor; spine lesions before the age of 30 are typically benign except for a few sarcomas such as osteosarcoma and Ewing sarcoma.[64] Another principle that aides in differentiation is lesion location; posterior spinal lesions are generally benign whereas lesions that arise within the vertebral body are frequently malignant, with hemangiomas an exception.[65]

One of the most important methods in determining whether a lesion in the spine is malignant or benign is anatomic imaging (CT scanning, MR imaging, etc), although these modalities present problems owing to overlapping imaging characteristics shared by benign and malignant lesions.[65] As an example, benign spinal lesions typically present with sclerotic, well-defined borders as opposed to aggressive tumors, which tend to present with a wider zone of transition and lamellated or sunburst periosteal reactions.[65] Additional important characteristics include increased adjacent marrow edema with aggressive tumors and increased fatty components with benign tumors.[66]

Interestingly, vertebral body malignancies tend to demonstrate greater FDG uptake, providing information crucial in differentiating a malignant lesion from a benign spinal lesion.[67–69] Alongside

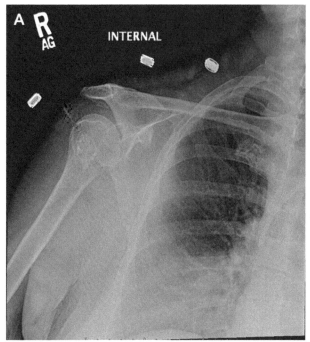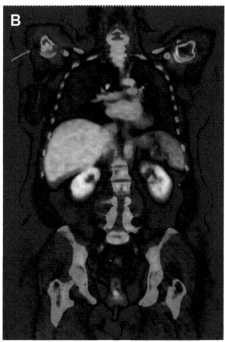

Fig. 6. Enchondroma. Anteroposterior radiograph of the right shoulder (*A*) demonstrates an intramedullary sclerotic lesion in the right proximal humerus (*arrow*) with chondroid matrix no resonant transition and no cortical aggressive extension. This is consistent with a low-grade cartilaginous tumor, such as an enchondroma. Coronal PET/CT scan (*B*) again demonstrates a focal sclerotic lesion within the right proximal humerus (*arrow*), with mild associated hypermetabolic activity These finals are suggestive of a low-grade cartilaginous tumor, such as enchondroma.

anatomic imaging, FDG PET scanning is a very promising option in the diagnosis of spinal malignancy. However, there are varying levels of FDG uptake among benign spinal lesions, with some of the more aggressive benign lesions showing comparable uptake to highly aggressive malignant neoplasms.[65] As mentioned elsewhere in this article, imaging characteristic overlap in classical imaging modalities poses a problem in lesional differentiation, which follows in hybrid modalities. For example, in 7% of lesions occurring in the spine, the majority occur in the sacrum with giant cell tumors being a common benign culprit. These tumors often exhibit an aggressive level of activity, which contributes to difficulty in differentiation from malignant lesions.[70–72] These benign tumors demonstrate aggressive features, such as endosteal scalloping and cortical destruction, which contributes to the difficulty in differentiating these from more malignant lesions on anatomic imaging alone. Furthermore, their high avidity for FDG limits the overall role of FDG PET/CT scanning in distinguishing them from malignancy.[67–69,73]

Another important example occurs in cases of eosinophilic granuloma, a benign form of Langerhans cell histiocytosis that is common in children and can present with vertebral body collapse when involving the spine. In cases of eosinophilic granuloma, the sole use of FDG PET scanning fails as a useful diagnostic option because the associated high histiocyte count leads to high FDG uptake, which also can occur with giant cell tumors.[65] However, hybrid imaging can provide a viable option in some instances, helping to differentiate nonaggressive benign lesions from malignant ones. Specifically, hybrid imaging is best used when benign tumors of similar histopathology are compared, such as enchondroma (**Fig. 6**) and chondrosarcoma.[8,68,69,74–76]

SUMMARY

Within the last decade, there have been significant strides in the use of hybrid imaging, such as PET/CT scanning and PET/MR imaging, for the provision of not only anatomic information, but also molecular and metabolic information of musculoskeletal disease processes. Hybrid imaging demonstrates strengths in using the specific metabolic features of a process in unison with anatomic information in helping differentiate between other etiologies, which may seem to be similar on standard imaging alone. Hybrid imaging can also provide important information regarding the monitoring of cancer progression and treatment response. However, the use of hybrid imaging in differentiation among different types of lesions is not always conclusive, such as in the differentiation of aggressive benign lesions from malignant lesions. For this reason, there should be strong consideration regarding the clinical viability of hybrid imaging as an option in diagnosis to maximize efficacy and efficiency in making imaging diagnosis. In recent years, the use of hybrid imaging has also extended from the realm of benign tumors, malignancies, and metastases to nononcologic applications. These new applications include the earlier diagnosis as well as a more thorough evaluation of the progression of common musculoskeletal processes, such as OA and RA. Research in this realm is promising yet sparse, warranting a call for further studies to accrue more data and better understand the complete role that hybrid imaging can play in the evaluation and treatment of multiple musculoskeletal pathologies.

REFERENCES

1. Behzadi AH, Raza SI, Carrino JA, et al. Applications of PET/CT and PET/MR imaging in primary bone malignancies. PET Clin 2018;13(4):623–34.
2. Hillner BE, Siegel BA, Liu D, et al. Impact of positron emission tomography/computed tomography and positron emission tomography (PET) alone on expected management of patients with cancer: initial results from the National Oncologic PET Registry. J Clin Oncol 2008;26(13):2155–61.
3. Lakkaraju A, Patel CN, Bradley KM, et al. PET/CT in primary musculoskeletal tumours: a step forward. Eur Radiol 2010;20(12):2959–72.
4. Gholamrezanezhad A, Basques K, Batouli A, et al. Non-oncologic Applications of PET/CT and PET/MR in musculoskeletal, orthopedic, and rheumatologic imaging: general considerations, techniques, and radiopharmaceuticals. J Nucl Med Technol 2017. https://doi.org/10.2967/jnmt.117.198663.
5. Angelini A, Castellucci P, Ceci F. Future perspective of the application of positron emission tomography-computed tomography-MR imaging in musculoskeletal disorders. PET Clin 2019;14(1):183–91.
6. Gholamrezanezhad A, Guermazi A, Salavati A, et al. Evolving Role of PET-Computed Tomography and PET-MR imaging in assessment of musculoskeletal disorders and its potential revolutionary impact on day-to-day practice of related disciplines. PET Clin 2018;13(4):xiii–xiv.
7. Katal S, Gholamrezanezhad A, Kessler M, et al. PET in the diagnostic management of soft tissue sarcomas of musculoskeletal origin. PET Clin 2018; 13(4):609–21.
8. Gholamrezanejhad A, Mirpour S, Mariani G. Future of nuclear medicine: SPECT versus PET. J Nucl Med 2009;50(7):16N–8N.
9. Gholamrezanezhad A, Basques K, Batouli A, et al. Clinical nononcologic applications of PET/CT and PET/MRI in musculoskeletal, orthopedic, and rheumatologic imaging. AJR Am J Roentgenol 2018; 210(6):W245–63.
10. Al-Zaghal A, Ayubcha C, Kothekar E, et al. Clinical applications of positron emission tomography in the evaluation of spine and joint disorders. PET Clin 2019;14(1):61–9.
11. Pawaskar A, Basu S, Jahangiri P, et al. In vivo molecular imaging of musculoskeletal inflammation and infection. PET Clin 2019;14(1):43–59.
12. Biswal S, Resnick DL, Hoffman JM, et al. Molecular imaging: integration of molecular imaging into the musculoskeletal imaging practice. Radiology 2007; 244(3):651–71.
13. Yoder JS, Kogan F, Gold GE. Applications of PET-computed tomography-magnetic resonance in the management of benign musculoskeletal disorders. PET Clin 2019;14(1):1–15.
14. Brady Z, Taylor ML, Haynes M, et al. The clinical application of PET/CT: a contemporary review. Australas Phys Eng Sci Med 2008;31(2):90–109.
15. Griffeth LK. Use of PET/CT scanning in cancer patients: technical and practical considerations. Proc (Bayl Univ Med Cent) 2005;18(4):321–30.
16. Kooraki S, Assadi M, Gholamrezanezhad A. Hot topics of research in musculoskeletal imaging: PET/MR Imaging, MR fingerprinting, dual-energy CT scan, ultrashort echo time. PET Clin 2019;14(1): 175–82.
17. Eiber M, Takei T, Souvatzoglou M, et al. Performance of whole-body integrated 18F-FDG PET/MR in comparison to PET/CT for evaluation of malignant bone lesions. J Nucl Med 2014;55(2):191–7.
18. Schmidkonz C, Ellmann S, Ritt P, et al. Hybrid Imaging (PET-computed tomography/PET-MR imaging) of bone metastases. PET Clin 2019;14(1):121–33.
19. Samarin A, Hüllner M, Queiroz MA, et al. 18F-FDG-PET/MR increases diagnostic confidence in detection of bone metastases compared with 18F-FDG-PET/CT. Nucl Med Commun 2015;36(12):1165–73.
20. Fransen M, Simic M, Harmer AR. Determinants of MSK health and disability: lifestyle determinants of symptomatic osteoarthritis. Best Pract Res Clin Rheumatol 2014;28(3):435–60.
21. Nguyen U-SDT, Zhang Y, Zhu Y, et al. Increasing prevalence of knee pain and symptomatic knee osteoarthritis: survey and cohort data. Ann Intern Med 2011;155(11):725–32.
22. Luyten FP, Denti M, Filardo G, et al. Definition and classification of early osteoarthritis of the knee.

Knee Surg Sports Traumatol Arthrosc 2012;20(3): 401–6.

23. Kellgren JH, Lawrence JS. Radiological assessment of osteo-arthrosis. Ann Rheum Dis 1957;16(4): 494–502.

24. Kogan F, Fan AP, McWalter EJ, et al. PET/MRI of metabolic activity in osteoarthritis: a feasibility study. J Magn Reson Imaging 2017;45(6):1736–45.

25. Parsons MA, Moghbel M, Saboury B, et al. Increased 18F-FDG uptake suggests synovial inflammatory reaction with osteoarthritis: preliminary in-vivo results in humans. Nucl Med Commun 2015;36(12):1215–9.

26. Nakamura H, Masuko K, Yudoh K, et al. Positron emission tomography with 18F-FDG in osteoarthritic knee. Osteoarthritis Cartilage 2007;15(6):673–81.

27. Draper CE, Quon A, Fredericson M, et al. Comparison of MRI and 18F-NaF PET/CT in patients with patellofemoral pain. J Magn Reson Imaging 2012; 36(4):928–32.

28. Scott DL, Symmons DP, Coulton BL, et al. Long-term outcome of treating rheumatoid arthritis: results after 20 years. Lancet 1987;1(8542):1108–11.

29. Watt I. Basic differential diagnosis of arthritis. Eur Radiol 1997;7(3):344–51.

30. McQueen FM, Stewart N, Crabbe J, et al. Magnetic resonance imaging of the wrist in early rheumatoid arthritis reveals a high prevalence of erosions at four months after symptom onset. Ann Rheum Dis 1998;57(6):350–6.

31. Nissilä M, Isomäki H, Kaarela K, et al. Prognosis of inflammatory joint diseases. A three-year follow-up study. Scand J Rheumatol 1983;12(1):33–8.

32. Möttönen TT. Prediction of erosiveness and rate of development of new erosions in early rheumatoid arthritis. Ann Rheum Dis 1988;47(8):648–53.

33. van der Heijde DM, van Leeuwen MA, van Riel PL, et al. Biannual radiographic assessments of hands and feet in a three-year prospective followup of patients with early rheumatoid arthritis. Arthritis Rheum 1992;35(1):26–34.

34. van der Heijde DM. Joint erosions and patients with early rheumatoid arthritis. Br J Rheumatol 1995; 34(Suppl 2):74–8.

35. Polisson RP, Schoenberg OI, Fischman A, et al. Use of magnetic resonance imaging and positron emission tomography in the assessment of synovial volume and glucose metabolism in patients with rheumatoid arthritis. Arthritis Rheum 1995;38(6): 819–25.

36. Palmer WE, Rosenthal DI, Schoenberg OI, et al. Quantification of inflammation in the wrist with gadolinium-enhanced MR imaging and PET with 2-[F-18]-fluoro-2-deoxy-D-glucose. Radiology 1995; 196(3):647–55.

37. Carey K, Saboury B, Basu S, et al. Evolving role of FDG PET imaging in assessing joint disorders: a

systematic review. Eur J Nucl Med Mol Imaging 2011;38(10):1939–55.

38. Boutry N, Morel M, Flipo R-M, et al. Early rheumatoid arthritis: a review of MRI and sonographic findings. AJR Am J Roentgenol 2007;189(6):1502–9.

39. Miese F, Scherer A, Ostendorf B, et al. Hybrid 18F-FDG PET-MRI of the hand in rheumatoid arthritis: initial results. Clin Rheumatol 2011;30(9):1247–50.

40. Kubota K, Ito K, Morooka M, et al. Whole-body FDG-PET/CT on rheumatoid arthritis of large joints. Ann Nucl Med 2009;23(9):783–91.

41. Kumar NS, Shejul Y, Asopa R, et al. Quantitative Metabolic Volumetric Product on 18Fluorine-2fluoro-2-deoxy-D-glucose-positron emission tomography/computed tomography in assessing treatment response to disease-modifying antirheumatic drugs in rheumatoid arthritis: multiparametric analysis integrating American College of Rheumatology/European League Against Rheumatism criteria. World J Nucl Med 2017;16(4):293–302.

42. Kanis JA. Diagnosis of osteoporosis and assessment of fracture risk. Lancet 2002;359(9321): 1929–36.

43. Consensus development conference: diagnosis, prophylaxis, and treatment of osteoporosis. Am J Med 1993;94(6):646–50.

44. Austin AG, Raynor WY, Reilly CC, et al. Evolving role of MR imaging and PET in assessing osteoporosis. PET Clin 2019;14(1):31–41.

45. Chang G, Honig S, Brown R, et al. Finite element analysis applied to 3-T MR imaging of proximal femur microarchitecture: lower bone strength in patients with fragility fractures compared with control subjects. Radiology 2014;272(2): 464–74.

46. Uchida K, Nakajima H, Miyazaki T, et al. Effects of alendronate on bone metabolism in glucocorticoid-induced osteoporosis measured by 18F-fluoride PET: a prospective study. J Nucl Med 2009;50(11): 1808–14.

47. Blake GM, Siddique M, Frost ML, et al. Imaging of site specific bone turnover in osteoporosis using positron emission tomography. Curr Osteoporos Rep 2014;12(4):475–85.

48. Siddique M, Blake GM, Frost ML, et al. Estimation of regional bone metabolism from whole-body 18F-fluoride PET static images. Eur J Nucl Med Mol Imaging 2012;39(2):337–43.

49. Strobel K, Exner UE, Stumpe KDM, et al. The additional value of CT images interpretation in the differential diagnosis of benign vs. malignant primary bone lesions with 18F-FDG-PET/CT. Eur J Nucl Med Mol Imaging 2008;35(11):2000–8.

50. Marulanda GA, Henderson ER, Johnson DA, et al. Orthopedic surgery options for the treatment of primary osteosarcoma. Cancer Control 2008;15(1): 13–20.

51. Vander Griend RA. Osteosarcoma and its variants. Orthop Clin North Am 1996;27(3):575–81.

52. Franzius C, Sciuk J, Daldrup-Link HE, et al. FDG-PET for detection of osseous metastases from malignant primary bone tumours: comparison with bone scintigraphy. Eur J Nucl Med 2000;27(9):1305–11.

53. Daldrup-Link HE, Franzius C, Link TM, et al. Whole-body MR imaging for detection of bone metastases in children and young adults: comparison with skeletal scintigraphy and FDG PET. AJR Am J Roentgenol 2001;177(1):229–36.

54. Even-Sapir E, Metser U, Flusser G, et al. Assessment of malignant skeletal disease: initial experience with 18F-fluoride PET/CT and comparison between 18F-fluoride PET and 18F-fluoride PET/CT. J Nucl Med 2004;45(2):272–8.

55. Meyers PA, Schwartz CL, Krailo M, et al. Osteosarcoma: a randomized, prospective trial of the addition of ifosfamide and/or muramyl tripeptide to cisplatin, doxorubicin, and high-dose methotrexate. J Clin Oncol 2005;23(9):2004–11.

56. Charest M, Hickeson M, Lisbona R, et al. FDG PET/CT imaging in primary osseous and soft tissue sarcomas: a retrospective review of 212 cases. Eur J Nucl Med Mol Imaging 2009;36(12):1944–51.

57. Fuglø HM, Jørgensen SM, Loft A, et al. The diagnostic and prognostic value of 18F-FDG PET/CT in the initial assessment of high-grade bone and soft tissue sarcoma. A retrospective study of 89 patients. Eur J Nucl Med Mol Imaging 2012;39(9):1416–24.

58. Buchbender C, Heusner TA, Lauenstein TC, et al. Oncologic PET/MRI, part 2: bone tumors, soft-tissue tumors, melanoma, and lymphoma. J Nucl Med 2012;53(8):1244–52.

59. Cheon GJ, Kim MS, Lee JA, et al. Prediction model of chemotherapy response in osteosarcoma by 18F-FDG PET and MRI. J Nucl Med 2009;50(9):1435–40.

60. Ye Z, Zhu J, Tian M, et al. Response of osteogenic sarcoma to neoadjuvant therapy: evaluated by 18F-FDG-PET. Ann Nucl Med 2008;22(6):475–80.

61. Dimopoulos M, Terpos E, Comenzo RL, et al. International myeloma working group consensus statement and guidelines regarding the current role of imaging techniques in the diagnosis and monitoring of multiple Myeloma. Leukemia 2009;23(9):1545–56.

62. Bartel TB, Haessler J, Brown TLY, et al. F18-fluorodeoxyglucose positron emission tomography in the context of other imaging techniques and prognostic factors in multiple myeloma. Blood 2009;114(10):2068–76.

63. Zamagni E, Nanni C, Gay F, et al. 18F-FDG PET/CT focal, but not osteolytic, lesions predict the progression of smoldering myeloma to active disease. Leukemia 2016;30(2):417–22.

64. Wang K, Allen L, Fung E, et al. Bone scintigraphy in common tumors with osteolytic components. Clin Nucl Med 2005;30(10):655–71.

65. Batouli A, Gholamrezanezhad A, Petrov D, et al. Management of primary osseous spinal tumors with PET. PET Clin 2019;14(1):91–101.

66. Rodallec MH, Feydy A, Larousserie F, et al. Diagnostic imaging of solitary tumors of the spine: what to do and say. Radiographics 2008;28(4):1019–41.

67. Schulte M, Brecht-Krauss D, Heymer B, et al. Grading of tumors and tumorlike lesions of bone: evaluation by FDG PET. J Nucl Med 2000;41(10):1695–701.

68. Costelloe CM, Chuang HH, Chasen BA, et al. Bone windows for distinguishing malignant from benign primary bone tumors on FDG PET/CT. J Cancer 2013;4(7):524–30.

69. Aoki J, Watanabe H, Shinozaki T, et al. FDG PET of primary benign and malignant bone tumors: standardized uptake value in 52 lesions. Radiology 2001;219(3):774–7.

70. Wafaie A, El-Liethy N, Kassem H, et al. A comparison between FDG PET/CT, CT and MRI in detection of spinal metastases and its impact on clinical management. Egypt J Nucl Med 2013;8(8):30–44.

71. Hart RA, Boriani S, Biagini R, et al. A system for surgical staging and management of spine tumors. A clinical outcome study of giant cell tumors of the spine. Spine 1997;22(15):1773–82 [discussion: 1783].

72. Laredo JD, el Quessar A, Bossard P, et al. Vertebral tumors and pseudotumors. Radiol Clin North Am 2001;39(1):137–63, vi.

73. Tian R, Su M, Tian Y, et al. Dual-time point PET/CT with F-18 FDG for the differentiation of malignant and benign bone lesions. Skeletal Radiol 2009;38(5):451–8.

74. Costelloe CM, Chuang HH, Madewell JE. FDG PET/CT of primary bone tumors. AJR Am J Roentgenol 2014;202(6):W521–31.

75. Feldman F, Van Heertum R, Saxena C, et al. 18FDG-PET applications for cartilage neoplasms. Skeletal Radiol 2005;34(7):367–74.

76. Aoki J, Watanabe H, Shinozaki T, et al. FDG-PET in differential diagnosis and grading of chondrosarcomas. J Comput Assist Tomogr 1999;23(4):603–8.

Potential Applications of PET/CT/MR Imaging in Inflammatory Diseases
Part I: Musculoskeletal and Gastrointestinal Systems

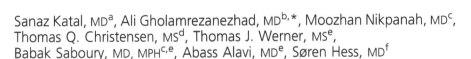

Sanaz Katal, MD[a], Ali Gholamrezanezhad, MD[b],*, Moozhan Nikpanah, MD[c],
Thomas Q. Christensen, MS[d], Thomas J. Werner, MS[e],
Babak Saboury, MD, MPH[c,e], Abass Alavi, MD[e], Søren Hess, MD[f]

KEYWORDS

- FDG • PET/CT • PET/MR imaging • Infection • Inflammation • Musculoskeletal disease
- Gastrointestinal disease

KEY POINTS

- Evidence is mounting for the use of combined fludeoxyglucose (FDG)-PET/computed tomography for selected indications in musculoskeletal and gastrointestinal inflammation.
- Combined FDG-PET/MR imaging especially has considerable potential in musculoskeletal and gastrointestinal inflammatory diseases due to exceptional soft tissue contrast and reduced radiation dose.
- Potential indications for PET-based imaging in musculoskeletal disorders include infection, joint prosthetic disease, articular and periarticular inflammation, osteoarthritis, metabolic bone disease, trauma, and pain syndromes.
- Potential indications for PET-based imaging in gastrointestinal inflammation include extra-intestinal disease extent, disease monitoring, response evaluation, and differentiation of stenosis etiology.

INTRODUCTION

During the first decades of fludeoxyglucose (FDG)-PET, the relative nonspecificity and the incidental false positive findings in patients with cancer caused by infectious or inflammatory processes were considered a nuisance. However, the usefulness and benefits have now been recognized outside the realm of malignancies: it is well known that molecular and cellular processes of inflammation create potential grounds for molecular targeted imaging, and the role of FDG-PET in the diagnosis and assessment of inflammation has been established in a multitude of clinical domains.[1–3] The fundamental basis for increased cellular uptake of FDG, the so-called Warburg

Sources of Funding: None.
Declaration of conflict of interest: None.
[a] Department of Nuclear Medicine/PET-CT, Kowsar Hospital, Shiraz, Iran; [b] Department of Radiology, Keck School of Medicine, University of Southern California (USC), Health Sciences Campus, 1500 San Pablo Street, Los Angeles, California 90033, USA; [c] Department of Radiology and Imaging Sciences, Clinical Center, National Institutes of Health, 9000 Rockville Pike, Bethesda, MD 20892, USA; [d] Department of Clinical Engineering, Region of Southern Denmark, Esbjerg, Denmark 5000; [e] Department of Radiology, Hospital of the University of Pennsylvania, 3400 Spruce St, Philadelphia, PA 19104, USA; [f] Department of Radiology and Nuclear Medicine, Hospital of South West Jutland, University Hospital of Southern Denmark, Esbjerg, Denmark 6700
* Corresponding author.
E-mail address: ali.gholamrezanezhad@med.usc.edu

effect, originally adhered to cancer cells, but increased glycolytic activity also occurs in activated inflammatory cells such as neutrophils and macrophages. The result is an increased cellular influx of FDG with subsequent metabolic trapping just like in malignant cells, for example, lymphocytes switch to glycolysis on activation and may increase uptake as much as 20-fold within 24 hours; this so-called respiratory burst and the speed with which it occurs is a key in understanding the potential of FDG-PET/computed tomography (CT) as an in vivo, noninvasive marker of disease extent and disease status in inflammatory diseases.[4]

The developments and implementation of PET/MR imaging has hitherto proceeded at much slower pace than PET/CT, with a current ratio of 1:50 in the United States. Reasons for this include significantly higher acquisition costs, higher operational costs with a need for additional training, and higher complexity, for example, electromagnetic interference creates PET artifacts and reduced signal-to-noise ratios. To the patient, MR imaging scans are usually considered less comfortable than either PET or CT with smaller bore diameter, noise, claustrophobia, and longer acquisition times. The latter, however, may be considered advantageous regarding PET, as it allows better count rates and superior image quality even with lesser radiopharmaceutical doses.[5,6] The gain from adding MR imaging to PET is especially obvious in musculoskeletal and gastrointestinal inflammatory diseases, that is, exceptional soft tissue contrast and reduced radiation dose.

A specific challenge with systemic inflammatory diseases is treatment and especially monitoring treatment response, not least in an era with an increasing use of novel biologic medicine. Biologic medicines may be more effective than standard treatment like steroids or methotrexate, but costs are many-fold higher and potential side effects more severe. This necessitates better and more rapid methods to evaluate treatment response so that ineffective medicine can be discontinued in a timely fashion. Generally speaking, response evaluation requires more objective parameters than visual assessment alone; although the literature remains to sparse to speculate on the true contribution of PET/CT or PET/MR imaging, it is reasonable to hypothesize that the continuous refinement of the quantitative potentials of both PET and MR imaging will significantly broaden their uses also in inflammatory disorders, and this may be increasingly important as inflammatory diseases often affect younger individuals, and therefore lower radiation is especially desirable for serial examinations, for example, response evaluation.

This article outlines the current potential for hybrid molecular imaging in the musculoskeletal system and the gastrointestinal tract with special focus on the potential for fused PET/CT/MR imaging.

MUSCULOSKELETAL DISORDERS

Potential clinical applications of PET/CT/MR imaging for nononcologic musculoskeletal disorders are described in the following sections, that is, musculoskeletal infections, joint prostheses, degeneration, inflammation, metabolic bone disorders, periarticular disorders, amyloid arthropathy, trauma, and pain syndromes.

Musculoskeletal Infection

Osteomyelitis is an increasingly common pathology that remains a major source of morbidity and mortality worldwide. A major challenge in the clinical management of osteomyelitis is to make a timely diagnosis to provide accurate and appropriate therapeutic management to prevent threatening complications. Although the diagnostic approach to osteomyelitis mainly relies on radiographic features, it is well known that radiographs are not sensitive enough in the early stages of the disease. In fact, osteolytic lesions and periosteal reaction as the main radiographic features of osteomyelitis may take several days to appear on radiographs. MR imaging has been shown to be a highly accurate and sensitive modality, even in early stages of osteomyelitis. The main features of osteomyelitis in MR imaging are decreased T1 and increased T2 and proton density signal intensity. Contrast administration is not indicated in most cases. The high accuracy of FDG-PET/CT in detecting and defining the extent of osteomyelitis has also been well documented. In a meta-analysis by Termaat and colleagues,[7] the sensitivity and specificity of FDG-PET for the detection of chronic osteomyelitis in the appendicular and axial skeleton was 91% and 96%, respectively, which was the highest among all other imaging modalities. Similarly, in another study, by Wang and colleagues,[8] FDG-PET/CT demonstrated the highest diagnostic value in patients with suspected osteomyelitis (**Fig. 1**).

Recently, hybrid FDG-PET/MR imaging has been shown to represent an important modality in the diagnostic workup of musculoskeletal infections. The advantage of MR imaging compared with CT for the detection of osteomyelitis makes PET/MR imaging superior over PET/CT,

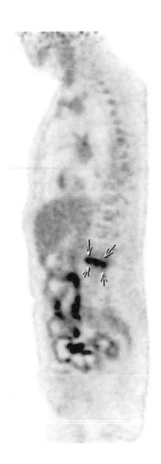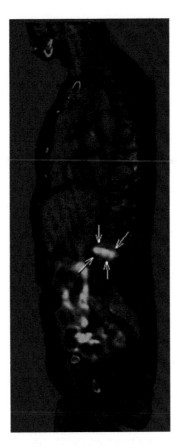

Fig. 1. Spondylodiscitis. Sagittal PET image (*left*) and sagittal fused PET/CT image (*right*) show intense FDG uptake in lumbar vertebrae at L2/L3, consistent with spondylodiscitis (*arrows*). A subsequent MR imaging scan confirmed the diagnosis. (*From* Hess S, Hansson SH, Pedersen KT, Basu S, Høilund-Carlsen PF. FDG-PET/CT in infectious and inflammatory diseases. PET Clinics 2014;9(4):497-519.)

specifically in vertebral osteomyelitis/spondylodiscitis.[9] FDG-PET/CT performs better than MR imaging in the early phase,[10] whereas MR imaging is better at assessing soft tissue abscesses associated with osteomyelitis and also for surgery planning, thus, hybrid FDG-PET/MR imaging is potentially even more valuable. Hulsen and colleagues[11] proposed FDG-PET/MR imaging to hold at least the equal diagnostic value as FDG-PET/CT in chronic osteomyelitis. When infection sites are assessed metabolically by FDG, findings correlate with MR imaging findings of marrow edema and soft tissue characteristics, which helps in accurate debridement planning. Other PET radiotracers such as ^{11}C-methionine, ^{11}C-PK11195, and ^{68}Ga-citrate have also been tested in osteomyelitis, but with lower efficacy than FDG.[12] Similarly, [124]I-FIAU has been evaluated in some studies as a promising PET agent for the detection of musculoskeletal bacterial infection, targeting microorganism thymidine kinase.[13] However, although results are interesting, a lack of sufficient data and failure to translate the promising preclinical and preliminary human results has hitherto halted further clinical implementation.

Joint Prosthesis

As a promising diagnostic tool, FDG-PET/CT has been investigated for the evaluation of infectious prosthetic complications after arthroplasty (**Fig. 2**). A meta-analysis by Hao and colleagues[14] on 14 studies demonstrated high pooled specificity and sensitivity (87%) for FDG-PET or FDG-PET/CT in cases suspicious for prosthetic infection. Furthermore, the pooled results of per prosthesis–based analyses were higher for hip than knee (88% and 88% vs 72% and 80%, respectively). Aside from diagnosis, FDG-PET/CT offers additional information on the exact site and extension of infection (**Figs. 3** and **4**), presence of periosteal reaction or osteolysis, the stability of prosthesis or joint, and the integrity of surrounding soft tissue,[15] all of which are of added value in guiding the orthopedic surgeons in the optimal management. The value of PET in these settings becomes even more important, as MR imaging is limited by significant susceptibility artifact limiting the evaluation of underlying bone and surrounding soft tissues.

In terms of interpretation criteria, Reinartz and colleagues[16] suggested standardized uptake

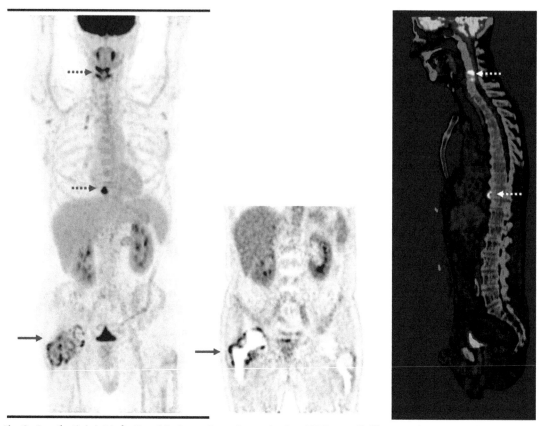

Fig. 2. Prosthetic joint infection. Maximum intensity projection PET image (*left*), coronal PET image (*middle*), and fused sagittal PET/CT image (*right*) show intense FDG uptake around the right hip prosthesis (*solid arrows*) and, furthermore, anteriorly in thoracic vertebrae Th9/Th10 and cervical vertebrae C3/C4 consistent with spondylodiscitis at 2 different levels (*dotted arrows*). MIP, Maximum intensity projection. (*From* Hess S, Hansson SH, Pedersen KT, Basu S, Høilund-Carlsen PF. FDG-PET/CT in infectious and inflammatory diseases. PET Clinics 2014;9(4):497-519.)

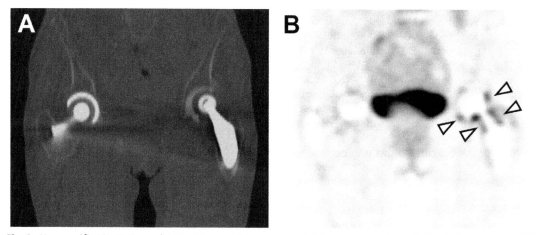

Fig. 3. Nonspecific 18F-FDG uptake in a 66-year-old woman with bilateral asymptomatic total hip prostheses. This patient underwent 18F FDG-PET to evaluate a lung lesion. Coronal PET image (*B*) shows nonspecific 18F-FDG uptake around the neck of the left hip prosthesis (*arrowheads*), with corresponding CT image (*A*). (*From* Kwee M and Kwee T. 18F-FDG PET for Diagnosing Infections in Prosthetic Joints. PET Clin 2020; 15(2):197-205; with permission.)

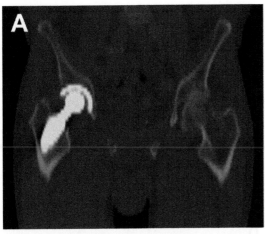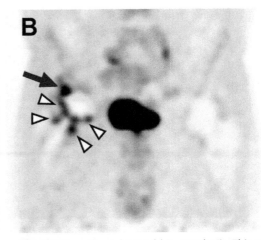

Fig. 4. Nonspecific 18F-FDG uptake in a 70-year-old man with asymptomatic right total hip prosthesis. This patient underwent 18F FDG-PET to identify the cause of fever of unknown origin. Coronal PET image (*B*) shows nonspecific 18F-FDG uptake around the neck (*arrowheads*) and nonspecific 18F-FDG uptake at lateral side of the acetabular cup (*arrow*), with corresponding CT image (*A*). (*From* Kwee M and Kwee T. 18F-FDG PET for Diagnosing Infections in Prosthetic Joints. PET Clin 2020; 15(2):197-205; with permission.)

value (SUV)mean thresholds of 3, 5, and 5.9 in prostheses without an infection, prostheses with aseptic loosening, and infected prostheses, respectively. In other studies, FDG uptake at the bone-prosthesis surface has been offered as the diagnostic standard in prosthesis infection (**Fig. 5**).[17] On the other hand, physiologic FDG uptake of noninfected prostheses has been described by Gelderman and colleagues[18] as diffuse heterogeneous FDG uptake pattern with median SUVmax values of approximately 2.5, and the highest FDG uptake around the neck of the prosthesis.

Inflammatory Arthropathies

Several studies have demonstrated that FDG precisely outlines the inflammatory activity in articular and extra-articular locations of different rheumatic diseases with strong correlations between FDG uptake and clinical and serologic values.[19,20] Lee and colleagues[21] studied 91 patients with rheumatoid arthritis (RA) and demonstrated a significant correlation between the number of inflamed joints on PET and the number of clinically swollen or tender joints as well as erythrocyte sedimentation rate and disease activity score. FDG/PET also offers early disease detection and monitoring of response to therapy in RA.[22–24] Moreover, different metabolic patterns of the disease in FDG-PET studies may potentially serve as a diagnostic guide to differentiate various inflammatory rheumatic conditions.[23,25]

Aside from FDG and NaF, several novel PET tracers have also been investigated for imaging

RA; for example, ^{11}C-choline, ^{11}C-PK11195, [11]CD-deprenyl, and ^{68}Ga-PRGD2. In patients with RA, ^{11}C-choline and FDG both correlate with the volume of synovial tissue on MR imaging,[26] although ^{11}C-choline detects the affected joints in a shorter period of time (10 minutes).[27] ^{68}Ga-PRGD2 mainly illustrates synovial angiogenesis.[28] As such, it specifically accumulates in synovia with active inflammation, but compared with FDG, ^{68}Ga-PRGD2 reveals far less skeletal muscle uptake. Overall, a vast potential exists to develop tracers targeting specific molecular components of synovitis, which present a better understanding of the molecular basis of the disease.[29]

FDG-PET/MR imaging has also been proposed for imaging in RA, which offers major advantages, including detection of synovitis and marrow edema. Miese and colleagues[30] reported the feasibility of FDG-PET/MR imaging for imaging the hands in early RA; however, further studies using this hybrid modality are yet needed.

Periarticular/Juxta-Articular Inflammatory Pathologies

Periarticular pathologies (including tendinopathy, enthesopathy, and bursitis) have been encountered incidentally in patients undergoing oncologic PET scans.[31–33] This fact has been considered as an evidence for potential utility of PET in the evaluation of periarticular/juxta-articular inflammatory pathologies. In a study by Moon and colleagues[34] of 24 patients with shoulder lesions (including acromion spur, cuff tear, frozen shoulder, and calcific tendinitis), 9 patients showed increased

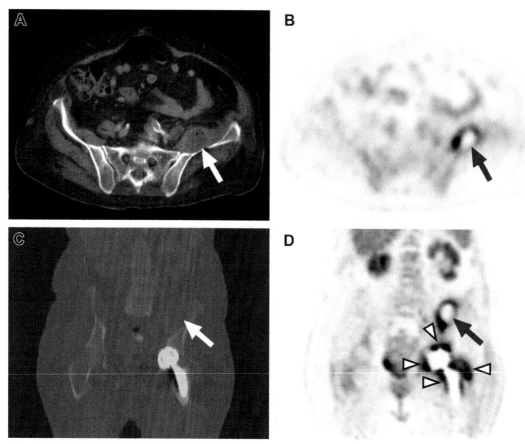

Fig. 5. Periprosthetic joint infection in an 80-year-old woman with painful left hip prosthesis. Axial (*A, B*) and coronal (*C, D*) CT and PET images are displayed. There is a fluid collection in the left iliacus (*arrows* [*A, C*]) muscle, which shows peripheral 18F-FDG uptake and no central 18F-FDG uptake (*arrows* [*B, D*]), compatible with an abscess. This abscess was not suspected clinically and extended caudally to the left hip joint. In addition, there is 18F-FDG uptake at the bone-prosthesis interface around the acetabular cup and at the proximal femoral stem (*arrowheads* [*D*]). (*From* Kwee M and Kwee T. 18F-FDG PET for Diagnosing Infections in Prosthetic Joints. PET Clin 2020; 15(2):197-205; with permission.)

FDG uptake about the shoulder girdle. Similarly, in patients with adhesive capsulitis,[27,35] FDG-PET uptake was noted in zones of inflammation and fibrosis (eg, along the inferior glenohumeral ligament and the axillary pouch).[27] In these conditions, PET findings could be superior to MR imaging abnormalities (including edema and loss of fat pad of the rotator interval and edema and thickening of the axillary pouch).[27]

Several cases have also been reported with Achilles tendonitis on PET scan.[29] Achilles pathologies may occur secondary to sports injuries, and local (such as retrocalcaneal bursa) or systemic (such as RA) inflammatory processes. Other incidental extra-articular pathologies found on PET include ischial tuberosity enthesopathy and iliopsoas bursitis.[36] Although PET/CT is not primarily established for this setting, especially if MR imaging is available and provides higher anatomic and

soft tissue resolution, these incidental benign musculoskeletal findings should be recognized, reported, and clinically correlated by the interpreting nuclear physicians.

Osteoarthritis

MR imaging alone has been used widely to study osteoarthritis (OA), yet cannot provide insights into the primary pathophysiological mechanisms. Although MR imaging can detect subtle changes of early OA (such as chondrosis and subchondral marrow edema), PET/CT/MR imaging can detect OA at a reversible stage before tissue loss and degeneration occurs. In accordance with the activated inflamed cells and bone remodeling, OA can be identified through both FDG-PET and NaF-PET. Draper and colleagues[37] found a correlation between increasing tracer uptake in patellofemoral

OA and increasing pain intensity using NaF-PET/CT. They also suggested that NaF-PET/CT may provide additional information in the diagnostic workup of patellofemoral pain compared with MR imaging.[38] Although cartilage damage and bone marrow edema in OA often correspond to areas of increased tracer uptake, metabolic changes can also occur in the lack of structural abnormalities found in MR imaging. Similarly, Kobayashi[39] reported that NaF-PET could detect bone abnormalities earlier than MR imaging in hip OA. However, it should be emphasized that novel MR imaging sequences, such as quantitative ultrashort echo time, have been very promising in early diagnosis of the disease and direct head-to-head comparison of these modalities is advised for future research.

Similar to NaF, FDG provides a potential added value in OA detection and progression. FDG-PET/MR imaging was able to recognize patients with degenerative facet joint arthropathy who may profit from CT-guided facet block injections; that is, patients with FDG-positive facet arthropathy had a significantly greater therapy response than those with FDG-negative findings.[40]

Metabolic Bone Disease

Metabolic bone disorders encompass a diverse class of diseases that involve homeostatic disruption of bone formation and resorption, for example, osteoporosis, osteomalacia, Paget disease, renal osteodystrophy, and parathyroid disorders. Although still evolving, PET/CT/MR imaging with NaF or FDG holds promise for the study of metabolic bone diseases,[41] not only for earlier detection and optimal treatment, but also the application of preventive measures.[42] Several studies have demonstrated the value of NaF-PET in the monitoring of therapy response in osteoporosis, specifically in postmenopausal women,[43,44] as the most common metabolic bone disorder. Similarly, NaF-PET has been successfully used to assess therapy response in other metabolic bone disorders, such as Paget disease.[45] In addition, FDG-PET is able to differentiate between osteoporotic fractures and pathologic fractures due to malignancies.[46] Last, NaF-uptake in PET studies of patients with renal osteodystrophy has been strongly correlated with markers of bone turnover.[47]

Amyloid Arthropathy

Amyloidosis results from abnormal extracellular deposition of protein and protein derivatives, interfering with normal tissue functions. In musculoskeletal involvement, amyloid may deposit in the joint, synovium, or periarticular soft tissues.

On FDG-PET, amyloid arthropathy is reported to demonstrate heterogeneous mild to moderate activity in periarticular, synovial, or intra-articular amyloid deposition.[35] It has been suggested that FDG-PET is potentially able to add valuable information when conventional radiological methods are inconclusive or contraindicated.[48] In a case series by Mekinian and colleagues,[49] FDG-avidity on PET was concordant with organ impairment in 86% cases and unmasked previously unknown nasopharyngeal and mesenteric lesions.

Traumatic Injuries, Fractures, and Complications

By far, radiographs and MR imaging are the mainstays of imaging in the setting of traumatic injuries. However, molecular imaging biomarkers like PET/MR imaging/CT with NaF or FDG provide more accurate and more in-depth insights into the pathogenesis of traumatic injuries to bone, cartilage, tendons, and ligaments, their recovery process, and posttraumatic complications.[50–52]

Within the realms of posttraumatic complications, Jeon and colleagues[53] assessed the potential role of NaF-PET/CT to evaluate ankle joint disability after trauma. They suggested that those regions with greater impairment displayed higher uptake of NaF, albeit the objective assessment of ankle range of motion was somewhat inconsistent. They subsequently proposed that bone PET/CT serves as an objective imaging marker for defining ankle joint disability after trauma. Animal studies have also shown the potential role of PET imaging as an indicator of nonunited fractures.[54] In a study by Wenter and colleagues,[55] FDG-PET was used with high accuracy to differentiate infected from noninfected nonunited fractures when other clinical results for local infection were inconclusive. Belehalli and colleagues[56] used FDG-PET/CT to evaluate the viability of the femoral head following acetabular fractures, which is beneficial for early detection of complications, such as avascular necrosis. The aforementioned studies suggest that FDG-PET or FDG-PET/CT offers additional value and represents a plausible alternative in traumatic injuries.

Pain Syndromes/Neuropathic Pain

Musculoskeletal pain syndromes are common disorders that have a tremendous impact on individuals and pose a high burden on social health services. However, an objective assessment of the pain remains a clinical challenge, as conventional structural imaging rarely captures the underlying pathologic alterations. Recently, neuro-functional imaging of pain with FDG-PET/MR imaging has been introduced to image inflamed overactive neurons in painful regions. In a study by Biswal and colleagues,[57] 5 of 6 of patients with chronic neuropathic lower extremity pain had foci of increased FDG uptake in the injured nerves and muscle, at the site of highest pain symptoms as well as in areas not associated with spine pain. The investigators suggested that FDG-PET can assist in localizing pain-related noci-ceptive activity. Interestingly, the abnormalities found on PET eventually alerted clinical management of their pain. Experimental nonhuman models have found similar results using PET in neuropathic pain.[58]

Recently, PET tracers beyond FDG have been investigated for this purpose. PET imaging of patients suffering from whiplash-associated pain disorders has revealed significantly elevated [11]CD-deprenyl uptake in the neck, serving as a marker of local persistent peripheral tissue inflammation.[59] In a study by Imamoto and colleagues,[60] ^{11}C-PK11195 PET imaged activated glia in the spinal cord of neuropathic pain. While these tracers hold a great promise for elucidating the underlying pathologies and may support the development of novel therapies, there remains a need for more studies in this field.

GASTROINTESTINAL INFLAMMATION

Imaging the bowel is challenging for several reasons, that is, an air-filled tubular organ with involuntary muscular movement and abundant bacterial flora may hamper the use of almost any modality due to a multitude of different potential artifacts. Coregistration may therefore be of particular importance to ensure comparable results under similar physiologic conditions and despite shifting organ position due to peristalsis or bladder filling.[6] Thus, to take full advantage of complementary imaging modalities, hybrid scanners may be especially interesting and FDG-PET/CT has already been suggested for various aspects of inflammatory bowel diseases (IBD) like ulcerative colitis, and Crohn's disease (CD), although the literature is still relatively sparse and of variable quality. Although some cases of IBD are encountered during workup in patients with nonspecific complaints or findings, such as fever of unknown origin, there is generally only limited diagnostic value in the primary diagnostic workup; endoscopic examination remains the mainstay with histopathologic confirmation. However, in the subsequent management, several domains holds

promise, for example, extra-intestinal disease extent (as many as 25% of patients with CD), for noninvasive disease monitoring (eg, patients with symptoms suggestive of disease flare), to monitor treatment response (especially with increasing use of biologic therapy with high costs and severe adverse effects), and to establish treatment strategy (eg, differentiating fibrostenotic stenoses requiring surgery from inflammatory stenoses requiring medical treatment)[61,62] (**Fig. 6**). These clinical domains may be especially desirable in children and adolescents in whom endoscopies sometimes necessitate general anesthesia.[63] Similarly, several MR imaging features of bowel inflammation (eg, intestinal wall hyperintensity on diffusion-weighted images and rapid gadolinium enhancement), the ability to differentiate the mucosa-submucosa complex and the muscularis propria layer, and the correlation between restricted diffusion at the terminal ileum and active inflammation have also been established with endoscopic confirmation,[6] and much like FDG-PET/CT MR imaging performs better in moderate to severe than mild cases.

With the often younger population of patients with IBD in mind, this disease complex may be one of the most interesting indications for hybrid PET/MR imaging, and several reports are emerging within several of the aforementioned subdomains. In 21 consecutive patients with CD, Domachevsky and colleagues[64] demonstrated the correlation between imaging and biomarkers with an increase in area under the curve from 0.63 to 0.92, with sensitivity and specificity of 83% and 100%, respectively, and concluded that FDG-PET/MR imaging significantly increased accuracy in discriminating active from nonactive

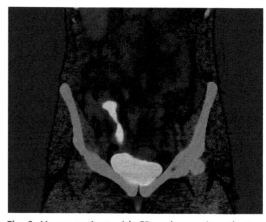

Fig. 6. Young patient with CD and stenosis at the terminal ileum. FDG-PET/CT clearly demonstrated a continuous active inflammatory component after initial treatment.

inflammation. This correlation may even be present in presymptomatic subclinical patients; Shih and colleagues[65] found correlating increased apparent diffusion coefficient (ADC) and SUVmax in bowel segments with corresponding endoscopic signs of active inflammation even in patients in perceived clinical and biochemical remission. The potential value has also been established for the important differentiation between purely fibrotic and inflammatory strictures, that is, Catalano and colleagues[66] performed preoperative FDG-PET/MR imaging in 19 patients with CD with strictures and found significant differences in PET and MR imaging–based parameters between fibrotic and inflammatory stenosis with the combined FDG-PET/MR imaging marker ADC $\times$ SUVmax being the best discriminator. Finally, Pellino and colleagues[67] compared the preoperative accuracy of MR imaging, FDG-PET/CT, and FDG-PET/MR imaging to detect disease sites and discriminate fibrotic from inflammatory strictures in 35 patients with CD with symptomatic small-bowel disease and scheduled for surgery. They found all 3 modalities equally accurate for detecting CD lesions, but FDG-PET/MR imaging more accurately detected extraluminal, distant disease and was better at discriminating fibrosis from inflammation in strictures. Overall, PET/MR imaging results impacted clinical management to a higher degree than PET/CT.

In a different, but comparable clinical entity with intra-abdominal inflammation, Thuermel and colleagues[68] found FDG-PET/MR imaging superior to clinical and biochemical markers to establish disease activity, extent, and vascular involvement in patients with retroperitoneal fibrosis: In 14 patients, FDG-PET/MR imaging demonstrated disease activity in 29% of scans with normal C-reactive protein and 50% of patients with normal erythrocyte sedimentation rate, and large-vessel vasculitis and aneurysm in 21% and 14%, respectively.

SUMMARY

The potential gain from FDG-PET/MR imaging over FDG-PET/CT is obvious and based on a sound rationale in both musculoskeletal inflammatory diseases and gastrointestinal inflammation, that is, the basic characteristics of increased FDG uptake in inflammatory tissue, better soft tissue contrast, and less radiation burden.[69–73] This is especially desirable in the younger populations that dominate these clinical domains. Despite several interesting results with alternative tracers, FDG remains the current mainstay, but regardless of tracer, the literature is even sparser with PET/

MR imaging than for PET/CT and further evaluations are necessary before FDG-PET/CT/MR imaging can be considered clinical routine to the benefit of patients who may require fewer sequential invasive endoscopic examinations.

REFERENCES

1. Gormsen LC, Hess S. Challenging but clinically useful: fluorodeoxyglucose PET/computed tomography in inflammatory and infectious diseases. PET Clin 2020;15(2):xi–xii.
2. Kung BT, Seraj SM, Zadeh MZ, et al. An update on the role of (18)F-FDG-PET/CT in major infectious and inflammatory diseases. Am J Nucl Med Mol Imaging 2019;9(6):255–73.
3. Alavi A, Hess S, Werner TJ, et al. An update on the unparalleled impact of FDG-PET imaging on the day-to-day practice of medicine with emphasis on management of infectious/inflammatory disorders. Eur J Nucl Med Mol Imaging 2020;47(1):18–27.
4. Sathekge M, Maes A, Wiele CVd. FDG-PET imaging in HIV infection and tuberculosis. Semin Nucl Med 2013;43(5):349–66.
5. Ehman EC, Johnson GB, Villanueva-Meyer JE, et al. PET/MRI: where might it replace PET/CT? J Magn Reson Imaging 2017;46(5):1247–62.
6. Sollini M, Berchiolli R, Kirienko M, et al. PET/MRI in infection and inflammation. Semin Nucl Med 2018; 48(3):225–41.
7. Termaat MF, Raijmakers PG, Scholten HJ, et al. The accuracy of diagnostic imaging for the assessment of chronic osteomyelitis: a systematic review and meta-analysis. J Bone Joint Surg Am 2005;87(11): 2464–71.
8. Wang GL, Zhao K, Liu ZF, et al. A meta-analysis of fluorodeoxyglucose-positron emission tomography versus scintigraphy in the evaluation of suspected osteomyelitis. Nucl Med Commun 2011;32(12): 1134–42.
9. Kouijzer IJE, Scheper H, de Rooy JWJ, et al. The diagnostic value of (18)F-FDG-PET/CT and MRI in suspected vertebral osteomyelitis - a prospective study. Eur J Nucl Med Mol Imaging 2018;45(5): 798–805.
10. Smids C, Kouijzer IJ, Vos FJ, et al. A comparison of the diagnostic value of MRI and (18)F-FDG-PET/CT in suspected spondylodiscitis. Infection 2017; 45(1):41–9.
11. Hulsen DJW, Geurts J, Arts JJ, et al. Hybrid FDG-PET/MR imaging of chronic osteomyelitis: a prospective case series. Eur J Hybrid Imaging 2019; 3(1):7.
12. Nielsen OL, Afzelius P, Bender D, et al. Comparison of autologous (111)In-leukocytes, (18)F-FDG, (11)C-methionine, (11)C-PK11195 and (68)Ga-citrate for diagnostic nuclear imaging in a juvenile porcine

haematogenous staphylococcus aureus osteomye-litis model. Am J Nucl Med Mol Imaging 2015;5(2): 169–82.

13. Diaz LA Jr, Foss CA, Thornton K, et al. Imaging of musculoskeletal bacterial infections by [124I]FIAU-PET/CT. PLoS One 2007;2(10):e1007.

14. Hao R, Yuan L, Kan Y, et al. 18F-FDG PET for diagnosing painful arthroplasty/prosthetic joint infection. Clinical and Translational Imaging 2017; 5(4):315–22. Available at: https://link.springer.com/ article/10.1007/s40336-017-0237-8.

15. Thapa P, Kalshetty A, Basu S. FDG PET/CT in assessment of prosthetic joint infection. In: Wagner T, Basu S, editors. PET/CT in infection and inflammation. Cham (Switzerland): Springer International Publishing; 2018. p. 43–54.

16. Reinartz P, Mumme T, Hermanns B, et al. Radionu-clide imaging of the painful hip arthroplasty: positron-emission tomography versus triple-phase bone scanning. J Bone Joint Surg Br 2005;87(4): 465–70.

17. Zhuang H, Duarte PS, Pourdehnad M, et al. The promising role of 18F-FDG PET in detecting infected lower limb prosthesis implants. J Nucl Med 2001; 42(1):44–8.

18. Gelderman SJ, Jutte PC, Boellaard R, et al. (18)F-FDG-PET uptake in non-infected total hip prosthe-ses. Acta Orthop 2018;89(6):634–9.

19. Beckers C, Ribbens C, Andre B, et al. Assess-ment of disease activity in rheumatoid arthritis with (18)F-FDG PET. J Nucl Med 2004;45(6): 956–64.

20. Hotta M, Minamimoto R, Kaneko H, et al. Fluoro-deoxyglucose PET/CT of arthritis in rheumatic dis-eases: a pictorial review. Radiographics 2020; 40(1):223–40.

21. Lee SJ, Jeong JH, Lee CH, et al. Development and validation of an (18) F-fluorodeoxyglucose-positron emission tomography with computed tomography-based tool for the evaluation of joint counts and disease activity in patients with rheu-matoid arthritis. Arthritis Rheumatol 2019;71(8): 1232–40.

22. Chaudhari AJ, Ferrero A, Godinez F, et al. High-res-olution (18)F-FDG PET/CT for assessing disease ac-tivity in rheumatoid and psoriatic arthritis: findings of a prospective pilot study. Br J Radiol 2016;89(1063): 20160138.

23. Vijayant V, Sarma M, Aurangabadkar H, et al. Poten-tial of (18)F-FDG-PET as a valuable adjunct to clin-ical and response assessment in rheumatoid arthritis and seronegative spondyloarthropathies. World J Radiol 2012;4(12):462–8.

24. Fosse P, Kaiser M-J, Namur G, et al. 18F- FDG PET/ CT joint assessment of early therapeutic response in rheumatoid arthritis patients treated with rituximab. Eur J Hybrid Imaging 2018;2(1):6.

25. Okabe T, Shibata H, Shizukuishi K, et al. F-18 FDG uptake patterns and disease activity of collagen vascular diseases-associated arthritis. Clin Nucl Med 2011;36(5):350–4.

26. Roivainen A, Parkkola R, Yli-Kerttula T, et al. Use of positron emission tomography with methyl-11C-choline and 2-18F-fluoro-2-deoxy-D-glucose in com-parison with magnetic resonance imaging for the assessment of inflammatory proliferation of syno-vium. Arthritis Rheum 2003;48(11):3077–84.

27. Roivainen A, Yli-Kerttula T. Whole-body distribution of (11)C-choline and uptake in knee synovitis. Eur J Nucl Med Mol Imaging 2006;33(11):1372–3.

28. Zhu Z, Yin Y, Zheng K, et al. Evaluation of synovial angiogenesis in patients with rheumatoid arthritis us-ing (6)(8)Ga-PRGD2 PET/CT: a prospective proof-of-concept cohort study. Ann Rheum Dis 2014;73(6): 1269–72.

29. Narayan N, Owen DR, Taylor PC. Advances in posi-tron emission tomography for the imaging of rheu-matoid arthritis. Rheumatology 2017;56(11): 1837–46.

30. Miese F, Scherer A, Ostendorf B, et al. Hybrid 18F-FDG PET-MRI of the hand in rheumatoid arthritis: initial results. Clin Rheumatol 2011;30(9):1247–50.

31. Salem U, Zhang L, Jorgensen JL, et al. Adhesive capsulitis mimicking metastasis on 18F-FDG-PET/ CT. Clin Nucl Med 2015;40(2):e145–7.

32. Vogel-Claussen J, Morrison W, Zoga A, et al. Calcific tendinosis: a potential mimicker of malignancy on PET. Radiol Case Rep 2006;1(2):38–41.

33. Huang SS, Yu JQ, Chamroonrat W, et al. Achilles tendonitis detected by FDG-PET. Clin Nucl Med 2006;31(3):147–8.

34. Moon YL, Lee SH, Park SY, et al. Evaluation of shoul-der disorders by 2-[F-18]-fluoro-2-deoxy-D-glucose positron emission tomography and computed to-mography. Clin Orthop Surg 2010;2(3):167–72.

35. White ML, Johnson GB, Howe BM, et al. Spectrum of benign articular and periarticular findings at FDG PET/CT. Radiographics 2016;36(3):824–39.

36. Flachra M, Flachra RJ, Twomey M, et al, editor. Inci-dental benign musculoskeletal findings on PET-CT: an educational pictorial review. 21st annual confer-ence of the European Society of Musculoskeletal Radiology; Riga, Latvia, June 26–28, 2014.

37. Draper CE, Fredericson M, Gold GE, et al. Patients with patellofemoral pain exhibit elevated bone meta-bolic activity at the patellofemoral joint. J Orthop Res 2012;30(2):209–13.

38. Draper CE, Quon A, Fredericson M, et al. Compari-son of MRI and (1)(8)F-NaF PET/CT in patients with patellofemoral pain. J Magn Reson Imaging 2012; 36(4):928–32.

39. Kobayashi N, Inaba Y, Tateishi U, et al. Comparison of 18F-fluoride positron emission tomography and magnetic resonance imaging in evaluating early-

stage osteoarthritis of the hip. Nucl Med Commun 2015;36(1):84–9.

40. Gholamrezanezhad A, Basques K, Batouli A, et al. Clinical nononcologic applications of PET/CT and PET/MRI in musculoskeletal, orthopedic, and rheumatologic imaging. AJR Am J Roentgenol 2018; 210(6):W245–63.

41. Kogan F, Fan AP, Gold GE. Potential of PET-MRI for imaging of non-oncologic musculoskeletal disease. Quant Imaging Med Surg 2016;6(6):756–71.

42. Yoder JS, Kogan F, Gold GE. PET-MRI for the study of metabolic bone disease. Curr Osteoporos Rep 2018;16(6):665–73.

43. Blake GM, Park-Holohan SJ, Fogelman I. Quantitative studies of bone in postmenopausal women using (18)F-fluoride and (99m)Tc-methylene diphosphonate. J Nucl Med 2002;43(3):338–45.

44. Hawkins RA, Choi Y, Huang SC, et al. Evaluation of the skeletal kinetics of fluorine-18-fluoride ion with PET. J Nucl Med 1992;33(5):633–42.

45. Devogelaer JP. Modern therapy for Paget's disease of bone: focus on bisphosphonates. Treat Endocrinol 2002;1(4):241–57.

46. Schmitz A, Risse JH, Textor J, et al. FDG-PET findings of vertebral compression fractures in osteoporosis: preliminary results. Osteoporos Int 2002; 13(9):755–61.

47. Messa C, Goodman WG, Hoh CK, et al. Bone metabolic activity measured with positron emission tomography and [18F]fluoride ion in renal osteodystrophy: correlation with bone histomorphometry. J Clin Endocrinol Metab 1993;77(4):949–55.

48. Kecler-Pietrzyk A, Kok HK, Lyburn ID, et al. Dialysis related amyloid arthropathy on (1)(8)FDG PET-CT. Ulster Med J 2014;83(2):117–8.

49. Mekinian A, Jaccard A, Soussan M, et al. 18F-FDG PET/CT in patients with amyloid light-chain amyloidosis: case-series and literature review. Amyloid 2012;19(2):94–8.

50. Menendez MI, Hettlich B, Wei L, et al. Feasibility of Na(18)F PET/CT and MRI for noninvasive in vivo quantification of knee pathophysiological bone metabolism in a canine model of post-traumatic osteoarthritis. Mol Imaging 2017;16. 1536012117714575.

51. El-Haddad G, Kumar R, Pamplona R, et al. PET/MRI depicts the exact location of meniscal tear associated with synovitis. Eur J Nucl Med Mol Imaging 2006;33(4):507–8.

52. Magnussen RA, Binzel K, Zhang J, et al. ACL graft metabolic activity assessed by (18)FDG PET-MRI. Knee 2017;24(4):792–7.

53. Jeon TJ, Kim S, Park J, et al. Use of (18)F-sodium fluoride bone PET for disability evaluation in ankle trauma: a pilot study. BMC Med Imaging 2018;18(1):34.

54. Hsu WK, Feeley BT, Krenek L, et al. The use of 18F-fluoride and 18F-FDG PET scans to assess fracture healing in a rat femur model. Eur J Nucl Med Mol Imaging 2007;34(8):1291–301.

55. Wenter V, Albert NL, Brendel M, et al. [(18)F]FDG PET accurately differentiates infected and non-infected non-unions after fracture fixation. Eur J Nucl Med Mol Imaging 2017;44(3):432–40.

56. Belehalli P, Kumar M, Prakash B, et al. Positron emission tomography-computed tomography in the assessment of viability of femoral head in acetabular fractures. Int Orthop 2014;38(5):1057–62.

57. Biswal S, Behera D, Yoon DH, et al. [18F]FDG PET/MRI of patients with chronic pain alters management: early experience. EJNMMI Phys 2015;2(Suppl 1):A84.

58. Behera D, Jacobs KE, Behera S, et al. (18)F-FDG PET/MRI can be used to identify injured peripheral nerves in a model of neuropathic pain. J Nucl Med 2011;52(8):1308–12.

59. Linnman C, Appel L, Fredrikson M, et al. Elevated [11C]-D-deprenyl uptake in chronic Whiplash Associated Disorder suggests persistent musculoskeletal inflammation. PLoS One 2011;6(4):e19182.

60. Imamoto N, Momosaki S, Fujita M, et al. [11C]PK11195 PET imaging of spinal glial activation after nerve injury in rats. Neuroimage 2013;79: 121–8.

61. Brodersen JB, Hess S. FDG-PET/CT in inflammatory bowel disease: is there a future? PET Clin 2020; 15(2):153–62.

62. Christlieb SB, Hess S, Høilund-Carlsen PF. Feasibility of FDG PET in inflammatory bowel disease. Curr Mol Imaging 2014;3(3):195–205.

63. Malham M, Hess S, Nielse RG, et al. PET/CT in the diagnosis of inflammatory bowel disease in pediatric patients: a review. Am J Nucl Med Mol Imaging 2014;4(3):225–30.

64. Domachevsky L, Leibovitzh H, Avni-Biron I, et al. Correlation of 18F-FDG PET/MRE metrics with inflammatory biomarkers in patients with crohn's disease: a pilot study. Contrast Media Mol Imaging 2017;2017:7167292.

65. Shih IL, Wei SC, Yen RF, et al. PET/MRI for evaluating subclinical inflammation of ulcerative colitis. J Magn Reson Imaging 2018;47(3):737–45.

66. Catalano OA, Gee MS, Nicolai E, et al. Evaluation of quantitative PET/MR enterography biomarkers for discrimination of inflammatory strictures from fibrotic strictures in Crohn disease. Radiology 2016;278(3): 792–800.

67. Pellino G, Nicolai E, Catalano OA, et al. PET/MR versus PET/CT imaging: impact on the clinical management of Small-Bowel Crohn's disease. J Crohns Colitis 2016;10(3):277–85.

68. Thuermel K, Einspieler I, Wolfram S, et al. Disease activity and vascular involvement in retroperitoneal fibrosis: first experience with fully integrated 18F-fluorodeoxyglucose positron emission tomography/ magnetic resonance imaging compared to clinical

and laboratory parameters. Clin Exp Rheumatol 2017;35(Suppl 103 (1)):146–54.

69. Gholamrezanejhad A, Mirpour S, Mariani G. Future of nuclear medicine: SPECT versus PET. J Nucl Med 2009;50(7):16N–8N.

70. Kooraki S, Assadi M, Gholamrezanezhad A. Hot Topics of Research in Musculoskeletal Imaging: PET/MR Imaging, MR Fingerprinting, Dual-energy CT Scan, Ultrashort Echo Time. PET Clin 2019; 14(1):175–82. https://doi.org/10.1016/j.cpet.2018.08.014.

71. Gholamrezanezhad A, Basques K, Batouli A, et al. Non-oncologic Applications of PET/CT and PET/MR in Musculoskeletal, Orthopedic, and Rheumatologic Imaging: General Considerations, Techniques, and Radiopharmaceuticals [published online ahead of print, 2017 Nov 10]. J Nucl Med Technol. 2017; jnmt.117.198663. https://doi.org/10.2967/jnmt.117.198663

72. Gholamrezanezhad A, Moinian D, Eftekhari M, Mirpour S, Hajimohammadi H. The prevalence and significance of increased gastric wall radiotracer uptake in sestamibi myocardial perfusion SPECT. Int J Cardiovasc Imaging 2006;22(3-4):435–41. https://doi.org/10.1007/s10554-005-9055-6.

73. Izadyar S, Gholamrezanezhad A. Bone scintigraphy elucidates different metabolic stages of melorheostosis. Pan Afr Med J 2012;11:21.

Potential Applications of PET Scans, CT Scans, and MR Imaging in Inflammatory Diseases

Part II: Cardiopulmonary and Vascular Inflammation

Moozhan Nikpanah, MD[a], Sanaz Katal, MD[b], Thomas Q. Christensen, MS[c],
Thomas J. Werner, MS[d], Søren Hess, MD[e,f], Ashkan A. Malayeri, MD[a],
Ali Gholamrezanezhad, MD[g], Abass Alavi, MD[d],
Babak Saboury, MD, MPH[a,d,*]

KEYWORDS

• PET • PET/CT • PET/MR • MRI • Vasculitis • Cardiopulmonary inflammation

KEY POINTS

• PET with fludeoxyglucose F 18 has a prominent role in detection and quantification of inflammatory processes, assessing the extent of involvement and global evaluation of the affected patients.
• Hybrid functional and anatomic imaging modalities in evaluation of systemic vascular, cardiac, and pulmonary inflammatory disorders can provide the opportunities for simultaneous imaging of structural pathologies and underlying metabolic and molecular processes of these multisystemic diseases.
• Literature is still sparse, and much is still unclarified, especially concerning PET/MR imaging owing to the inherent challenges of imaging in quantification of inflammation.

INTRODUCTION

As described in Part I of this double article, "Potential Applications of PET/CT/MR imaging in Inflammatory Diseases Pt. I", the nonspecificity of fludeoxyglucose F 18 (FDG), which was originally considered a drawback, now forms the basis of PET-hybrid imaging in systemic inflammatory disorders—the targets are molecular and cellular processes of inflammation, that is, the so-called respiratory burst based on the same principles as the Warburg effect in malignant cells,[1–4] but,

Sources of funding: None.
Declaration of conflict of interest: None.
[a] Department of Radiology and Imaging Sciences, Clinical Center, National Institutes of Health, 9000 Rockville Pike, Bethesda, MD 20892, USA; [b] Department of Nuclear Medicine/PET-CT, Kowsar Hospital, Shiraz, Iran; [c] Department of Clinical Engineering, Region of Southern Denmark, Esbjerg, Denmark 5000; [d] Department of Radiology, Hospital of the University of Pennsylvania, 3400 Spruce St, Philadelphia, PA 19104, USA; [e] Department of Radiology and Nuclear Medicine, Hospital of South West Jutland, University Hospital of Southern Denmark, Esbjerg, Denmark 6700; [f] Department of Regional Health Research, Faculty of Health Sciences, University of Southern Denmark, Odense, Denmark; [g] Department of Radiology, Keck School of Medicine, University of Southern California (USC), Health Sciences Campus, 1500 San Pablo Street, Los Angeles, California 90033, USA
* Corresponding author. 9000 Rockville Pike, Bethesda, MD 20892.
E-mail address: babak.saboury@nih.gov

PET Clin 15 (2020) 559–576
https://doi.org/10.1016/j.cpet.2020.06.010
1556-8598/20/Published by Elsevier Inc.

as mentioned, clinical implementation is still lacking despite the obvious potential from exceptional soft tissue contrast and decreased radiation dose.[5,6]

Some features of inflammatory diseases make them particularly interesting in the era of FDG and PET-based imaging. First, many inflammatory diseases including vasculitides are inherently systemic diseases, but present with relatively nonspecific symptoms and signs with few organ-specific diagnostic clues, for example, fever and general malaise. Thus, a high sensitivity whole-body scan is a desirable first-line imaging modality, and it is perhaps not surprising that the most investigated clinical entities include the highly heterogeneous groups of unclarified fever of unknown origin and systemic bacteremia to find the focal origin.[7] In these domains, the upfront implementation of routine whole-body FDG-PET/MR imaging is probably not yet warranted or logistically feasible. Nonetheless, the potential to supplement the initial whole-body FDG-PET/computed tomography (CT) scan with focused PET/MR imaging of suspicious findings is not far-fetched in our time with novel fast reconstruction algorithms that allows for almost instantaneous image interpretation. The same is probably true for other whole-body disorders, where the FDG-PET/CT scan is finding its place, but where the literature is still lacking, for example, in human immunodeficiency virus infection, where studies have demonstrated correlation between FDG uptake pattern in lymph nodes, disease stage, and viral load.[8,9]

A specific challenge is the effect of treatment on FDG-uptake, which not only is exploited in monitoring treatment response, but also may cause false-negative findings if patient preparation is not controlled sufficiently, especially in vasculitides. Thus, steroid-naïve patients are preferable, but if this is not possible, scans should be performed within 3 days of treatment initiation or steroids should be discontinued for at least 2 weeks in any patients treated with doses of more than 10 mg/d.[10]

This article outlines the current potential for hybrid molecular imaging in cardiopulmonary and vascular inflammation with a special focus on the potential for fused FDG-PET/CT/MR imaging.

BRIDGING THE GAP: PET WITH FLUDEOXYGLUCOSE F 18/MR IMAGING AS THE MODALITY OF CHOICE FOR IMAGING VASCULITIDES

Systemic vasculitides are multisystemic diseases defined by inflammation in the walls of blood vessels of varying size, type, and location.[11]

Categorization of noninfectious vasculitides is mainly based on the predominant size of the affected vessels, namely, large, medium, or small vessel size (**Fig. 1**).[11] An important point in this classification is that overlaps exist within the size of the involved arteries, because arteries of any size can be affected by any of the 3 major categories of vasculitis.[11]

Patients affected by systemic vasculitis might show a wide range of clinical presentations, from organ-specific manifestations to generalized symptoms.[12] In numerous instances, patients are diagnosed when showing late manifestations of the disease, although early diagnosis and therapy for systemic vasculitides can prevent life-threatening complications leading to organ failure.[12] Moreover, even though inflammatory markers are mostly elevated in these patients, no particular laboratory test has been found useful as a solo biomarker for diagnostic confirmation.[12] Additionally, systemic vasculitides can be mimicked by several inflammatory, infectious, and neoplastic diseases.[13] Therefore, tissue biopsy has been considered the gold standard in vasculitis diagnosis. However, sampling errors, invasiveness, and infeasibility of performing biopsy in some instances emphasizes the need for a robust method for making the diagnosis, evaluating disease extension, and assessing the therapeutic response.[12]

Because vasculitis involves various regions of arteries simultaneously, understanding the extent and activity of the disease is essential for appropriate clinical response. Imaging has shown a critical role in the detection of vascular abnormalities, assessing the extent of involvement and global evaluation of the affected patients and has helped broaden our knowledge of these disorders. Structural imaging modalities predominantly used for assessment of vasculitis include doppler ultrasound imaging, MR imaging, CT scan, and angiography. Ultrasound imaging, CT scans, and MR imaging detect vessel wall and luminal changes associated with vasculitis,[14] whereas angiography lacks the ability to evaluate vessel wall alterations, but may detect vascular stenosis and occlusions to guide interventional procedures.[15]

All modalities contribute to various aspects of disease management in vasculitis, but each demonstrates specific advantages and disadvantages. MR imaging has exquisite soft tissue contrast that makes it useful for detecting edema, deep vascular involvement, and perivascular changes.[15,16] CT angiography is particularly useful for large vessel vasculitis (LVV) owing to its spatial resolution, and additionally for detecting and evaluation of pulmonary changes and osseous lesions

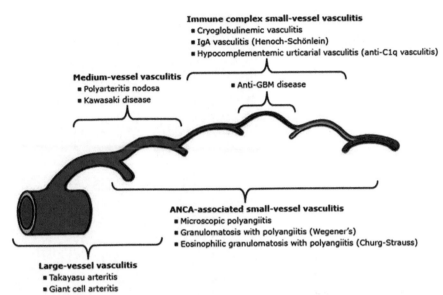

Fig. 1. This diagram demonstrates (from left to right) the aorta, large artery, medium artery, small artery/arteriole, capillary, venule, and vein. Vasculitides are a group of disorders with a common pathogenetic process: inflammation centered on the vessel wall. Vessels could be classified into 3 categories based on their luminal diameter and wall structure: large vessels, medium vessels, and small vessels. The distribution of vessel involvement is depicted in this figure. It is important to remember all 3 major categories of vasculitides can affect any size artery and there is substantial overlap with respect to arterial involvement. It is fair to say that LVV affects large arteries more often than other vasculitides; the same can be said for medium vessel vasculitis. Small vessel vasculitis predominantly affects small vessels; however, medium arteries and veins may be affected. A subgroup of small vessel vasculitides, immune complex small vessel vasculitis, rarely affects arteries. ANCA, antineutrophil cytoplasmic antibody; Anti-GBM, antiglomerular basement membrane. (*Reproduced from* Jennette JC, Falk RJ, Bacon PA, Basu N, Cid MC, Ferrario F, et al. 2012 Revised International Chapel Hill Consensus Conference Nomenclature of Vasculitides. Arthritis Rheum. 2013;65(1):1–11.)

associated with some vasculitides, although iodinated contrast and radiation exposure are of concern in serial imaging.[16,17]

Although FDG-PET has been shown to provide information about vascular inflammation, these findings should be interpreted by the experts who master nuances of diagnostic molecular imaging and understand the pitfalls; pattern recognition is only rarely useful alone and extreme caution should be exercised because increased metabolic activity could be attributed to other subclinical or secondary processes such as hypoxia, vascular remodeling, or atherosclerosis.[18] We review applications of combined FDG-PET/MR imaging in diagnosis, assessment and follow-up of large, medium, and small vessel vasculitis, and speculate on the future role of this modality for management of patients within the spectrum of these disorders.

Large Vessel Vasculitis

LVV mainly affects arteries comprising intima, media and adventitia.[19] Giant cell arteritis (GCA) and Takayasu arteritis (TAK) are well-known forms of LVV, characterized by involvement of the aorta and its major branches.[11] Several studies have reported approximate sensitivity of 89.5% and 87% for GCA and TAK respectively, using FDG-PET/CT scanning.[18,20–24]

The role of PET/MR imaging as a potential tool to assess inflammatory processes in LVV has been investigated by previous studies. Einspieler and colleagues[14] evaluated 12 patients with LVV including 10 GCA and 2 TAK cases with FDG-PET/MR imaging and reported a significant correlation between C-reactive protein levels and disease activity on PET ($P = 0.0067$) and FDG-PET/MR imaging ($P<.0001$). In a retrospective study of 23 patients with LVV evaluated by FDG-PET/MR imaging, Padoan and colleagues[25] reported increased maximum standard uptake values in patients with different types of LVV, that is, GCA, TAK, and isolated aortitis. Laurent and colleagues[20] evaluated the application of FDG-PET/MR imaging in 13 patients with LVV and found vascular wall inflammatory patterns on PET/MR imaging to correlate highly with disease activity in all patients with TAK and 50% of patients with GCA (**Figs. 2** and **3**). The authors highlighted the role of PET/MR imaging evaluation of LVV in characterizing disease burden.

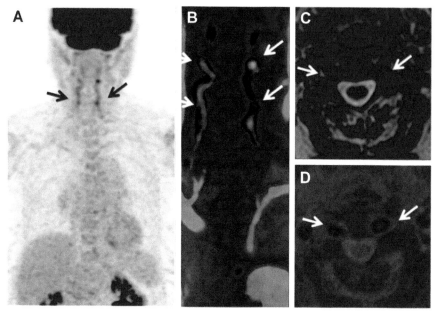

Fig. 2. Female with temporal headaches and elevated acute-phase reactants; clinical diagnosis of GCA. PET/MR imaging showed significant FDG uptake in bilateral vertebral arteries (*arrows*). (*A*) Maximum intensity projection, and (*B*) fused MR angiography/PET scan. There is arterial wall thickening (*arrows*) on (*C*) MR axial T2-weighted image, and (*D*) fused T2-weighted/PET scan. (*Reproduced from* Laurent C, Ricard L, Fain O, Buvat I, Adedjouma A, Soussan M, et al. PET/MRI in large-vessel vasculitis: clinical value for diagnosis and assessment of disease activity. Sci Rep. 2019 Aug 27;9(1):1–7.)

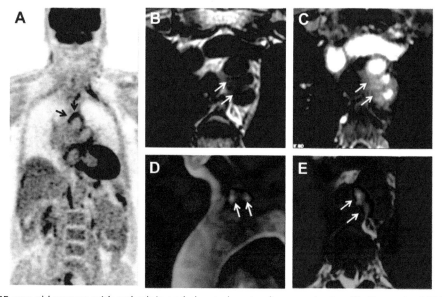

Fig. 3. A 45-year-old woman with arthralgia and elevated acute phase reactants with diagnosis of TAK. PET/MR imaging showed an increased FDG uptake in aortic arch and at the origin of supra-aortic vessels associated with arterial wall thickening on T2-weighted image (*B*, *arrows*) and wall enhancement (*C*, *arrows*). (*A*) Coronal PET scan, (*B*) T2-weighted image, (*C*) postcontrast T1-weighted image, (*D*) fused MR-angiography/PET scan, and (*E*) fused PET/T2-weighted image. (*Reproduced from* Laurent C, Ricard L, Fain O, Buvat I, Adedjouma A, Soussan M, et al. PET/MR imaging in large-vessel vasculitis: clinical value for diagnosis and assessment of disease activity. Sci Rep. 2019 Aug 27;9(1):1–7.)

Giant cell arteritis

GCA is a chronic vasculitis defined by granulomatous inflammation of large and medium vessels, including cranial arteries (known as temporal arteritis).[26] GCA is the most common systemic vasculitis and seen mainly in the elderly white population.[27] The incidence of GCA increases with aging in individuals older than 50 years with a peak at 70 to 79 years of age.[28] GCA has a broad range of clinical manifestations from constitutional symptoms to new-onset headaches, jaw claudication, amaurosis fugax, and permanent vision loss.[29–33] GCA diagnosis might be challenging, especially in cases with typical clinical features of GCA, but negative results of temporal artery biopsy. Evaluating arterial involvement is of high importance for diagnosis confirmation in these patients.[20]

The role of MR imaging as a noninvasive imaging modality has been probed in the diagnosis and management of GCA with key features reported as arterial wall thickening and mural contrast enhancement of occipital and superficial temporal arteries (**Fig. 4**).[27] Bley and colleagues[34] evaluated temporal arteries in 16 patients with biopsy-confirmed GCA by high-resolution

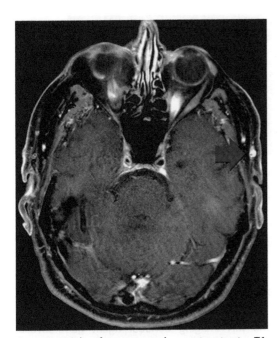

Fig. 4. Axial, fat-suppressed, postcontrast T1-weighted brain MR image in a patient with GCA. The *red arrow* shows concentric enhancement and mural thickening of the left superficial temporal artery. (*Reproduced from* Halbach, C., McClelland, C. M., Chen, J., Li, S., & Lee, M. S. (2018). Use of noninvasive imaging in giant cell arteritis. The Asia-Pacific Journal of Ophthalmology, 7(4), 260-264.)

contrast-enhanced MR imaging and confirmed visualization of mural inflammatory changes even in small arteries. The authors suggested T1-weighted sequences of up to 6 minutes can provide a sufficient signal-to-noise ratio for the detection of mural contrast enhancement that is a common sign of acute inflammatory change. They also investigated the use of unenhanced images without fat suppression that did not show diagnostic usefulness.[34] In addition to commonly used sequences of MR imaging, functional sequences such as diffusion-weighted imaging have also been shown effective in detection of GCA-associated vascular inflammation (**Fig. 5**). Diffusion-weighted imaging is based on measuring random motion of water molecules known as Brownian motion. Owing to strong infiltration of vessel walls in patients with active vasculitis, diffusion-weighted imaging potentially reveals increased cellularity by measuring restricted water diffusion.[35]

Studies have proven the value of FDG-PET scans to detect involvements in the aorta, carotid, subclavian, brachiocephalic, and iliofemoral arteries.[36] In a study by Hautzel and colleagues[37] the authors reported high sensitivity (89%) and specificity (95%) for FDG-PET scans in diagnosing associated aortic involvement in GCA. In a study by Meller and colleagues,[38] the authors compared the performance of FDG-PET with MR imaging in 76 vascular regions from 14 patients undergoing PET and MR imaging clinically suspected for GCA; MR imaging and PET scans were comparable in early stages of aortitis, but 29 vascular regions were discordantly found positive on either MR imaging or PET scans, emphasizing the improved diagnostic capacity of a combined system.[17]

Takayasu arteritis

TAK, identified by granulomatous panarteritis, is a rare form of LVV that predominantly affects women younger than 40 years of age.[39] Diagnosis is challenging owing to nonspecific primary symptoms like low-grade fever and fatigue. Later in the disease course, the onset of vascular involvement, which predominantly includes the aortic arch and its main branches, as well as the renal, mesenteric, and pulmonary arteries, leads clinicians toward the diagnosis.[17,39] However, the diagnosis of TAK needs histopathologic confirmation, which is not feasible in all patients.[40]

Similar to GCA, MR imaging is an excellent tool in patients with TAK to evaluate both the vessel lumen and wall for edema, particularly in the aorta and its large branches. It could also be a useful supplement in follow-up for vascular anatomic

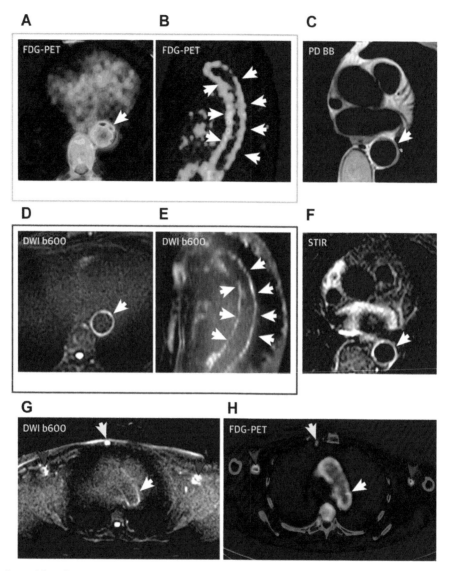

Fig. 5. Patient with active GCA. Increased FDG uptake of the descending aorta in axial (*A*) and sagittal (*B*) planes. Mural changes in black-blood (BB) (*C*) and fluid-suppressed (*D*) sequences. High b-value diffusion-weighted images demonstrate restricted diffusion in axial (*D*) and sagittal (*E*) planes. Axial short T1 inversion recovery (STIR) image (*F*) shows hyperintensity of the vessel wall. Axial plane at the level of aortic arch demonstrates mural restricted diffusion (*G*) as well as increased FDG uptake (*H*). Similar correspondence was noticed between FDG uptake and hyperintensity on DWI in arteries smaller than the aorta, for example the right and left subclavian arteries (*red arrowheads*) and the right mammarian artery (*yellow arrows*). White arrows demonstrate the aorta. DWI, diffusion-weighted imaging. (*Reproduced from* Ironi G, Tombetti E, Napolitano A, Campolongo M, Fallanca F, Incerti E, et al. Diffusion-Weighted Magnetic Resonance Imaging Detects Vessel Wall Inflammation in Patients With Giant Cell Arteritis. JACC Cardiovasc Imaging. 2018 Dec 3;11(12):1879–82.)

changes. Desai and colleagues[41] suggested hyperenhancement on delayed phase contrast-enhanced MR imaging might be useful in identifying inflammation in aortic wall. However, it has been argued that gadolinium contrast enhancement could potentially indicate fibrosis as this is observed in patients in stable remission. Papa and colleagues[42] reported the effectiveness of

the MR imaging contrast agent gadofosveset that, in contrast with gadolinium, does not enhance fibrous tissue, and they found a correlation between vessel wall enhancement and active disease, a finding that warrants wider evaluation. However, studies have reported a potential for false-positive cases with MR imaging. In a study of 24 patients with TAK, Tso and colleagues[43] found vessel wall edema measured by increased MR signal intensity in 94% of patients with active disease and more than 50% of patients with inactive disease or uncertain activity status inferred from clinical judgment (**Fig. 6**).

FDG-PET has shown usefulness for early disease diagnosis in patients with TAK, in treatment follow-up, and detecting active disease. In a study by Tezuka and colleagues,[44] FDG-PET/CT scanning was useful for detecting inflammation not only in patients with active TAK, but also in relapsing individuals receiving immunosuppressive agents. The reported sensitivity and specificity of FDG-PET for the initial assessment of active vasculitis covers a wide range. A meta-analysis calculated a pooled sensitivity and specificity of 70.1% and 77.2%, respectively, from retrospective studies and small case series and speculated that inclusion of treated cases contributed to inferior accuracy of this modality in TAK.[42,45] Tsuchiya and colleagues[46] reported the extent and distribution of extravascular findings on FDG-PET/CT scans in patients with TAK in regions such as the thyroid glands, lymph nodes, and bone marrow of the vertebrae and pelvis. Even though these findings cannot be attributed to known pathophysiologic processes of the disease, it can increase our understanding of the mechanisms of inflammation in TA.

Medium Vessel Vasculitis

Polyarteritis nodosa

Polyarteritis nodosa (PAN) is a systemic necrotizing vasculitis mainly involving medium size muscular arteries; small muscular arteries may also be affected.[11] PAN has a relative average age at onset of 50 years with peak in the fifth and sixth decades of life.[47,48] PAN is a multisystemic disease mainly marked by renal, nervous system, gastrointestinal, and cutaneous involvement, but for undetermined reasons spares the lungs.[47,49]

Even though the evaluation of medium arteries is mainly performed with angiography, the tissue effect of vascular injury and resultant manifestations have specific presentation in structural, physiologic, and molecular imaging. MR imaging can detect intracerebral hemorrhage and intracranial aneurysms, and aneurysms of other arteries such as hepatic, mesenteric, and renal arteries

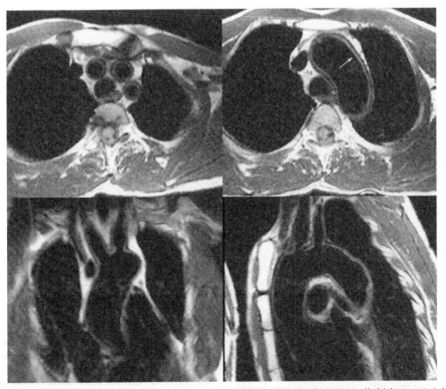

Fig. 6. Patient with TAK. Magnetic resonance images demonstrate increased aortic wall thickness. Axial (*top*) and longitudinal-oblique (*bottom*) images of the thoracic aorta reveal abnormal aortic wall thickening and ectatic changes (*arrow*). (*Reproduced from* Tso E, Flamm SD, White RD, Schvartzman PR, Mascha E, Hoffman GS. Takayasu arteritis: Utility and limitations of magnetic resonance imaging in diagnosis and treatment. Arthritis Rheum. 2002;46(6):1634–42.)

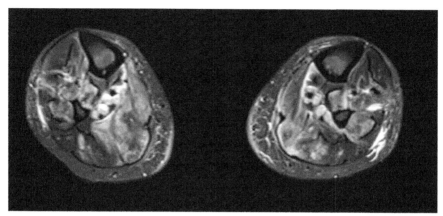

Fig. 7. Axial short T1 inversion recovery MR image in a patient with PAN showing bilateral diffuse hyperintensity in all 4 compartments of the lower legs compatible with myositis; deep fascial and intermuscular edema are also noted. (*Reproduced from* Ganeshanandan, L. R., Brusch, A. M., Dyke, J. M., & McLean-Tooke, A. P. (2019, December). Polyarteritis nodosa isolated to muscles-A case series with a review of the literature. In Seminars in Arthritis and Rheumatism. WB Saunders.)

(microaneurysms create the appearance, which is the origin of naming, *nodosa*[50]). In some cases, the affected vessels are below the spatial resolution of MR imaging; however, the downstream effect of vascular damage could be assessed by this modality, considering its high soft tissue contrast resolution; MR imaging is particularly useful for the assessment of subcutaneous fat, muscle, and visceral involvement (**Fig. 7**).[51–53] In a study on MR imaging findings of muscle involvement in patients with PAN by Kang and colleagues,[54] the authors concluded that the differential diagnosis can be considered in cases with patchy diffuse muscle signal changes. The authors also reported fascial and periosteal involvement and enhancing lesions on vessels on contrast-enhanced images.

FDG-PET scans can detect signs of vasculitis in PAN (**Fig. 8**).[55–57] FDG-PET scanning is also a useful modality for nonvascular findings of PAN. Previous studies have found FDG-PET scans to be sensitive for detecting disseminated spots throughout subcutaneous tissue and muscle associated with cutaneous PAN, a rare manifestation sometimes referred to as leopard skin appearance.[58] Cutaneous PAN is characterized by necrotizing vasculitis of medium and small arteries of the skin and is also associated with extracutaneous findings, such as fever, malaise, and neuropathy, but no visceral involvement.[59]

Kawasaki disease

Kawasaki disease (KD; mucocutaneous lymph node syndrome) is one of the most prevalent forms of vasculitis in children younger than 5 years, barely affecting adults.[60,61] KD affects small and medium size vessels and presents as an acute

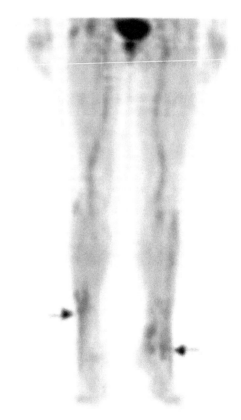

Fig. 8. FDG PET scan of a 60-year-old woman with PAN who presented with myalgia of the lower legs, skin ulcerations on both legs, livedo reticularis, and mild polyneuropathy. (*Reproduced from* Bleeker-Rovers CP, Bredie SJ, Van Der Meer JW, Corstens 0 FH, Oyen WJ. F-18-fluorodeoxyglucose positron emission tomography in diagnosis and follow-up of patients with different types of vasculitis. Neth J Med. 2003;61(10):323–9.)

febrile illness with symptoms of acute inflammation; typical clinical manifestations include cervical lymphadenopathy, bilateral nonexudative conjunctivitis, mucositis, rash, and edema of the extremities.[57,58] KD is a self-limited disease that evolves over 10 to 12 days without therapy.[61] However, affected children are highly vulnerable to life-threatening cardiovascular complications, the most concerning of which is coronary artery abnormalities, leading to coronary artery aneurysms, arrhythmias, myocardial ischemia, and infarction.[62]

MR imaging has been shown to be useful in the identification of coronary artery aneurysms in KD. In addition to coronary artery abnormalities, MR imaging provides clinically relevant information regarding myocardial inflammation, infarction, and ischemia.[63] In a previous study, Tacke and colleagues[64] evaluated the performance of MR imaging in assessment of 63 patients with KD. The authors concluded comparable performance to echocardiography for long term surveillance of patients with KD in identifying coronary artery pathology, ischemia, and myocardial infarction (**Fig. 9**).[64]

There is limited information about the use of FDG-PET imaging in patients with KD. There have been reports of persistent coronary arterial inflammation in patients with KD long after onset of the disease.[65,66] Hauser and colleagues[67] used ^{13}N-ammonia-PET for noninvasive assessment of regional myocardial blood flow and coronary flow reserve in follow-up of the functionality of the coronary arteries in patients with normal epicardial coronary arteries after the onset of KD. The authors reported a significant decrease in coronary flow reserve and attenuation of myocardial blood flow after vasodilation in children with angiographically normal epicardial coronary arteries, and this lack in vasoreactivity could indicate residual damage of the coronary arteries.[67]

Small Vessel Vasculitis

Small vessel vasculitides are characterized by involvement of arterioles, capillaries, and venules that are smaller in size compared with arteries, but otherwise similar to other types of vasculitides; overlaps exist and small vessel vasculitis might also involve medium size vessels.[68]

Small vessel vasculitides are mainly categorized on the basis of involvement of immune complexes. The main 2 categories are pauci-immune (antineutrophil cytoplasmic antibody [ANCA]-associated) small vessel vasculitis and immune complex small vessel vasculitis.[68]

A variety of immune mechanisms are thought to be involved in the inflammatory responses in small vessel vasculitis that mainly occur in vessels with substantial trafficking of cells and fluids between tissue and blood. The endothelia of these vessels are particularly responsive to proinflammatory signals, increasing the probability of association with cascades of events including endothelial damage, thrombosis, ischemia, and tissue necrosis.[69,70]

Even though imaging is limited with regard to direct assessment of these very small vessels, it plays a significant role in assessment of metabolic processes and tissue damages as a result of small-vessel vasculitis.[71] MR imaging is particularly useful for revealing intra-abdominal involvements such as ischemia, bowel wall hemorrhage, and edema. Additionally, it can help with otorhinolaryngologic involvement, such as mucosal inflammation and granulomatous tissue in the paranasal sinus, mastoid, middle ear, and orbit. On MR imaging, early granulomatous tissue shows nonspecific hypointense signal on T1-weighted images and hyperintense signal on T2-weighted images

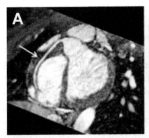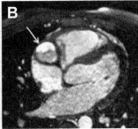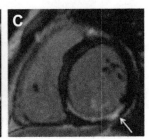

Fig. 9. Cardiac MR images of 3 patients with KD. The coronary artery could be normal (*A; arrow* shows right coronary artery) or markedly abnormal (*B, arrow* shows a giant aneurysm of the right coronary artery with thrombosis). Subsequent myocardial ischemic defects could be the result of coronary artery involvement (*C, arrow* shows basal inferoseptal-inferior myocardial infarction). (*Reproduced from* Tacke Carline E., Kuipers Irene M., Groenink Maarten, Spijkerboer Anje M., Kuijpers Taco W. Cardiac Magnetic Resonance Imaging for Noninvasive Assessment of Cardiovascular Disease During the Follow-Up of Patients With Kawasaki Disease. Circ Cardiovasc Imaging. 2011 Nov 1;4(6):712–20.)

in paranasal sinuses, whereas chronic granulomatous inflammation appears hypointense on both T1- and T2-weighted images and shows less enhancement (**Fig. 10**).[17,71]

ANCA-associated vasculitis is characterized by inflammatory infiltrates that could be a good target for FDG uptake.[72,73] However, data regarding evaluation of disease extent using FDG-PET scans is limited. Ito and colleagues explored the usefulness of FDG-PET/CT imaging in the diagnosis and follow-up of patients with granulomatosis with polyangiitis. The authors showed the feasibility of FDG-PET/CT scans by retrospective review of 8 patients. FDG-PET/CT imaging improved the detection of upper respiratory tract and lung lesions in comparison with noncontrast CT scans and provided complementary information to indicate biopsy site.[74] Soussan and colleagues[73] reviewed FDG-PET/CT imaging in 16 patients with ANCA-associated vasculitis, including 10 granulomatosis with polyangiitis, 2 eosinophilic granulomatosis with polyangiitis, and 4 microscopic polyangiitis. The authors concluded that FDG-PET/CT imaging accurately identifies organ impairments in granulomatosis with polyangiitis, but does not bring additional value to usual screening (**Fig. 11**). The authors did not identify any uptake in the skin, joint, eye, or large vessels.[73] The same group reported 2 cases of asymptomatic aortic arch involvement in ANCA-associated vasculitis diagnosed with FDG-PET/CT imaging.[75] Finally, a small retrospective study

from Frary and colleagues[76] found FDG-PET/CT scans to have high accuracy and predictive values for differentiating disease relapse of ANCA-associated vasculitides from infection and malignancies, 2 important differential diagnoses with often indistinguishable symptoms and signs.

Role of FDG-PET scans in other forms of small vessel vasculitis is not well-determined by means of large cohort investigations; however, small studies and case reports show the potential of this modality in providing complementary information in identifying the extent of the disease and disease activity beyond usual screening.[77,78]

CARDIOPULMONARY INFLAMMATION

FDG-PET/CT imaging is already used to assess inflammation in the heart and lungs, for example, in infectious endocarditis and sarcoidosis, but additional challenges arise with imaging these organs including with PET/MR imaging. First, with regard to the heart, specific preparation is necessary to suppress physiologic activity and glucose consumption, for example, prolonged fasting, low-carbohydrate–high-fat dietary restraints, and pretreatment with heparin.[10] Also, artifacts from motion or cardiac devices may interfere with image quality, and devices' noncompliance with MR imaging magnetism may hamper use overall.[6] In the lungs, the low tissue proton density generates fewer MR imaging signals and results in many tissue-to-air interfaces, which render attenuation correction of the PET images more difficult and create more attenuation artifacts that will impact quantification.[79] If these issues were to be resolved, PET/MR imaging might have a more promising potential for the correction of respiratory motion and misalignment artifacts from simultaneous dynamic acquisition of PET and MR imaging signals,[79,80] which could greatly improve the quantification potential in the lung.

Cardiac Sarcoidosis

Sarcoidosis is a systemic non-necrotizing granulomatous inflammatory disease with multiple organ involvement and heterogeneous clinical presentation.[81] It primarily affects the lungs and lymph nodes, but may affect every organ, and whole-body FDG-PET/CT imaging may aid in establishing disease extent, including extrapulmonary sarcoidosis, the location of biopsy accessible lymph nodes, occult lesions, or multiorgan involvement. Some studies have found potential for the evaluation of treatment response.[2,3] With the abovementioned caveats in mind, it remains to be seen if PET/MR imaging adds further to the diagnostic

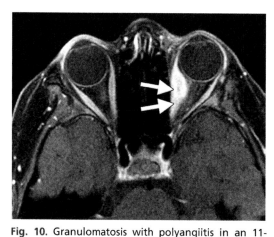

Fig. 10. Granulomatosis with polyangiitis in an 11-year-old boy with left orbital pain and fever. Axial postcontrast MR image of the orbits shows hyperenhancement of the enlarged left medial rectus muscle with surrounding fat stranding (*arrows*). (*Reproduced from* Khanna G, Sargar K, Baszis KW. Pediatric Vasculitis: Recognizing Multisystemic Manifestations at Body Imaging. RadioGraphics. 2015 May 1;35(3):849–65.)

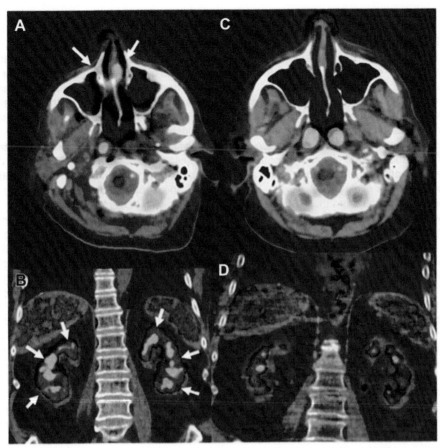

Fig. 11. A 67-year-old woman with a granulomatosis with polyangiitis. FDG-PET/CT scan shows increased FDG up-take in sinonasal and kidney locations (*A, B, arrows*). A follow-up FDG-PET/CT scan, although the patient achieved remission, showed resolution of hypermetabolic activities in both locations (*C, D*). (*Reproduced from* Soussan M, Abisror N, Abad S, Nunes H, Terrier B, Pop G, et al. FDG-PET/CT in patients with ANCA-associated vasculitis: Case-series and literature review. Autoimmun Rev. 2014 Feb 1;13(2):125–31.)

strategy in pulmonary and systemic sarcoidosis per se, but in cardiac sarcoidosis represent an important entity, where PET/MR imaging may find a considerable place.

Almost 25% of deaths attributable to sarcoidosis is related to cardiac involvement; cardiac granulomas are found in about one-fourth of the patients with sarcoidosis on autopsy. The involvement of the heart is underdiagnosed, although cardiac involvement plays a very important role in the course of the disease. Sudden cardiac death may be the first sign of cardiac sarcoidosis and historically, an electrocardiogram has been strongly considered in all patients with suspected cardiac involvement.

There are multiple reasons for the underdiagnosing of cardiac sarcoidosis. First, the manifestations are very nonspecific (conductive aberrancy and/or cardiomyopathy). Second, conventional diagnosis by endomyocardial biopsy has a low diagnostic yield because the technique is not optimal for the pathologic involvement; that is, most lesions are in left ventricle, whereas the biopsies are obtained from right ventricle and, in addition, a random sampling of the patchy involvement of myocardium leads to sampling error and a low yield with a high false-negative rate. Finally, histologic diagnosis based on the Dallas criteria is disputable.[82] Also, isolated cardiac sarcoidosis is not a very clear concept in the literature. The prevalence of cardiac involvement among patients with systemic sarcoidosis ranges from 25% (in the United States) to 60% (in Japan); however, the prevalence of isolated cardiac sarcoidosis is not known.[83] Reported rates of isolated cardiac sarcoidosis among patients with cardiac sarcoidosis have similar ranges from 25% to 55%.[84] Considering the importance of this clinical condition and limitations of traditional diagnostic methods, FDG-PET/CT imaging has gained extensive attention in recent years to address this unmet need.[85–92]

MR imaging has been used to detect the sequelae of chronic inflammatory changes of myocarditis by using delayed postcontrast sequences. Late gadolinium enhancement demonstrates entrapment of extravasated contrast in the fibrous tissue representing the scar. This finding in itself is quite nonspecific; however, by attention to the pattern of myocardial involvement (subepicardial vs subendocardial and transmural) as well as location of involvement (such as the junction of right and left ventricles), diagnosticians can narrow the differential diagnosis and favor sarcoidosis over other etiologies.

It is important to understand that FDG-PET and delayed postcontrast MR imaging provide complementary information regarding sarcoidosis biology.[93] PET FDG avidity demonstrates active inflammation, whereas late gadolinium enhancement lesions on MR imaging show chronic sequelae. Wicks and colleagues[94] investigated 51 patients suspected of having cardiac sarcoidosis and showed that the presence of late gadolinium enhancement and FDG uptake on PET/MR imaging identified patients at greater risk of adverse events and suggested that both PET scans and cardiac MR imaging should be considered in the assessment of disease presence, stage, and prognosis. To explore the usefulness of hybrid FDG-PET/MR imaging to detect cardiac sarcoidosis, Dweck and colleagues[95] evaluated 25 suspected patients. Eight patients were MR+ PET+ (**Fig. 12**), suggestive of cardiac sarcoidosis; 1 patient was MR+ PET−, consistent with inactive cardiac sarcoidosis; and 8 were MR− PET−, with no imaging evidence of cardiac sarcoidosis; and finally 8 patients were MR− PET+ with 2 distinctive patterns: global myocardial uptake (n = 6) and focal-on-diffuse uptake (n = 2).

In conclusion, the excitement about the application of PET/MR to diagnose and characterize myocarditis is profound and some clinicians believe that by this application, "cardiac PET/MR imaging entered the clinical arena! Finally."[96]

Chronic Obstructive Pulmonary Disease

Chronic obstructive pulmonary disease (COPD) is a major health care issue worldwide and, although the initial diagnoses can be obtained relatively simple through spirometric examinations, several aspects of the disease complex point toward a potential role for FDG-PET/CT imaging to increase our basic knowledge of the disease and perhaps impact future clinical strategies. Thus, FDG-PET/CT imaging has shown some ability to separate different phenotypes on the basis of FDG uptake

patterns, to identify patients with increased use of accessory breathing muscles, and to identify patients with right heart strain—different features within the disease spectrum that may affect prognosis and treatment strategy.[97] However, changes are often subtle and quantitative measures are usually warranted; most of the scarce literature on FDG in COPD focuses on quantification.

Most studies use the Patlak-Gjede graphical analysis technique[98,99] based on tracer kinetic modeling. By modeling the FDG uptake as an irreversible compartmental model the net influx rate of FDG, the K_i, can be derived as a parameter for the rate of tissue FDG metabolism.

Jones and colleagues[100] used this method to show increased FDG uptake in the lungs of 6 patients with COPD compared with patients with chronic asthma and age-matched controls. Subramanian and colleagues[101] later reinforced these quantitative results in 10 patients with COPD who displayed higher FDG uptake in the lungs compared with healthy controls and patients with COPD with α1-antitrypsin deficiency, especially in the upper zone of the lungs. The reproducibility of this method was highlighted by Chen and colleagues[102] in abstract form; they compared 10 patients with COPD with healthy age-matched controls and scanned each object 3 times during a 7-week period. They found significantly higher FDG uptake in patients with COPD compared with controls, irrespective of the examination time point.[102]

The lungs give rise to multiple challenges for quantitation, especially the fact that uptake areas consist of very small regions (in terms of PET resolution) surrounded by air with no uptake. Hence, activity spillover from partial volume effects will be a considerable problem in quantitation, and blood in the lungs will lead to an increased background signal.[103,104] Also, the fraction of air and blood in the lungs changes in patients with COPD furthering the need for correction of these parameters in quantification.[103] Coello and colleagues[105] proposed a tracer kinetic modeling method that took into account air and blood volume in the lungs. After applying the corrections, they were not able to see a significant difference between 10 patients with COPD and a healthy control group.[105]

Recently, Vass and colleagues[106] tested the reproducibility for tracer kinetic modeling by applying the same methodology for the same reconstructed images with 2 different processing pipelines for 10 patients with COPD compared with patients with COPD with α1-antitrypsin deficiency and a healthy control group. They found no significant differences between

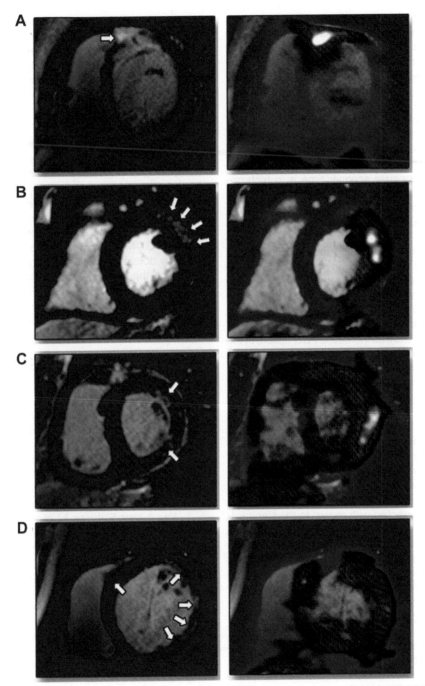

Fig. 12. MR+ PET+ patients with imaging evidence of acute coronary syndrome on hybrid CMR/PET. Late gadolinium enhancement (LGE) cardiac magnetic resonance (CMR) images on the left with hybrid FDG CMR/PET images on the *right*. (*A*) Subepicardial (near transmural) LGE in the basal anteroseptum extending in to the right ventricular free wall with increased FDG uptake localizing to exactly the same region on fused CMR/PET scan (maximum standardized uptake value, 3.4; maximum tissue-to-background ratio, 2.3; maximum target-to-normal myocardium ratio, 2.0). (*B*) Subepicardial LGE in the basal anterolateral wall with increased FDG uptake colocalizing to exactly that region on CMR/PET scan. (*C*) Patchy midwall LGE in the anterolateral wall with matched increased FDG uptake on CMR/PET scan. (*D*) Multifocal LGE in the lateral wall with matched increased FDG uptake on CMR/PET scan. (*Reproduced from* Dweck, Marc R., Ronan Abgral, Maria Giovanna Trivieri, Philip M. Robson, Nicolas Karakatsanis, Venkatesh Mani, Anna Palmisano, et al. 2018. Hybrid Magnetic Resonance Imaging and Positron Emission Tomography With Fluorodeoxyglucose to Diagnose Active Cardiac Sarcoidosis. JACC. Cardiovascular Imaging 11 (1): 94–107.)

the groups, but some variations in individual patients between the 2 processing pipelines. They found blood region of interest methodology, input function modeling, and time delay estimation to be key factors influencing the outcome.[106]

To derive parameters from tracer kinetic modeling, patients need to have a dynamic PET scan, which means they will have to be injected directly on the scan bed and scanned continuously for 60 to 90 minutes. This factor limits the clinical usefulness, because scanner time is in high demand with static PET scans as the routine. Static scans are often quantified using the standardized uptake value, but reproducibility has often been discussed.[107]

Torigian and colleagues[108] showed that the PET standardized uptake value in patients with COPD correlated positively with emphysema severity from CT scans in 49 patients, but only if partial volume correction was used. In a recent study by Garpered and colleagues,[109] 33 patients and current smokers showed increased FDG uptake in the lungs compared with never smokers, but this was only statistically significant when the data were corrected for air fraction.

COPD may harbor an element of systemic inflammation with increased cardiovascular risk. Coulson and colleagues[110] examined aortic wall uptake in 7 patients with COPD compared with 5 patients with metabolic syndrome, and 7 former smokers without COPD. Aortic uptake was quantified using target-to-background ratio where the standardized uptake value of the Volume of Interest (VOI) is corrected with regard to the standardized uptake value of arterial blood. The authors found aortic uptake in patients with COPD was lower than in patients with the metabolic syndrome but higher than the former smoker controls. This finding was further investigated by Fisk and colleagues,[111] who compared 85 patients with COPD with groups of 12 consisting of patients with COPD with α1-antitrypsin deficiency, smokers without COPD, and never smokers. Using the target-to-background ratio of the aortic walls, they found significantly greater FDG uptake in both COPD with and without α1-antitrypsin deficiency compared with the groups of smokers and never smokers. These findings indicate that aortic inflammation is related to COPD in itself, regardless of smoking history.[111]

Recently, Kothekar and colleagues[112] linked an increased uptake in respiratory muscles in 33 patients with COPD with pulmonary function test results, showing that increased uptake significantly correlated with COPD severity, albeit mainly based on a visual grading score and with supporting

standardized uptake value quantitation only to a small extent. This finding was previously observed in studies by Aydin and colleagues[113] and Osman and colleagues,[114] and it might hold potential to stratify patients with COPD according to respiratory strain.

SUMMARY

The use of FDG-PET/CT imaging in cardiac, vascular, and pulmonary inflammation in some ways represents the extremes, that is, from well-established indications like large vessel vasculitis to the hitherto strictly exploratory uses like COPD. The potential for PET/CT scans and PET/CT/MR imaging is undoubtedly present in these domains, albeit probably to varying degree, but the literature is still sparse and much is still unclarified, especially with regards to PET/MR imaging owing to the inherent challenges of imaging in quantification of the heart and lungs.

REFERENCES

1. Gormsen LC, Hess S. Challenging but clinically useful: fluorodeoxyglucose PET/computed tomography in inflammatory and infectious diseases. PET Clin 2020;15(2):xi–xii.
2. Kung BT, Seraj SM, Zadeh MZ, et al. An update on the role of (18)F-FDG-PET/CT in major infectious and inflammatory diseases. Am J Nucl Med Mol Imaging 2019;9(6):255–73.
3. Alavi A, Hess S, Werner TJ, et al. An update on the unparalleled impact of FDG-PET imaging on the day-to-day practice of medicine with emphasis on management of infectious/inflammatory disorders. Eur J Nucl Med Mol Imaging 2020;47(1):18–27.
4. Sathekge M, Maes A, Wiele CVd. FDG-PET imaging in HIV infection and tuberculosis. Semin Nucl Med 2013;43(5):349–66.
5. Ehman EC, Johnson GB, Villanueva-Meyer JE, et al. PET/MRI: where might it replace PET/CT? J Magn Reson Imaging 2017;46(5):1247–62.
6. Sollini M, Berchiolli R, Kirienko M, et al. PET/MRI in infection and inflammation. Semin Nucl Med 2018; 48(3):225–41.
7. Hess S. FDG-PET/CT in fever of unknown origin, bacteremia, and febrile neutropenia. PET Clin 2020;15(2):175–85.
8. Scharko AM, Perlman SB, Pyzalski RW, et al. Whole-body positron emission tomography in patients with HIV-1 infection. Lancet 2003; 362(9388):959–61.
9. Brust D, Polis M, Davey R, et al. Fluorodeoxyglucose imaging in healthy subjects with HIV infection:

impact of disease stage and therapy on pattern of nodal activation. AIDS 2006;20(7):985–93.

10. Hess S, Scholtens AM, Gormsen LC. Patient preparation and patient-related challenges with FDG-PET/CT in infectious and inflammatory disease. PET Clin 2020;15(2):125–34.

11. Jennette JC, Falk RJ, Bacon PA, et al. 2012 revised International Chapel Hill consensus conference nomenclature of vasculitides. Arthritis Rheum 2013;65(1):1–11.

12. Danve A, O'Dell J. The role of 18F fluorodeoxyglucose positron emission tomography scanning in the diagnosis and management of systemic vasculitis. Int J Rheum Dis 2015;18(7):714–24.

13. Molloy ES, Langford CA. Vasculitis mimics. Curr Opin Rheumatol 2008;20(1):29–34.

14. Einspieler I, Thürmel K, Pyka T, et al. Imaging large vessel vasculitis with fully integrated PET/MRI: a pilot study. Eur J Nucl Med Mol Imaging 2015;42(7):1012–24.

15. Pipitone N, Versari A, Salvarani C. Role of imaging studies in the diagnosis and follow-up of large-vessel vasculitis: an update. Rheumatology 2008;47(4):403–8.

16. Prieto-Gonzalez S, Espigol-Frigole G, Garcia-Martinez A, et al. The expanding role of imaging in systemic vasculitis. Rheum Dis Clin North Am 2016;42(4):733–51.

17. Schmidt WA. Use of imaging studies in the diagnosis of vasculitis. Curr Rheumatol Rep 2004;6(3):203–11.

18. Grayson PC, Alehashemi S, Bagheri AA, et al. 18F-Fluorodeoxyglucose–Positron emission tomography as an imaging biomarker in a prospective, longitudinal cohort of patients with large vessel vasculitis. Arthritis Rheumatol 2018;70(3):439–49.

19. Schmidt WA. Imaging in vasculitis. Best Pract Res Clin Rheumatol 2013;27(1):107–18.

20. Laurent C, Ricard L, Fain O, et al. PET/MRI in large-vessel vasculitis: clinical value for diagnosis and assessment of disease activity. Sci Rep 2019;9(1):12388.

21. Soussan M, Nicolas P, Schramm C, et al. Management of large-vessel vasculitis with FDG-PET: a systematic literature review and meta-analysis. Medicine (Baltimore) 2015;94(14):e622.

22. Incerti E, Tombetti E, Fallanca F, et al. 18F-FDG PET reveals unique features of large vessel inflammation in patients with Takayasu's arteritis. Eur J Nucl Med Mol Imaging 2017;44(7):1109–18.

23. Andrews J, Al-Nahhas A, Pennell DJ, et al. Noninvasive imaging in the diagnosis and management of Takayasu's arteritis. Ann Rheum Dis 2004;63(8):995–1000.

24. Walter MA, Melzer RA, Schindler C, et al. The value of [18F]FDG-PET in the diagnosis of large-vessel vasculitis and the assessment of activity and extent of disease. Eur J Nucl Med Mol Imaging 2005;32(6):674–81.

25. Padoan R, Crimì F, Felicetti M, et al. Fully integrated 18F-FDG PET/MR in large vessel vasculitis. Q J Nucl Med Mol Imaging. October 2019.

26. Younger DS. Epidemiology of the vasculitides. Neurol Clin 2019;37(2):201–17.

27. Halbach C, McClelland CM, Chen J, et al. Use of noninvasive imaging in giant cell arteritis. Asia Pac J Ophthalmol (Phila) 2018;7(4):260–4.

28. Gonzalez-Gay MA, Vazquez-Rodriguez TR, Lopez-Diaz MJ, et al. Epidemiology of giant cell arteritis and polymyalgia rheumatica. Arthritis Rheum 2009;61(10):1454–61.

29. Salvarani C, Pipitone N, Versari A, et al. Clinical features of polymyalgia rheumatica and giant cell arteritis. Nat Rev Rheumatol 2012;8(9):509–21.

30. Calamia KT, Hunder GG. Giant cell arteritis (temporal arteritis) presenting as fever of undetermined origin. Arthritis Rheum 1981;24(11):1414–8.

31. Gonzalez-Gay MA, Barros S, Lopez-Diaz MJ, et al. Giant cell arteritis: disease patterns of clinical presentation in a series of 240 patients. Medicine (Baltimore) 2005;84(5):269–76.

32. Myklebust G, Gran JT. A prospective study of 287 patients with polymyalgia rheumatica and temporal arteritis: clinical and laboratory manifestations at onset of disease and at the time of diagnosis. Br J Rheumatol 1996;35(11):1161–8.

33. Gonzalez-Gay MA, Garcia-Porrua C, Llorca J, et al. Visual manifestations of giant cell arteritis. Trends and clinical spectrum in 161 patients. Medicine (Baltimore) 2000;79(5):283–92.

34. Bley TA, Wieben O, Uhl M, et al. High-resolution MRI in giant cell arteritis: imaging of the wall of the superficial temporal artery. AJR Am J Roentgenol 2005;184(1):283–7.

35. Ironi G, Tombetti E, Napolitano A, et al. Diffusion-weighted magnetic resonance imaging detects vessel wall inflammation in patients with giant cell arteritis. JACC Cardiovasc Imaging 2018;11(12):1879–82.

36. Blockmans D, Stroobants S, Maes A, et al. Positron emission tomography in giant cell arteritis and polymyalgia rheumatica: evidence for inflammation of the aortic arch. Am J Med 2000;108(3):246–9.

37. Hautzel H, Sander O, Heinzel A, Schneider M, Muller H-W. Assessment of Large-Vessel Involvement in Giant Cell Arteritis with 18F-FDG PET: Introducing an ROC-Analysis-Based Cutoff Ratio. Journal of Nuclear Medicine 2008;49(7):1107–13.

38. Meller J, Strutz F, Siefker U, et al. Early diagnosis and follow-up of aortitis with [(18)F]FDG PET and MRI. Eur J Nucl Med Mol Imaging 2003;30(5):730–6.

39. Mason JC. Takayasu arteritis–advances in diagnosis and management. Nat Rev Rheumatol 2010;6(7):406–15.

40. Barra L, Kanji T, Malette J, et al. Imaging modalities for the diagnosis and disease activity assessment of Takayasu's arteritis: a systematic review and meta-analysis. Autoimmun Rev 2018;17(2):175–87.

41. Desai MY, Stone JH, Foo TKF, et al. Delayed contrast-enhanced MRI of the aortic wall in Takayasu's arteritis: initial experience. AJR Am J Roentgenol 2005;184(5):1427–31.

42. Papa M, De Cobelli F, Baldissera E, et al. Takayasu arteritis: intravascular contrast medium for MR angiography in the evaluation of disease activity. AJR Am J Roentgenol 2012;198(3):W279–84.

43. Tso E, Flamm SD, White RD, et al. Takayasu arteritis: utility and limitations of magnetic resonance imaging in diagnosis and treatment. Arthritis Rheum 2002;46(6):1634–42.

44. Tezuka D, Haraguchi G, Ishihara T, et al. Role of FDG PET-CT in Takayasu arteritis: sensitive detection of recurrences. JACC Cardiovasc Imaging 2012;5(4):422–9.

45. Webb M, Chambers A, AL-Nahhas A, et al. The role of 18F-FDG PET in characterising disease activity in Takayasu arteritis. Eur J Nucl Med Mol Imaging 2004;31(5):627–34.

46. Tsuchiya J, Tezuka D, Maejima Y, et al. Takayasu arteritis: clinical importance of extra-vessel uptake on FDG PET/CT. Eur J Hybrid Imaging 2019;3(1):12.

47. De Virgilio A, Greco A, Magliulo G, et al. Polyarteritis nodosa: a contemporary overview. Autoimmun Rev 2016;15(6):564–70.

48. Gonzalez-Gay MA, Garcia-Porrua C. Systemic vasculitis in adults in northwestern Spain, 1988-1997. Clinical and epidemiologic aspects. Medicine (Baltimore) 1999;78(5):292–308.

49. Stanson AW, Friese JL, Johnson CM, et al. Polyarteritis nodosa: spectrum of angiographic findings. Radiographics 2001;21(1):151–9.

50. Matteson EL. Historical perspective of vasculitis: polyarteritis nodosa and microscopic polyangiitis. Curr Rheumatol Rep 2002;4(1):67–74.

51. Eckel CG, Sibbitt RR, Sibbitt WL, et al. A possible role for MRI in polyarteritis nodosa: the "creeping fat" sign. Magn Reson Imaging 1988;6(6):713–5.

52. Hofman DM, Lems WF, Witkamp TD, et al. Demonstration of calf abnormalities by magnetic resonance imaging in polyarteritis nodosa. Clin Rheumatol 1992;11(3):402–4.

53. Ganeshanandan LR, Brusch AM, Dyke JM, McLean-Tooke APC. Polyarteritis nodosa isolated to muscles-A case series with a review of the literature. Semin Arthritis Rheum 2020;50(3):503–8.

54. Kang Y, Hong SH, Yoo HJ, et al. Muscle involvement in polyarteritis nodosa: report of eight cases

55. Bleeker-Rovers CP, Bredie SJ, Van Der Meer JW, et al. F-18-fluorodeoxyglucose positron emission tomography in diagnosis and follow-up of patients with different types of vasculitis. Neth J Med 2003;61(10):323–9.

56. Muratore F, Pipitone N, Salvarani C, et al. Imaging of vasculitis: state of the art. Best Pract Res Clin Rheumatol 2016;30(4):688–706.

57. Schollhammer R, Schwartz P, Jullie ML, et al. 18F-FDG PET/CT Imaging of popliteal vasculitis associated with polyarteritis nodosa. Clin Nucl Med 2017; 42(8):e385–7.

58. Shimizu M, Inoue N, Mizuta M, et al. Leopard skin appearance of cutaneous polyarteritis nodosa on 18Ffluorodeoxyglucose positron emission tomography. Rheumatology 2016;55(6):1090.

59. Kizawa T, Yoto Y, Mizukami M, et al. A case report of cutaneous polyarteritis nodosa in siblings. Mod Rheumatol 2018;28(6):1049–52.

60. Burns JC, Mason WH, Glode MP, et al. Clinical and epidemiologic characteristics of patients referred for evaluation of possible Kawasaki disease. J Pediatr 1991;118(5):680–6.

61. McCrindle Brian W, Rowley Anne H, Newburger Jane W, et al. Diagnosis, treatment, and long-term management of Kawasaki disease: a scientific statement for health professionals from the American Heart Association. Circulation 2017;135(17): e927–99.

62. Kato H. Cardiovascular complications in Kawasaki disease: coronary artery lumen and long-term consequences. Prog Pediatr Cardiol 2004;19(2): 137–45.

63. Dietz SM, Tacke CE, Kuipers IM, et al. Cardiovascular imaging in children and adults following Kawasaki disease. Insights Imaging 2015;6(6): 697–705.

64. Tacke CE, Kuipers IM, Groenink M, et al. Cardiac magnetic resonance imaging for noninvasive assessment of cardiovascular disease during the follow-up of patients with Kawasaki disease. Circ Cardiovasc Imaging 2011;4(6): 712–20.

65. Suda K, Tahara N, Honda A, et al. Statin reduces persistent coronary arterial inflammation evaluated by serial (1)(8)fluorodeoxyglucose positron emission tomography imaging long after Kawasaki disease. Int J Cardiol 2015;179:61–2.

66. Suda K, Tahara N, Kudo Y, et al. Persistent coronary arterial inflammation in a patient long after the onset of Kawasaki disease. Int J Cardiol 2012;154(2):193–4.

67. Hauser M, Bengel F, Kuehn A, et al. Myocardial blood flow and coronary flow reserve in children

with "normal" epicardial coronary arteries after the onset of Kawasaki disease assessed by positron emission tomography. Pediatr Cardiol 2004;25(2): 108–12.

68. Jennette JC, Falk RJ. Small-vessel vasculitis. N Engl J Med 1997;337(21):1512–23.

69. Jennette JC. Implications for pathogenesis of patterns of injury in small- and medium-sized-vessel vasculitis. Cleve Clin J Med 2002;69(Suppl 2): Sii33–8.

70. Passam FH, Diamantis ID, Perisinaki G, et al. Intestinal ischemia as the first manifestation of vasculitis. Semin Arthritis Rheum 2004;34(1):431–41.

71. Khanna G, Sargar K, Baszis KW. Pediatric vasculitis: recognizing multisystemic manifestations at body imaging. Radiographics 2015;35(3): 849–65.

72. Kallenberg CG. Pathogenesis of PR3-ANCA associated vasculitis. J Autoimmun 2008;30(1–2):29–36.

73. Soussan M, Abisror N, Abad S, et al. FDG-PET/CT in patients with ANCA-associated vasculitis: case-series and literature review. Autoimmun Rev 2014; 13(2):125–31.

74. Ito K, Minamimoto R, Yamashita H, et al. Evaluation of Wegener's granulomatosis using 18F-fluorodeoxyglucose positron emission tomography/ computed tomography. Ann Nucl Med 2013; 27(3):209–16.

75. Soussan M, Abad S, Mekinian A, et al. Detection of asymptomatic aortic involvement in ANCA-associated vasculitis using FDG PET/CT. Clin Exp Rheumatol 2013;31(1 Suppl 75):S56–8.

76. Frary EC, Hess S, Gerke O, et al. 18F-fluoro-deoxy-glucose positron emission tomography combined with computed tomography can reliably rule-out infection and cancer in patients with anti-neutrophil cytoplasmic antibody-associated vasculitis suspected of disease relapse. Medicine (Baltimore) 2017;96(30):e7613.

77. Nakazawa J, Watanabe A, Nakajima T, et al. [Henoch-Schonlein Purpura with lung abscess]. Kyobu Geka 2013;66(10):886–9.

78. Mooij CF, Hermsen R, Hoppenreijs EP, et al. Fludeoxyglucose positron emission tomography-computed tomography scan showing polyarthritis in a patient with an atypical presentation of Henoch-Schonlein vasculitis without clinical signs of arthritis: a case report. J Med Case Rep 2016; 10(1):159.

79. Lillington J, Brusaferri L, Klaser K, et al. PET/MRI attenuation estimation in the lung: a review of past, present, and potential techniques. Med Phys 2020;47(2):790–811.

80. Holman B, Cuplov V, Millner L, et al. Failure to account for density variation during respiration can significantly affect PET quantitation in the lung. J Nucl Med 2015;56(supplement 3):1770.

81. Iannuzzi MC, Rybicki BA, Teirstein AS. Sarcoidosis. N Engl J Med 2007;357(21):2153–65.

82. Friedrich MG, Sechtem U, Schulz-Menger J, et al. Cardiovascular magnetic resonance in myocarditis: a JACC White Paper. J Am Coll Cardiol 2009;53(17):1475–87.

83. Juneau D, Nery P, Russo J, et al. How common is isolated cardiac sarcoidosis? Extra-cardiac and cardiac findings on clinical examination and whole-body (18)F-fluorodeoxyglucose positron emission tomography. Int J Cardiol 2018;253: 189–93.

84. Okada DR, Bravo PE, Vita T, et al. Isolated cardiac sarcoidosis: a focused review of an under-recognized entity. J Nucl Cardiol 2018;25(4): 1136–46.

85. Genovesi D, Bauckneht M, Altini C, et al. The role of positron emission tomography in the assessment of cardiac sarcoidosis. Br J Radiol 2019;92(1100): 20190247.

86. Ramirez R, Trivieri M, Fayad ZA, et al. Advanced imaging in cardiac sarcoidosis. J Nucl Med 2019; 60(7):892–8.

87. Divakaran S, Stewart GC, Lakdawala NK, et al. Diagnostic accuracy of advanced imaging in cardiac sarcoidosis. Circ Cardiovasc Imaging 2019; 12(6):e008975.

88. Bois JP, Muser D, Chareonthaitawee P. PET/CT evaluation of cardiac sarcoidosis. PET Clin 2019; 14(2):223–32.

89. Miller EJ, Culver DA. Establishing an evidence-based method to diagnose cardiac sarcoidosis: the complementary use of cardiac magnetic resonance imaging and FDG-PET. Circ Cardiovasc Imaging 2018;11(1):e007408.

90. Lu Y, Patel DC, Sweiss N. Using and interpreting (18)F-FDG PET/CT images in patients referred for assessment of cardiac sarcoidosis: the devil is in the details. J Nucl Med 2017;58(12):2039.

91. Ohira H, Ardle BM, deKemp RA, et al. Inter- and intraobserver agreement of (18)F-FDG PET/CT image interpretation in patients referred for assessment of cardiac sarcoidosis. J Nucl Med 2017;58(8):1324–9.

92. Hulten E, Aslam S, Osborne M, et al. Cardiac sarcoidosis-state of the art review. Cardiovasc Diagn Ther 2016;6(1):50–63.

93. Van Schandevyl S, Waterschoot R, De Vos N, et al. Cardiac sarcoidosis: the complementary role of 18F-FDG PET and MRI. J Cardiovasc Med (Hagerstown) 2020;21(4):335–6.

94. Wicks EC, Menezes LJ, Barnes A, et al. Diagnostic accuracy and prognostic value of simultaneous hybrid 18F-fluorodeoxyglucose positron emission tomography/magnetic resonance imaging in cardiac sarcoidosis. Eur Heart J Cardiovasc Imaging 2018;19(7):757–67.

95. Dweck MR, Abgral R, Trivieri MG, et al. Hybrid magnetic resonance imaging and positron emission tomography with fluorodeoxyglucose to diagnose active cardiac sarcoidosis. JACC Cardiovasc Imaging 2018;11(1):94–107.

96. Rischpler C, Langwieser N, Nekolla SG. Cardiac PET/MRI enters the clinical arena! Finally. J Nucl Cardiol 2018;25(3):795–6.

97. Hess S, Henning Madsen P. Potential Applications of FDG-PET/CT in COPD: A Review of the Literature. Curr Mol Imaging. 2014;3(3):191-194.

98. Gjedde A. Calculation of cerebral glucose phosphorylation from brain uptake of glucose analogs in vivo: a re-examination. Brain Res 1982;257(2): 237–74.

99. Patlak CS, Blasberg RG. Graphical evaluation of blood-to-brain transfer constants from multiple-time uptake data. Generalizations. J Cereb Blood Flow Metab 1985;5(4):584–90.

100. Jones HA, Marino PS, Shakur BH, et al. In vivo assessment of lung inflammatory cell activity in patients with COPD and asthma. Eur Respir J 2003; 21(4):567–73.

101. Subramanian DR, Jenkins L, Edgar R, et al. Assessment of pulmonary neutrophilic inflammation in emphysema by quantitative positron emission tomography. Am J Respir Crit Care Med 2012;186(11):1125–32.

102. Chen DL, Azulay D-O, Atkinson JJ, et al. Reproducibility Of Positron Emission Tomography (PET)-Measured [18F]Fluorodeoxyglucose ([18F] FDG) Uptake As A Marker Of Lung Inflammation In Chronic Obstructive Pulmonary Disease (COPD). D99 ASSESSMENT OF LUNG INJURY AND INFLAMMATION. 2011.

103. Chen DL, Cheriyan J, Chilvers ER, et al. Quantification of Lung PET images: challenges and opportunities. J Nucl Med 2017;58(2):201–7.

104. Lambrou T, Groves AM, Erlandsson K, et al. The importance of correction for tissue fraction effects in lung PET: preliminary findings. Eur J Nucl Med Mol Imaging 2011;38(12):2238–46.

105. Coello C, Fisk M, Mohan D, et al. Quantitative analysis of dynamic (18)F-FDG PET/CT for measurement of lung inflammation. EJNMMI Res 2017; 7(1):47.

106. Vass LD, Lee S, Wilson FJ, et al. Reproducibility of compartmental modelling of (18)F-FDG PET/CT to evaluate lung inflammation. EJNMMI Phys 2019; 6(1):26.

107. Keyes JW Jr. SUV: standard uptake or silly useless value? J Nucl Med 1995;36(10):1836–9.

108. Torigian DA, Dam V, Chen X, et al. In vivo quantification of pulmonary inflammation in relation to emphysema severity via partial volume corrected (18)F-FDG-PET using computer-assisted analysis of diagnostic chest CT. Hell J Nucl Med 2013; 16(1):12–8.

109. Garpered S, Minarik D, Diaz S, et al. Measurement of airway inflammation in current smokers by positron emission tomography. Clin Physiol Funct Imaging 2019;39(6):393–8.

110. Coulson JM, Rudd JHF, Duckers JM, et al. Excessive aortic inflammation in chronic obstructive pulmonary disease: an 18F-FDG PET pilot study. J Nucl Med 2010;51(9):1357–60.

111. Fisk M, Cheriyan J, Mohan D, et al. Vascular inflammation and aortic stiffness: potential mechanisms of increased vascular risk in chronic obstructive pulmonary disease. Respir Res 2018;19(1):100.

112. Kothekar E, Borja AJ, Gerke O, et al. Assessing respiratory muscle activity with (18)F-FDG-PET/CT in patients with COPD. Am J Nucl Med Mol Imaging 2019;9(6):309–15.

113. Aydin A, Hickeson M, Yu JQ, et al. Demonstration of excessive metabolic activity of thoracic and abdominal muscles on FDG-PET in patients with chronic obstructive pulmonary disease. Clin Nucl Med 2005;30(3):159–64.

114. Osman MM, Tran IT, Muzaffar R, et al. Does 18F-FDG Uptake by Respiratory Muscles on PET/CT correlate with chronic obstructive pulmonary disease? J Nucl Med 2011;39(4):252–7.

Moving?

Make sure your subscription moves with you!

To notify us of your new address, find your **Clinics Account Number** (located on your mailing label above your name), and contact customer service at:

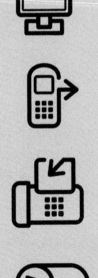

Email: journalscustomerservice-usa@elsevier.com

800-654-2452 (subscribers in the U.S. & Canada)
314-447-8871 (subscribers outside of the U.S. & Canada)

Fax number: 314-447-8029

Elsevier Health Sciences Division
Subscription Customer Service
3251 Riverport Lane
Maryland Heights, MO 63043

*To ensure uninterrupted delivery of your subscription, please notify us at least 4 weeks in advance of move.

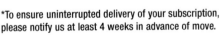

Printed and bound by CPI Group (UK) Ltd, Croydon, CR0 4YY

03/10/2024

01040372-0001